Targeting the Wnt Pathway in Cancer

D1615273

Kathleen H. Goss · Michael Kahn
Editors

Targeting the Wnt Pathway in Cancer

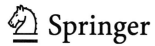 Springer

Editors
Kathleen H. Goss, Ph.D.
Department of Surgery
University of Chicago
5841 South Maryland Ave.
SBRI J557F/MC 5032
Chicago, IL 60637
kgoss@surgery.bsd.uchicago.edu

Michael Kahn, Ph.D.
Provost's Professor of Medicine
and Pharmacy
Eli and Edythe Broad Center
for Regenerative Medicine and Stem
Cell Research
University of Southern California
1425 San Pablo, ZNI-533
Los Angeles, CA 90033
kahnm@usc.edu

ISBN 978-1-4419-8022-9   e-ISBN 978-1-4419-8023-6
DOI 10.1007/978-1-4419-8023-6
Springer New York Dordrecht Heidelberg London

Library of Congress Control Number: 2011920692

Printed on acid-free paper

Springer is part of Springer Science+Business Media (www.springer.com)

Preface

The first hint that the Wnt signaling pathway might be involved in cancer came in the 1980s when one of the integration sites of the Mouse Mammary Tumor Virus (MMTV) was mapped to *Int-1*, later renamed *Wnt-1* for its homology to the *wingless* (*Wg*) *Drosophila* patterning gene. A second provocative link to cancer came in the mid-1990s when *adenomatous polyposis coli* (*APC*), a tumor suppressor gene already strongly associated with hereditary and sporadic colorectal cancer, was identified as a negative regulator of Wnt signaling. In the years that followed, researchers have uncovered many of the molecular details of pathway regulation and function in developmental systems and adult tissues and found a critical role for Wnt signaling in the stem cells of several tissue types. Moreover, Wnt pathway hyperactivation, or dysregulation of specific pathway components, has now been observed in almost 50% of all human cancers. Numerous genetic animal models have been generated and characterized that provide compelling evidence that pathway activation is necessary and sufficient for the pathogenesis of several tumor types. Importantly, these models also provide preclinical tools to test the efficacy of Wnt pathway antagonists in vivo.

Recently, a major focus in the field has been to develop specific and effective Wnt pathway inhibitors, including small molecules and antibodies, for potential clinical use for colorectal cancer and other tumor types. In fact, nearly all levels or components of the pathway have been targeted, including Wnt secretion, ligand binding, β-catenin stabilization, and of course, β-catenin transcriptional activity. While there have been several successes with impressive preclinical data that are currently leading to clinical trials, there remain several questions and concerns in regard to the safety of antagonizing this pathway for cancer treatment. One issue is the essential role of Wnt signaling in the maintenance and self-renewal of normal adult stem cells and the impact of systemic Wnt pathway inhibition on their number and function. Another challenge is the multifunctional nature of some Wnt pathway components. For example, β-catenin is the major effector of Wnt signaling; yet, its localization and activity at the adherens junctions of differentiated epithelial cells are essential for tissue homeostasis. Therefore, strategies to deplete β-catenin levels, rather than solely inhibit its transcriptional activity, may be problematic. A third formidable challenge is the extent by which the Wnt pathway cooperates with other signaling pathways to exert its biological effects. While this may result in far-reaching effects of Wnt pathway inhibition to cripple tumor cells, it also might lead to the ability of tumor cells to readily circumvent targeting of the Wnt pathway and develop therapy resistance. An additional challenge is that not all subtypes within tumor types demonstrate Wnt pathway activation. Therefore, it is critical to better understand which patient populations are most likely to respond and design clinical trials around these populations so that effectiveness of Wnt-directed therapies can be accurately evaluated. All of these challenges provide opportunities to better understand the nuances of Wnt signaling while moving toward the clinic with Wnt antagonists.

Each of the chapters of this book presents different aspects of Wnt signaling as they apply to translating basic research into Wnt-directed therapies for cancer patients. They are not comprehensive in their scope, but, instead, give a current snapshot of the state of the field, particularly focused on the importance of Wnt signaling in cancer and the approaches that have been taken to target the pathway therapeutically. Our goal was to highlight how far the field has come in these areas as well as underscore the challenges and opportunities that lie ahead in the next phase of translational studies with Wnt pathway inhibitors.

Chicago, IL   Kathleen H. Goss
Los Angeles, CA   Michael Kahn

Contents

Contributors

Masahiro Aoki
Department of Pharmacology, Graduate School of Medicine, Kyoto University, Yoshida-Konoé-che, Sakyo, Kyoto 606-8501, Japan

Alan R. Clarke
Cardiff School of Biosciences, Cardiff University, Museum Avenue, Cardiff, UK

Xiaolan Fan
Wenzhou Medical College, Wenzhou, Zhejiang, 325000, China

Kathleen H. Goss
Department of Surgery, University of Chicago, Chicago, IL 60637, USA

Aliaksei Holik
Cardiff School of Biosciences, Cardiff University, Museum Avenue, Cardiff, UK

Michael Kahn
Eli and Edythe Broad Center for Regenerative Medicine and Stem Cell Research at USC, University of Southern California, 1425 San Pablo Street,
Los Angeles, CA 90033, USA;
Department of Biochemistry and Molecular Biology Keck School of Medicine, University of Southern California, 1425 San Pablo Street,
Los Angeles, CA 90033, USA;
Department of Molecular Pharmacology and Toxicology, University of Southern California, 1425 San Pablo Street, Los Angeles, CA 90033, USA

Ho-Jin Lee
Department of Structural Biology, St. Jude Children's Research Hospital, 262 Danny Thomas Place, MS 311, Memphis, TN 38105-3678, USA

Xinhua Lin
Division of Developmental Biology, Cincinnati Children's Hospital Medical Center, and The Graduate Program in Molecular and Developmental Biology, University of Cincinnati College of Medicine, Cincinnati, OH 45229, USA;
State Key Laboratory of Biomembrane and Membrane Biotechnology, and Key Laboratory of stem cell, Institute of Zoology, Chinese Academy of Sciences, Beijing, 100101, China

Hue H. Luu
Department of Surgery, University of Chicago, Chicago, IL 60637, USA

Philipp C. Manegold
Eli and Edythe Broad Center for Regenerative Medicine and Stem Cell Research
at USC, University of Southern California, 1425 San Prblo Street,
Los Angeles, CA 90033, USA

Satdarshan P.S. Monga
Division of Experimental Pathology (EP), University of Pittsburgh School
of Medicine, 200 Lothrop Street S-421 BST, Pittsburgh, PA 15261, USA

Markus Müschen
Department of Laboratory Medicine, Department of Pathology and Department
of Medicine, UCSF School of Medicine, University of California San Francisco,
521 Parnassus Avenue, San Francisco, CA 94143, USA

Kari Nejak-Bowen
University of Pittsburgh School of Medicine, 200 Lothrop Street S-421 BST,
Pittsburgh, PA 15261, USA

Paul Polakis
Department of Research, Genentech, Inc, 1 DNA Way,
South San Francisco, CA 94080, USA

Jenifer R. Prosperi
Department of Surgery, University of Chicago, Chicago, IL 60637, USA

Miki Shitashige
Chemotherapy Division, National Cancer Center Research Institute,
5-1-1 Tsukiji, Chuo-ku, Tokyo 104-0045, Japan

Makoto Mark Taketo
Department of Pharmacology, Graduate School of Medicine, Kyoto University,
Yoshida-Konoé-cho, Sakyo, Kyoto 606-8501, Japan

Xiaofang Tang
Division of Developmental Biology, Cincinnati Children's Hospital Medical
Center, and The Graduate Program in Molecular and Developmental Biology,
University of Cincinnati College of Medicine, Cincinnati, OH 45229, USA

Jia-Ling Teo
Eli and Edythe Broad Center for Regenerative Medicine and Stem Cell Research
at USC, University of Southern California, 1425 San Prblo Street,
Los Angeles, CA 90033, USA

Michael Thompson
University of Pittsburgh School of Medicine,
200 Lothrop Street S-421 BST, Pittsburgh, PA 15261, USA

Tesshi Yamada
Chemotherapy Division, National Cancer Center Research Institute,
5-1-1 Tsukiji, Chuo-ku, Tokyo 104-0045, Japan

Xinxin Zhang
Department of Structural Biology, St. Jude Children's Research Hospital,
262 Danny Thomas Place, MS 311, Memphis, TN 38105, USA

Jie J. Zheng
Department of Structural Biology, St. Jude Children's Research Hospital,
262 Danny Thomas Place, MS 311, Memphis, TN 38105-3678, USA

Chapter 1
An Introduction to Wnt Signaling

Paul Polakis

Abstract This chapter provides a chronological outline of the landmark discoveries in developmental biology, genetics, cell biology, and biochemistry that have established our understanding of wnt signaling. Particular emphasis is placed on the role of wnt signaling in human cancer and the alterations in pathway components that contribute to aberrant signaling in this disease.

Keywords Wnt • Catenin • APC • Frizzled • Cancer

1.1 The War on Wnt

Targeted cancer drug therapy relies upon a detailed understanding of the molecular mechanisms by which various gene products contribute to the aberrant growth control of cancer cells. In the past couple of decades, we have accrued and assembled the parts and processes that define wnt signaling in sickness and in health. From this knowledge it is painfully apparent that β-catenin is indeed a human oncogene, yet specifically drugging it in a manner that warrants advance to clinical testing remains elusive. Alternatively, more blinded cell-based screens that read out wnt signaling can be performed, but the targets of any compounds netted need to be identified to improve upon compound activity and to anticipate potential toxicities. Thus in the war on cancer, as it applies specifically to wnt, we know the enemy well, we are poised for attack, yet lack the armament to prosecute it. In this chapter, I will review the research that has established our understanding of the wnt battlefield, which should serve as a reference for subsequent chapters on developing the weapons for this war.

P. Polakis (✉)
Department of Research, Genentech, Inc, 1 DNA Way,
South San Francisco, CA 94080, USA
e-mail: ppolakis@gene.com

K.H. Goss and M. Kahn (eds.), *Targeting the Wnt Pathway in Cancer*,
DOI 10.1007/978-1-4419-8023-6_1, © Springer Science+Business Media, LLC 2011

1.2   Wnt Signaling Regulates Genes

"What can be the nature of the generality of neoplastic changes? A favorite explanation has been oncogens cause alterations in the genes of the ordinary cells of the body. But numerous facts, when taken together, decisively exclude this explanation." This seemingly heretical statement was excerpted from a 1966 Nobel Lecture delivered by Peyton Rous, who was awarded the prize for discovering that viruses could cause cancer in animals. It is particularly ironic that only 9 years later Bishop and Varmus employed his namesake virus, the Rous Sarcoma virus, to demonstrate the cellular nature of retroviral oncogenes (Stehelin et al. 1975; Varmus et al. 1974). That our own normal genes can indeed turn against us, and that viruses can facilitate oncogenesis, is central to the history of wnt in cancer. In a landmark discovery in 1982, Varmus and Nusse found that the mouse mammary tumor virus (MMTV) promoted tumors by aberrantly activating a cellular gene they termed int1, short for integration1 (Nusse and Varmus 1982).

Our understanding of how int1 promotes tumor formation is rooted in genetic studies of embryonic development in flies and frogs. Working with *Drosophila*, Nusslein-Volhard and Wieschaus (Nusslein-Volhard and Wieschaus 1980) had identified a number of pattern-forming genes affecting segmentation, one of which had been previously termed wingless (wg) for its effects on wing development (Sharma and Chopra 1976). In addition to wing defects, larva with mutations in wg also displayed denticles on the normally naked posterior portion of the segments. This segment polarity readout became instrumental in the subsequent assembly of genes operating in the nascent wg signaling pathway (Klingensmith et al. 1994; Noordermeer et al. 1994; Siegfried et al. 1992; Wieschaus and Riggleman 1987). For example, deletion of zeste white 3, which encodes glycogen synthase kinase 3β, produced completely naked segments, lacking the normal anterior denticles, whereas loss-of-function mutations in armadillo or disheveled produced the opposing wg mutant phenotype.

A parallel manipulation of some of these same genes was carried out in vertebrates, where a primary outcome was the duplication of the body axis in *Xenopus* embryos. In one of the first such experiments, reported by McMahon and Moon, dorsal axis duplication was observed upon injection of mRNA transcribed from the proto-oncogene int1 (McMahon and Moon 1989). Subsequent studies involving interference with GSK3β or ectopic expression of mRNA coding for the armadillo homolog β-catenin also resulted in *Xenopus* embryo axis duplication (Dominguez et al. 1995; Guger and Gumbiner 1995). In this way, some of the most fundamental components of wnt signaling were revealed through developmental biology. However, knowledge relating to the functional relationships among these gene products was scant, and that which existed was difficult to reconcile with profound developmental outcomes that presumably required genetic programming. Indeed, the molecular cloning of vertebrate β-catenin in 1991 was the culmination of cell adhesion studies focused on the identification of proteins associated with the intracellular region of E-cadherin (McCrea et al. 1991).

Bejsovec and Martinez Arias, who linked wg activity to the expression of the segment polarity gene engrailed (Bejsovec and Martinez Arias 1991), established early support for wg as a signaling molecule controlling gene expression. Siegfried and Perrimon elaborated on this by showing that *Drosophila* GSK3β represses gene expression and that wg relieves this repression (Siegfried et al. 1992). How wg, a secreted molecule (van den Heuvel et al. 1989), achieved this was unclear, but another piece of the signaling puzzle was revealed by the observation that both wg and disheveled posttranscriptionally controlled the levels of armadillo protein (Riggleman et al. 1990). Mark Peifer later showed that GSK3β and wg impacted the intracellular distribution of armadillo in opposing manners and that this involved phosphorylation of armadillo (Peifer et al. 1994a, b). Thus, a secreted molecule influenced adjacent cells to activate genes by promoting the accumulation of what was then largely considered a cell adhesion molecule, armadillo/β-catenin.

While it was certainly appreciated that cell adhesion was important for cell signaling, mounting evidence suggested these two β-catenin-dependent activities were separable. Surprisingly, overexpression of cadherin in *Xenopus* suppressed rather than enhanced β-catenin activity in wnt signaling (Heasman et al. 1994). Moreover, armadillo accumulation in response to wg signaling occurred in the cytoplasm and, strikingly, certain deletion mutants of armadillo were found to independently support either signaling or cell adhesion (Orsulic and Peifer 1996; Peifer et al. 1994a). Speculation on a potential transcription factor that might transduce wnt signals ended when the labs of Clevers and Birchmeier independently reported on the functional association of β-catenin with mammalian LEF-1 and *Xenopus* XTCF-3, respectively (Behrens et al. 1996; Molenaar et al. 1996). These transcription factors belonged to a family of high mobility group proteins previously described in association with the T-cell receptor enhancer (Oosterwegel et al. 1991; Waterman et al. 1991).

1.3 Wnt Signaling Causes Human Cancer

While the elucidation of the wnt signaling pathway (Fig. 1.1) progressed on the back of developmental biology, its contribution to human cancer was gradually falling into place. Paramount to this connection was the discovery of defects in the adenomatous polyposis coli (APC) gene in patients with a familial predisposition to colorectal cancer (Groden et al. 1991; Nishisho et al. 1991). The APC gene was also found mutated in the majority of sporadic colorectal cancers (reviewed in (Polakis 2000)). Moreover, APC was also identified as the underlying cause of heritable intestinal cancers in the so-called Min mouse, previously derived by chemical mutagenesis (Moser et al. 1990; Su et al. 1992). The function of the APC gene remained entirely enigmatic for a couple of years until two labs, my own and that of Kinzler and Vogelstein, both pulled out β-catenin during unrelated fishing expeditions using APC protein as bait (Rubinfeld et al. 1993; Su et al. 1993). In both of these studies, the binding of β-catenin was mapped to the central region of the

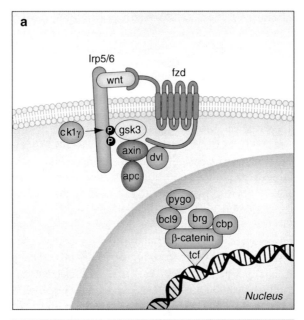

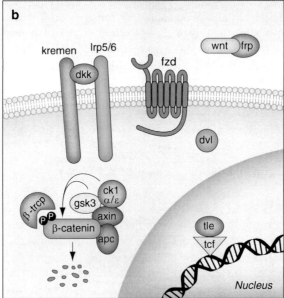

Fig. 1.1 Core components of wnt signaling. In the ON state (*top*) a wnt ligand bridges the fzd and LRP receptors bringing the dvl/axin complex into the proximity of the phosphorylated LRP cytoplasmic region that binds and inhibits gsk3. Inhibition of the destruction complex stabilizes β-catenin which enters the nucleus and interacts with TCF/LEF and recruits the indicated transcriptional coactivators. In the OFF state (*bottom*), where ligand is absent, or wnt is inhibited by frp binding or its LRP binding site is occupied by a dkk, the destruction complex is active and coordinates the phosphorylation, ubiquitination, and degradation of β-catenin by the proteosome. Dvl remains cytoplasmic and TCF is associated with TLE corepressors

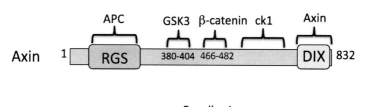

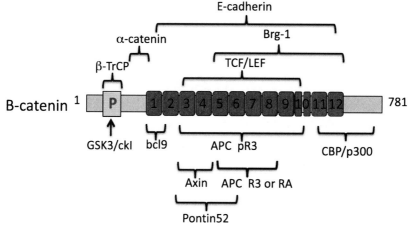

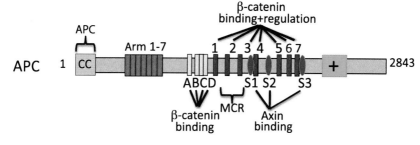

Fig. 1.2 Interaction maps for Axin, APC, and β–catenin. *Brackets* denote the region or domain to which each of the indicated binding partners associate. For Axin, the approximate amino acid positions comprising the binding site for GSK3 and β-catenin are indicated. For β-catenin, the *red boxes* indicate the 12 armadillo repeats and the *blue box* the site of phospho-dependent binding for β-TrCP. For APC, the 15- and 20-amino acid repeats are indicated as A–D and 1–7, respectively, and the Axin-binding sites as S1–S3. The coiled-coil (CC) oligomerization domain is in *blue* and the basic region (+) in *green*

2,843-amino acid APC polypeptide. This region contained a series of imperfectly repeated motifs of either 15 or 20 amino acids each (Fig. 1.2).

The association of the APC tumor suppressor with β-catenin cemented a link between wnt signaling and human cancer. However, these papers predated the finding that β-catenin associated with LEF/TCF, so the discussions remained focused on cadherin-based cell adhesion and how APC might influence it. A functional role for APC was uncovered in 1995 when my lab found that introduction of wild-type APC into APC mutant colorectal cancer cells resulted in the downregulation of β-catenin through a posttranslational mechanism (Munemitsu et al. 1995). Remarkably, the mapping of this activity to the APC polypeptide strongly coincided with structure that was commonly deleted by mutations associated with colorectal cancer. It was proposed that the genetic selection for APC mutants in colorectal cancer favored the disposal of its β-catenin regulatory activity (Polakis 1995). This hypothesis described counteracting forces wherein wnt, the oncogene, upregulated β-catenin (Hinck et al. 1994), and APC, the tumor suppressor, downregulated it.

During the next few years, a veritable explosion in our understanding of wnt signaling in cancer was played out. Arguably, the most formidable of these discoveries was the aforementioned identification of the LEF/TCF transcription factors as effectors of β-catenin (Behrens et al. 1996; Molenaar et al. 1996). Prior to this, β-catenin had been flirting with transcriptional activity by showing up in the nucleus in a number of studies (Funayama et al. 1995; Inomata et al. 1996; Schneider et al. 1996; Yost et al. 1996). Inomata proposed that this localization related to cancer, as β-catenin was found in the nucleus of APC mutant colorectal tumor cells, but not in corresponding normal epithelium (Inomata et al. 1996). This agreed well with concurrent embryonic development studies in which the nuclear localization of β-catenin occurred specifically in tissues when and where wnt was known to exert its pattern-forming activities (Schneider et al. 1996). Randall Moon's lab also reported on nuclear localization in *Xenopus* and added that this was negatively regulated by phosphorylation of N-terminal serine/threonine residues by GSK3β (Yost et al. 1996).

The potential significance of β-catenin N-terminal sequence had also surfaced previously in what should be considered the first demonstration of β-catenin itself as a proto-oncogene. In a random cDNA expression cloning effort to identify genes that could transform NIH3T3 cells, Robert Kay's lab pulled out an N-terminally truncated form of β-catenin (Whitehead et al. 1995). Subsequently, my lab reported that N-terminal truncation of β-catenin stabilized the protein by retarding its degradation rate (Munemitsu et al. 1996). Further adding to the intrigue, Paul Robbins happened upon a β-catenin N-terminal peptide while looking for melanoma-specific antigens recognized by lymphocytes (Robbins et al. 1996). This peptide, however, contained a phenylalanine substituted for serine-37, and thus represented the first cancer-associated mutation in β-catenin. Paul then collaborated with my lab to identify additional β-catenin N-terminal point mutations and truncations in a panel of melanoma cell lines (Rubinfeld et al. 1997). We showed that these mutations stabilized catenin by making them refractory to downregulation by APC. Concurrently, the labs of Clevers and Kinzler reported on similar mutants in colorectal cancers and showed that APC failed to downregulate their transcriptional output using an LEF/TCF reporter assay (Korinek et al. 1997; Morin et al. 1997). Subsequent studies identified these N-terminal mutants of β-catenin in a wide variety of human cancers at variable frequencies (rev. in Polakis 2000). Importantly, mutations in β-catenin were exclusive to those in APC, strongly supporting the proposal that the tumor-suppressive activity of APC is defined by its ability to downregulate β-catenin.

It was now apparent that β-catenin contained a regulatory motif in its N-terminal region and that phosphorylation of serine/threonine residues, therein, was critical for controlling its turnover. The degradation of β-catenin was facilitated by the ubiquitin-proteosome system, as first demonstrated by the Kemler lab (Aberle et al. 1997). A WD40/FBox-containing protein termed slimb was subsequently identified as a negative regulator of armadillo in *Drosophila*. Based on its homology to the cdc4p cell cycle regulator, it was proposed that slimb targeted armadillo for degradation by the ubiquitin-proteosome system (Jiang and Struhl 1998). A similar finding was later reported in *Xenopus*, where the cdc4p homolog was referred to as β-TrCP (Marikawa and Elinson 1998). The critical phosphorylation of β-catenin N-terminal sequence turned out to be essential for recognition by β-TrCP (Hart et al. 1998). Thus, mutations affecting the phosphorylation of serine/threonine residues encompassed by amino acid positions 33–45 prevented the targeted destruction of β-catenin by the proteosome. Yost et al. had previously identified GSK3β as a kinase that phosphorylates this region of β-catenin, which further explained the negative regulatory activity of this enzyme in wnt signaling (Yost et al. 1996). Surprisingly, a second kinase, casein kinase1, was found to function sequentially with GSK3β to complete the series of phosphorylations (Amit et al. 2002; Liu et al. 2002; Yanagawa et al. 2002). This was surprising because previous reports had positioned CK1 as a positive regulator of wnt signaling (Peters et al. 1999; Sakanaka et al. 1999).

Colorectal cancer could now in part be attributed to runaway nuclear activity of β-catenin resulting from inactivation of APC or activation of β-catenin. Accordingly, the target genes activated by β-catenin were keenly sought after. Two of the earliest target genes identified were cyclin D1 and c-myc, both proto-oncogenes and master regulators of cell growth control (He et al. 1998; Tetsu and McCormick 1999). Numerous additional targets have been identified and a list compiled by the Nusse Lab and posted on their Wnt Home Page can be perused at (http://www.stanford. edu/%7ernusse/wntwindow.html).

1.4   Downregulation of Wnt Signaling

In 1997 and 1998, negative regulators of wnt signaling were identified in perfusion. Perhaps most intriguing was the discovery of the Axins. Axin1 was originally identified by the Costantini lab as a product of the fused locus in mice (Zeng et al. 1997). Homozygous mutations in the fused locus led to embryonic axial duplication, suggesting that Axin repressed an axis-forming activity. Indeed, dorsal injection of Axin mRNA ventralized *Xenopus* embryos and the addition of β-catenin mRNA rescued this effect. This strongly suggested Axin was a negative regulator of the wnt signaling pathway positioned upstream of β-catenin. Shortly thereafter, several papers were published in which Axin was confirmed as a negative regulator of β-catenin (Behrens et al. 1998; Hart et al. 1998; Ikeda et al. 1998; Itoh et al. 1998).

Together, these studies supported a role for Axin as a multidomain organizer of the β-catenin destruction complex (Fig. 1.2). Distinct binding sites for APC, β-catenin, and GSK3β were localized on Axin and its ability to downregulate β-catenin protein and signaling was demonstrated (Fig. 1.2). Additional interactions of Axin with CK1, disheveled, and the LRP5/6 wnt coreceptors were also established (Amit et al. 2002; Kishida et al. 1999; Liu et al. 2002; Mao et al. 2001; Smalley et al. 1999). The Birchmeier lab mapped three binding sites for Axin on APC that were interspersed among the 20-amino acid repeat motifs (Behrens et al. 1998). Remarkably, the most N-terminal of these binding sites resided just C-terminal to the boundary of the APC mutational cluster region (Fig. 1.2). This suggested that genetic selection in cancer was actually driven by pressure to eliminate all of the Axin-binding sites on APC. Mouse models of APC-mediated tumorigenesis reported by the Fodde lab were highly consistent with this hypothesis (Smits et al. 1999). More recently, WTX, a tumor suppressor implicated in pediatric kidney cancers, was identified as additional component of the β-catenin destruction complex (Major et al. 2007). WTX binds both β-catenin and β-TrCP and facilitates the ubiquitination of β-catenin.

The importance of Axins as negative regulators of wnt signaling was made more poignant by the discovery of inactivating mutations in the genes coding for them. This was first noted for Axin1 in primary hepatocellular cancers where polypeptide chain terminating mutations were identified in the context of loss of heterozygosity (Satoh et al. 2000). Concurrently, a point mutation affecting Leucine-396, which resided in the well-defined GSK3β binding motif of Axin1, was identified and shown to ablate GSK3β binding (Webster et al. 2000). Truncating mutations in Axin2 were also found in colorectal cancer (Liu et al. 2000). Numerous mutations in the Axins in a variety of cancers have since been reported (rev (Polakis 2007)) including germline mutations in Axin2 that predispose to colorectal cancer (Lammi et al. 2004). Thus, Axins exhibit all the hallmarks of classical tumor suppressors. However, it is interesting to note that Axin2 mutations in colorectal cancers sometimes occur concomitantly with mutations in APC (Thorstensen et al. 2005). This implies that additional gain in wnt signaling can be selected for beyond that which occurs by APC mutation alone. This is relevant to drug discovery as new compounds appear to inhibit wnt signaling through elevation of Axin levels and therefore could be beneficial even in cancers with compromised APC (Chen et al. 2009; Huang et al. 2009).

Many inhibitors of wnt signaling reside outside of the cell and affect ligand–receptor interactions. Among these are the frizzled-related proteins (FRP) (Finch et al. 1997; Leyns et al. 1997; Rattner et al. 1997), so named because of their distinct homology to frizzled, the long sought-after wnt receptor that was finally identified just prior to the cloning of FRP (Bhanot et al. 1996). The inhibitory activity of FRP, as well as WIF (Hsieh et al. 1999), a structurally unrelated secreted inhibitor, is attributed to their direct binding to wnt ligands in a manner competitive with frizzled binding. An additional secreted wnt antagonist, dickkopf, discovered by the Niehrs lab, does not bind wnts, but rather binds to and interferes with the wnt coreceptors LRP5 and LRP6 (Glinka et al. 1998). Subsequently, additional secreted antagonists, SOST and the related Wise protein, were also found to exert their effects by binding to LRP5/6 (Itasaki et al. 2003; Li et al. 2005).

As was the case for APC and the Axins, one might anticipate that the secreted antagonists would ultimately be defined as tumor suppressors in familial or sporadic cancers. Although evidence for their downregulation or epigenetic silencing has been reported (Sato et al. 2007; Suzuki et al. 2004), inactivating mutations in the genes coding for these proteins have never been associated with cancer. Interestingly, biallelic germline defects in SOST exist in humans and are associated with increased bone density, as are other wnt components, but not with cancer (rev. in Hoeppner et al. 2009). Conceptually, clonal selection for genetic defects in secreted antagonists would need to overcome the paracrine influence from neighboring wild-type cells, perhaps precluding their outgrowth. However, the target of the secreted antagonist could acquire a functional gain should a mutation render it refractory to the secreted antagonist. Accordingly, an aberrantly spliced internally truncated LRP5 receptor insensitive to dkk1 has recently been associated with parathyroid and breast tumors (Bjorklund et al. 2007, 2009).

1.5 Interactions at the Cell Surface

Although the regulation of β-catenin was considered a nexus in wnt signaling, the means by which an extracellular ligand achieved this awaited the discovery of the frizzled wnt receptors (Bhanot et al. 1996), and later, the LDL receptor-related proteins (LRPs) as coreceptors (Pinson et al. 2000; Tamai et al. 2000; Wehrli et al. 2000). The discovery by Dianqing Wu's lab that Axin was recruited to the cytoplasmic face of LRP5 upon wnt stimulation was particularly enlightening (Mao et al. 2001). This was shown later to require phosphorylation of a repeated motif in LRP5/6 by both casein kinase 1γ and GSK3β (Davidson et al. 2005; Zeng et al. 2005). A recent study indicates that these phosphorylated motifs in LRP5/6 bind to and inhibit the activity of GSK3β associated with Axin and may serve to bridge the association of Axin with the receptor (Piao et al. 2008). This finally accounts for the inactivation of GSK3β by wnt, which had been presumed for many years based on developmental genetics, yet remained mechanistically elusive. The recruitment of Axin to the plasma membrane is in turn facilitated by disheveled (dvl), which was first identified by the Perrimon lab as an essential component of wg signaling in *Drosophila* (Siegfried et al. 1994). Disheveled forms higher order oligomeric assemblies in the cytoplasm that associate with Axin and localize to the plasma membrane in response to wnt signaling (Schwarz-Romond et al. 2007). This localization is dependent upon frizzled and purportedly involves direct binding of the dvl PDZ domain to intracellular sequence of the frizzled receptor (Wong et al. 2003). Conceivably, a mutant deregulated frizzled receptor could contribute to tumorgenesis, as previously found for the fzd relative smoothened in the hedgehog pathway (Xie et al. 1998). However, mutant frizzled receptors have not been linked to cancer.

1.6   Interactions in the Nucleus

Gene regulation typically involves assembly of multiprotein complexes at promotor/ enhancer elements in target genes. Accordingly, a plethora of transcriptional cofactors have been tied to the β-catenin-TCF/LEF nuclear complex. Among the first of these cofactors to be identified were the groucho/TLE family of corepressors that bind directly to the *Drosophila* and vertebrate family of TCF proteins (Cavallo et al. 1998; Levanon et al. 1998; Roose et al. 1998). When associated with corepressors, TCF acts to suppress gene expression, which explains why mutation of TCF-binding sites can sometimes lead to activation of wg/wnt target genes (Brannon et al. 1999; Riese et al. 1997). During active wnt signaling, β-catenin displaces Groucho/TLE from TCF/LEF proteins by direct competition for an overlapping binding site on TCF/LEF (Daniels and Weis 2005). Transcriptional coactivators also functionally associate with the β-catenin nuclear complex as first demonstrated for the CREB-binding protein (CBP) and its homolog p300, by the Moon and Kemler labs (Hecht et al. 2000; Takemaru and Moon 2000). These coactivators bind directly to C-terminal sequence in β-catenin, possess intrinsic acetyl transferase activity, and contain docking sites for the recruitment of numerous additional transcriptional cofactors.

An additional coactivator of armadillo-dependent transcription, *Pygopus*, was isolated in genetic modifier screens in *Drosophila* by several labs (Belenkaya et al. 2002; Kramps et al. 2002; Parker et al. 2002; Thompson et al. 2002). The presence of a PHD-finger domain in *Pygopus* was consistent with a role in chromatin remodeling. *Pygopus* does not bind directly to armadillo but is bridged by legless, which associates with sequence in the first armadillo repeat of the armadillo protein (Stadeli and Basler 2005). Although Pygo and legless mutants closely phenocopy wg/arm defects in developing *Drosophila* embryos, this is not observed when their homologs, pygo1 and pygo2 or bcl9 and bcl9-2, are disrupted in mice (Brack et al. 2009). Nevertheless, these genes are clearly important for wnt signaling in vertebrates, but appear to play a more restricted role than that observed in flies.

Gene activation involves the acetylation and methylation of nucleosomal histones as well as the unwinding of DNA catalyzed by ATP-dependent helicases. The Kemler lab established the first connection to helicases when they fished out the Tat-interacting protein Pontin52/TIP49a from human cell extracts using β-catenin protein as bait (Bauer et al. 1998). TIP49 was later found in complexes with chromatin remodeling and histone-modifying cofactors and interference with its activity inhibited β-catenin-dependent transformation (Feng et al. 2003). An additional chromatin remodeling factor, Brg-1, was also found to functionally interact directly with β-catenin (Barker et al. 2001). More recently, the Jones lab reported that the C-terminal transactivation domain of β-catenin binds to chromatin-modifying complexes containing catalytic subunits harboring acetyl transferase and histone methlyase activities (Sierra et al. 2006). Beta-catenin recruits these activities to the promotor of the wnt target gene c-Myc, where they promote H3K4 methylation. This fascinating study also shows that the APC tumor suppressor is recruited to the myc gene in temporal manner consistent with downregulation of transcription.

1.7 Wnt and Stem Cells

Wnt signaling was once principally regarded as a developmental activity orchestrating embryonic patterning and cell type specification. Apart from its role in cancer, the utility of wnt signaling in adult tissues had gone vastly underappreciated. More recent studies, however, have delineated a crucial contribution of wnt signaling in the maintenance of regenerative tissues in the adult. In short, wnt seems essential for the regulation of the progenitor/stem cell compartment in the intestine, blood, skin, and other regenerating adult tissues (rev in (Reya and Clevers 2005)). This was first made apparent in the intestine by the Clevers lab reporting the complete depletion of the progenitor cell compartment in newborn TCF4-/- mice (Korinek et al. 1998). Later elaborations on this work include lineage tracing marked by the wnt target gene LGR5 (Barker et al. 2007). This elegant study inarguably identifies an early progenitor/stem cell population reliant upon wnt signaling that gives rise to all of the differentiated cell types in the gut. It is noteworthy that specific deletion of the APC tumor suppressor from these cells resulted in a florid tumor phenotype not observed upon deletion of APC from cells that have exited this progenitor compartment (Barker et al. 2009). Regulation of hematopoietic progenitors by wnt signaling has also been established (Austin et al. 1997; Reya et al. 2003; Willert et al. 2003). This was followed by a report linking hematopoietic cancer stem cells in chronic myelogenous leukemia to the activation of β-catenin-dependent signaling (Jamieson et al. 2004). Similar parallels have been drawn between wnt signaling in stem/progenitor cell populations in the skin and their role in certain skin cancers (Blanpain et al. 2004; Lo Celso et al. 2004; Malanchi et al. 2008). A requirement for wnt signaling in the maintenance of cancer stem cells, particularly that driven by receptors, has obvious therapeutic appeal.

1.8 Structural Biology

The mutations in APC, β-catenin, and the Axins all strongly implicate β-catenin itself as a potential therapeutic drug target in cancers harboring these defects. Therefore, a drug that disrupts the association between β-catenin and TCF/LEF transcription factors would be desirable. However, the structural biology underlying this interaction presents some rather formidable obstacles. When the Weis lab first disclosed the crystal structure of the armadillo repeat containing region of β-catenin, it was of intense interest as numerous structure–function studies had demonstrated the importance of these repeats in various β-catenin interactions (Huber et al. 1997). Three helices comprise each of the 12 arm repeats that in turn form a superhelix that presents a positively charged groove along the length of the structure. As speculated by Weis, this groove provides sites for overlapping electrostatic interactions with APC, TCF/LEF, or cadherins (Fig. 1.2). The structure of the β-catenin/xTCF3 complex reported by Xu was highly illuminating as it revealed extensive interactions spanning arm repeats 3–10 with a total buried interface of approximately 5,000 A^2 (Graham et al. 2000). Based on the accompanying mutational analysis, Xu surmised that TCF, APC, cadherin, and Axin shared common contact sites for their interactions with β-catenin. This was corroborated by subsequent crystal structures of these complexes solved by the Weis and Xu labs (Eklof Spink et al. 2001; Huber and Weis 2001; Xing et al. 2003). Although we can remain optimistic that a compound that disrupts the β-catenin-TCF complex will someday be developed, the nature of this interaction is clearly not optimal for such an approach. Moreover, such a compound would also have to avoid simultaneous disruption of the other three complexes sharing common interaction sites. For example, experimental disruption of the cadherin-β-catenin complex in mice leads to severe intestinal inflammation and ultimately neoplasia (Hermiston and Gordon 1995). The Xu lab more recently described the structure of the β-catenin-bcl-9 interface, which appears somewhat more amenable to disruption by small molecules (Sampietro et al. 2006).

1.9   Conclusion

It is now apparent that aberrant wnt signaling contributes to a significant proportion of human cancers. The most transparent examples of this are those cancers harboring functionally relevant mutations in wnt pathway genes. Attacking these cancers will likely require drugs that operate inside the cell and downstream of β-catenin. The good news is that these patients can be readily identified, and in colorectal cancer, where mutations are extremely common, a diagnostic might not even be required in clinical testing. Deregulated wnt signaling is also apparent in some cancers lacking pathway mutations. This raises hope for therapeutics that function outside the cell by interfering with ligand–receptor interactions. However, innovative diagnostics will be required to identify these patients. Finally, the potential for wnt signaling in the maintenance of cancer stem cells is particularly exciting. Here a therapeutic could be beneficial in the adjuvant setting, where standard care reduces the bulk tumor and wnt inhibitors retard residual progenitors from reinitiating outgrowth.

References

Aberle H, Bauer A, Stappert J, Kispert A and Kemler R. (1997) Beta-catenin is a target for the ubiquitin-proteasome pathway Embo J 16:3797–804

Amit S, Hatzubai A, Birman Y, et al. (2002) Axin-mediated CKI phosphorylation of beta-catenin at Ser 45: a molecular switch for the Wnt pathway Genes Dev 16:1066–76

Austin TW, Solar GP, Ziegler FC, Liem L and Matthews W. (1997) A role for the Wnt gene family in hematopoiesis: expansion of multilineage progenitor cells Blood 89:3624–35

Barker N, Hurlstone A, Musisi H, et al. (2001) The chromatin remodelling factor Brg-1 interacts with beta-catenin to promote target gene activation Embo J 20:4935–43

Barker N, Ridgway RA, van Es JH, *et al.* (2009) Crypt stem cells as the cells-of-origin of intestinal cancer Nature 457:608–11

Barker N, van Es JH, Kuipers J, *et al.* (2007) Identification of stem cells in small intestine and colon by marker gene Lgr5 Nature 449:1003–7

Bauer A, Huber O and Kemler R. (1998) Pontin52, an interaction partner of beta-catenin, binds to the TATA box binding protein Proc Natl Acad Sci U S A 95:14787–92

Behrens J, Jerchow BA, Wurtele M, *et al.* (1998) Functional interaction of an axin homolog, conductin, with beta-catenin, APC, and GSK3beta Science 280:596–9

Behrens J, von Kries JP, Kuhl M, *et al.* (1996) Functional interaction of beta-catenin with the transcription factor LEF-1 Nature 382:638–42

Bejsovec A and Martinez Arias A. (1991) Roles of wingless in patterning the larval epidermis of Drosophila Development 113:471–85

Belenkaya TY, Han C, Standley HJ, *et al.* (2002) pygopus Encodes a nuclear protein essential for wingless/Wnt signaling Development 129:4089–101

Bhanot P, Brink M, Samos CH, *et al.* (1996) A new member of the frizzled family from Drosophila functions as a Wingless receptor Nature 382:225–30

Bjorklund P, Akerstrom G and Westin G. (2007) An LRP5 receptor with internal deletion in hyperparathyroid tumors with implications for deregulated WNT/beta-catenin signaling PLoS Med 4:e328

Bjorklund P, Svedlund J, Olsson AK, Akerstrom G and Westin G. (2009) The internally truncated LRP5 receptor presents a therapeutic target in breast cancer PLoS One 4:e4243

Blanpain C, Lowry WE, Geoghegan A, Polak L and Fuchs E. (2004) Self-renewal, multipotency, and the existence of two cell populations within an epithelial stem cell niche Cell 118:635–48

Brack AS, Murphy-Seiler F, Hanifi J, *et al.* (2009) BCL9 is an essential component of canonical Wnt signaling that mediates the differentiation of myogenic progenitors during muscle regeneration Dev Biol 335:93–105

Brannon M, Brown JD, Bates R, Kimelman D and Moon RT. (1999) XCtBP is a XTcf-3 co-repressor with roles throughout Xenopus development Development 126:3159–70

Cavallo RA, Cox RT, Moline MM, *et al.* (1998) Drosophila Tcf and Groucho interact to repress Wingless signalling activity Nature 395:604–8

Chen B, Dodge ME, Tang W, *et al.* (2009) Small molecule-mediated disruption of Wnt-dependent signaling in tissue regeneration and cancer Nat Chem Biol 5:100–7

Daniels DL and Weis WI. (2005) Beta-catenin directly displaces Groucho/TLE repressors from Tcf/Lef in Wnt-mediated transcription activation Nat Struct Mol Biol 12:364–71

Davidson G, Wu W, Shen J, *et al.* (2005) Casein kinase 1 gamma couples Wnt receptor activation to cytoplasmic signal transduction Nature 438:867–72

Dominguez I, Itoh K and Sokol SY. (1995) Role of glycogen synthase kinase 3 beta as a negative regulator of dorsoventral axis formation in Xenopus embryos Proc Natl Acad Sci U S A 92:8498–502

Eklof Spink K, Fridman SG and Weis WI. (2001) Molecular mechanisms of beta-catenin recognition by adenomatous polyposis coli revealed by the structure of an APC-beta-catenin complex Embo J 20:6203–12

Feng Y, Lee N and Fearon ER. (2003) TIP49 regulates beta-catenin-mediated neoplastic transformation and T-cell factor target gene induction via effects on chromatin remodeling Cancer Res 63:8726–34

Finch PW, He X, Kelley MJ, *et al.* (1997) Purification and molecular cloning of a secreted, Frizzled-related antagonist of Wnt action Proc Natl Acad Sci U S A 94:6770–5

Funayama N, Fagotto F, McCrea P and Gumbiner BM. (1995) Embryonic axis induction by the armadillo repeat domain of beta-catenin: evidence for intracellular signaling J Cell Biol 128:959–68

Glinka A, Wu W, Delius H, *et al.* (1998) Dickkopf-1 is a member of a new family of secreted proteins and functions in head induction Nature 391:357–62

Graham TA, Weaver C, Mao F, Kimelman D and Xu W. (2000) Crystal structure of a beta-catenin/Tcf complex Cell 103:885–96

Groden J, Thliveris A, Samowitz W, *et al.* (1991) Identification and characterization of the familial adenomatous polyposis coli gene Cell 66:589–600

Guger KA and Gumbiner BM. (1995) beta-Catenin has Wnt-like activity and mimics the Nieuwkoop signaling center in Xenopus dorsal-ventral patterning Dev Biol 172:115–25

Hart MJ, de los Santos R, Albert IN, Rubinfeld B and Polakis P. (1998) Downregulation of beta-catenin by human Axin and its association with the APC tumor suppressor, beta-catenin and GSK3 beta Curr Biol 8:573–81

He TC, Sparks AB, Rago C, *et al.* (1998) Identification of c-MYC as a target of the APC pathway Science 281:1509–12

Heasman J, Crawford A, Goldstone K, *et al.* (1994) Overexpression of cadherins and underexpression of beta-catenin inhibit dorsal mesoderm induction in early Xenopus embryos Cell 79:791–803

Hecht A, Vleminckx K, Stemmler MP, van Roy F and Kemler R. (2000) The p300/CBP acetyltransferases function as transcriptional coactivators of beta-catenin in vertebrates Embo J 19:1839–50

Hermiston ML and Gordon JI. (1995) Inflammatory bowel disease and adenomas in mice expressing a dominant negative N-cadherin Science 270:1203–7

Hinck L, Nelson WJ and Papkoff J. (1994) Wnt-1 modulates cell-cell adhesion in mammalian cells by stabilizing beta-catenin binding to the cell adhesion protein cadherin J Cell Biol 124:729–41

Hoeppner LH, Secreto FJ and Westendorf JJ. (2009) Wnt signaling as a therapeutic target for bone diseases Expert Opin Ther Targets 13:485–96

Hsieh JC, Kodjabachian L, Rebbert ML, *et al.* (1999) A new secreted protein that binds to Wnt proteins and inhibits their activities Nature 398:431–6

Huang SM, Mishina YM, Liu S, *et al.* (2009) Tankyrase inhibition stabilizes axin and antagonizes Wnt signalling Nature 461:614–20

Huber AH and Weis WI. (2001) The structure of the beta-catenin/E-cadherin complex and the molecular basis of diverse ligand recognition by beta-catenin Cell 105:391–402

Huber AH, Nelson WJ and Weis WI. (1997) Three-dimensional structure of the armadillo repeat region of beta-catenin Cell 90:871–82

Ikeda S, Kishida S, Yamamoto H, *et al.* (1998) Axin, a negative regulator of the Wnt signaling pathway, forms a complex with GSK-3beta and beta-catenin and promotes GSK-3beta-dependent phosphorylation of beta-catenin Embo J 17:1371–84

Inomata M, Ochiai A, Akimoto S, Kitano S and Hirohashi S. (1996) Alteration of beta-catenin expression in colonic epithelial cells of familial adenomatous polyposis patients Cancer Res 56:2213–7

Itasaki N, Jones CM, Mercurio S, *et al.* (2003) Wise, a context-dependent activator and inhibitor of Wnt signalling Development 130:4295–305

Itoh K, Krupnik VE and Sokol SY. (1998) Axis determination in Xenopus involves biochemical interactions of axin, glycogen synthase kinase 3 and beta-catenin Curr Biol 8:591–4

Jamieson CH, Ailles LE, Dylla SJ, *et al.* (2004) Granulocyte-macrophage progenitors as candidate leukemic stem cells in blast-crisis CML N Engl J Med 351:657–67

Jiang J and Struhl G. (1998) Regulation of the Hedgehog and Wingless signalling pathways by the F-box/WD40-repeat protein Slimb Nature 391:493–6

Kishida S, Yamamoto H, Hino S, *et al.* (1999) DIX domains of Dvl and axin are necessary for protein interactions and their ability to regulate beta-catenin stability Mol Cell Biol 19:4414–22

Klingensmith J, Nusse R and Perrimon N. (1994) The Drosophila segment polarity gene dishevelled encodes a novel protein required for response to the wingless signal Genes Dev 8:118–30

Korinek V, Barker N, Moerer P, *et al.* (1998) Depletion of epithelial stem-cell compartments in the small intestine of mice lacking Tcf-4 Nat Genet 19:379–83

Korinek V, Barker N, Morin PJ, *et al.* (1997) Constitutive transcriptional activation by a beta-catenin-Tcf complex in APC-/- colon carcinoma Science 275:1784–7

Kramps T, Peter O, Brunner E, *et al.* (2002) Wnt/wingless signaling requires BCL9/ legless-mediated recruitment of pygopus to the nuclear beta-catenin-TCF complex Cell 109:47–60

Lammi L, Arte S, Somer M, *et al.* (2004) Mutations in AXIN2 cause familial tooth agenesis and predispose to colorectal cancer Am J Hum Genet 74:1043–50

Levanon D, Goldstein RE, Bernstein Y, *et al.* (1998) Transcriptional repression by AML1 and LEF-1 is mediated by the TLE/Groucho corepressors Proc Natl Acad Sci U S A 95: 11590–5

Leyns L, Bouwmeester T, Kim SH, Piccolo S and De Robertis EM. (1997) Frzb-1 is a secreted antagonist of Wnt signaling expressed in the Spemann organizer Cell 88:747–56

Li X, Zhang Y, Kang H, *et al.* (2005) Sclerostin binds to LRP5/6 and antagonizes canonical Wnt signaling J Biol Chem 280:19883–7

Liu C, Li Y, Semenov M, *et al.* (2002) Control of beta-catenin phosphorylation/degradation by a dual-kinase mechanism Cell 108:837–47

Liu W, Dong X, Mai M, *et al.* (2000) Mutations in AXIN2 cause colorectal cancer with defective mismatch repair by activating beta-catenin/TCF signalling Nat Genet 26:146–7

Lo Celso C, Prowse DM and Watt FM. (2004) Transient activation of beta-catenin signalling in adult mouse epidermis is sufficient to induce new hair follicles but continuous activation is required to maintain hair follicle tumours Development 131:1787–99

Major MB, Camp ND, Berndt JD, *et al.* (2007) Wilms tumor suppressor WTX negatively regulates WNT/beta-catenin signaling Science 316:1043–6

Malanchi I, Peinado H, Kassen D, *et al.* (2008) Cutaneous cancer stem cell maintenance is dependent on beta-catenin signalling Nature 452:650–3

Mao J, Wang J, Liu B, *et al.* (2001) Low-density lipoprotein receptor-related protein-5 binds to Axin and regulates the canonical Wnt signaling pathway Mol Cell 7:801–9

Marikawa Y and Elinson RP. (1998) beta-TrCP is a negative regulator of Wnt/beta-catenin signaling pathway and dorsal axis formation in Xenopus embryos Mech Dev 77:75–80

McCrea PD, Turck CW and Gumbiner B. (1991) A homolog of the armadillo protein in Drosophila (plakoglobin) associated with E-cadherin Science 254:1359–61

McMahon AP and Moon RT. (1989) Ectopic expression of the proto-oncogene int-1 in Xenopus embryos leads to duplication of the embryonic axis Cell 58:1075–84

Molenaar M, van de Wetering M, Oosterwegel M, *et al.* (1996) XTcf-3 transcription factor mediates beta-catenin-induced axis formation in Xenopus embryos Cell 86:391–9

Morin PJ, Sparks AB, Korinek V, *et al.* (1997) Activation of beta-catenin-Tcf signaling in colon cancer by mutations in beta-catenin or APC Science 275:1787–90

Moser AR, Pitot HC and Dove WF. (1990) A dominant mutation that predisposes to multiple intestinal neoplasia in the mouse Science 247:322–4

Munemitsu S, Albert I, Rubinfeld B and Polakis P. (1996) Deletion of an amino-terminal sequence beta-catenin in vivo and promotes hyperphosporylation of the adenomatous polyposis coli tumor suppressor protein Mol Cell Biol 16:4088–94

Munemitsu S, Albert I, Souza B, Rubinfeld B and Polakis P. (1995) Regulation of intracellular beta-catenin levels by the adenomatous polyposis coli (APC) tumor-suppressor protein Proc Natl Acad Sci U S A 92:3046–50

Nishisho I, Nakamura Y, Miyoshi Y, *et al.* (1991) Mutations of chromosome 5q21 genes in FAP and colorectal cancer patients Science 253:665–9

Noordermeer J, Klingensmith J, Perrimon N and Nusse R. (1994) dishevelled and armadillo act in the wingless signalling pathway in Drosophila Nature 367:80–3

Nusse R and Varmus HE. (1982) Many tumors induced by the mouse mammary tumor virus contain a provirus integrated in the same region of the host genome Cell 31:99–109

Nusslein-Volhard C and Wieschaus E. (1980) Mutations affecting segment number and polarity in Drosophila Nature 287:795–801

Oosterwegel MA, van de Wetering ML, Holstege FC, *et al.* (1991) TCF-1, a T cell-specific transcription factor of the HMG box family, interacts with sequence motifs in the TCR beta and TCR delta enhancers Int Immunol 3:1189–92

Orsulic S and Peifer M. (1996) An in vivo structure-function study of armadillo, the beta-catenin homologue, reveals both separate and overlapping regions of the protein required for cell adhesion and for wingless signaling J Cell Biol 134:1283–300

Parker DS, Jemison J and Cadigan KM. (2002) Pygopus, a nuclear PHD-finger protein required for Wingless signaling in Drosophila Development 129:2565–76

Peifer M, Pai LM and Casey M. (1994) Phosphorylation of the Drosophila adherens junction protein Armadillo: roles for wingless signal and zeste-white 3 kinase Dev Biol 166:543–56

Peifer M, Sweeton D, Casey M and Wieschaus E. (1994) wingless signal and Zeste-white 3 kinase trigger opposing changes in the intracellular distribution of Armadillo Development 120:369–80

Peters JM, McKay RM, McKay JP and Graff JM. (1999) Casein kinase I transduces Wnt signals Nature 401:345–50

Piao S, Lee SH, Kim H, et al. (2008) Direct inhibition of GSK3beta by the phosphorylated cytoplasmic domain of LRP6 in Wnt/beta-catenin signaling PLoS One 3:e4046

Pinson KI, Brennan J, Monkley S, Avery BJ and Skarnes WC. (2000) An LDL-receptor-related protein mediates Wnt signalling in mice Nature 407:535–8

Polakis P. (1995) Mutations in the APC gene and their implications for protein structure and function Curr Opin Genet Dev 5:66–71

Polakis P. (2000) Wnt signaling and cancer Genes Dev 14:1837–51

Polakis P. (2007) The many ways of Wnt in cancer Curr Opin Genet Dev 17:45–51

Rattner A, Hsieh JC, Smallwood PM, et al. (1997) A family of secreted proteins contains homology to the cysteine-rich ligand-binding domain of frizzled receptors Proc Natl Acad Sci U S A 94:2859–63

Reya T and Clevers H. (2005) Wnt signalling in stem cells and cancer Nature 434:843–50

Reya T, Duncan AW, Ailles L, et al. (2003) A role for Wnt signalling in self-renewal of haematopoietic stem cells Nature 423:409–14

Riese J, Yu X, Munnerlyn A, et al. (1997) LEF-1, a nuclear factor coordinating signaling inputs from wingless and decapentaplegic Cell 88:777–87

Riggleman B, Schedl P and Wieschaus E. (1990) Spatial expression of the Drosophila segment polarity gene armadillo is posttranscriptionally regulated by wingless Cell 63:549–60

Robbins PF, El-Gamil M, Li YF, et al. (1996) A mutated beta-catenin gene encodes a melanoma-specific antigen recognized by tumor infiltrating lymphocytes J Exp Med 183:1185–92

Roose J, Molenaar M, Peterson J, et al. (1998) The Xenopus Wnt effector XTcf-3 interacts with Groucho-related transcriptional repressors Nature 395:608–12

Rubinfeld B, Robbins P, El-Gamil M, et al. (1997) Stabilization of beta-catenin by genetic defects in melanoma cell lines Science 275:1790–2

Rubinfeld B, Souza B, Albert I, et al. (1993) Association of the APC gene product with beta-catenin Science 262:1731–4

Sakanaka C, Leong P, Xu L, Harrison SD and Williams LT. (1999) Casein kinase iepsilon in the wnt pathway: regulation of beta-catenin function Proc Natl Acad Sci U S A 96:12548–52

Sampietro J, Dahlberg CL, Cho US, et al. (2006) Crystal structure of a beta-catenin/BCL9/Tcf4 complex Mol Cell 24:293–300

Sato H, Suzuki H, Toyota M, et al. (2007) Frequent epigenetic inactivation of DICKKOPF family genes in human gastrointestinal tumors Carcinogenesis 28:2459–66

Satoh S, Daigo Y, Furukawa Y, et al. (2000) AXIN1 mutations in hepatocellular carcinomas, and growth suppression in cancer cells by virus-mediated transfer of AXIN1 Nat Genet 24:245–50

Schneider S, Steinbeisser H, Warga RM and Hausen P. (1996) Beta-catenin translocation into nuclei demarcates the dorsalizing centers in frog and fish embryos Mech Dev 57:191–8

Schwarz-Romond T, Fiedler M, Shibata N, et al. (2007) The DIX domain of Dishevelled confers Wnt signaling by dynamic polymerization Nat Struct Mol Biol 14:484–92

Sharma RP and Chopra VL. (1976) Effect of the Wingless (wg1) mutation on wing and haltere development in Drosophila melanogaster Dev Biol 48:461–5

Siegfried E, Chou TB and Perrimon N. (1992) wingless signaling acts through zeste-white 3, the Drosophila homolog of glycogen synthase kinase-3, to regulate engrailed and establish cell fate Cell 71:1167–79

Siegfried E, Wilder EL and Perrimon N. (1994) Components of wingless signalling in Drosophila Nature 367:76–80

Sierra J, Yoshida T, Joazeiro CA and Jones KA. (2006) The APC tumor suppressor counteracts beta-catenin activation and H3K4 methylation at Wnt target genes Genes Dev 20:586–600

Smalley MJ, Sara E, Paterson H, *et al.* (1999) Interaction of axin and Dvl-2 proteins regulates Dvl-2-stimulated TCF-dependent transcription Embo J 18:2823–35

Smits R, Kielman MF, Breukel C, *et al.* (1999) Apc1638T: a mouse model delineating critical domains of the adenomatous polyposis coli protein involved in tumorigenesis and development Genes Dev 13:1309–21

Stadeli R and Basler K. (2005) Dissecting nuclear Wingless signalling: recruitment of the transcriptional co-activator Pygopus by a chain of adaptor proteins Mech Dev 122:1171–82

Stehelin D, Varmus HE and Bishop JM. (1975) Detection of nucleotide sequences associated with transformation by avian sarcoma viruses Bibl Haematol 539–41

Su LK, Kinzler KW, Vogelstein B, *et al.* (1992) Multiple intestinal neoplasia caused by a mutation in the murine homolog of the APC gene Science 256:668–70

Su LK, Vogelstein B and Kinzler KW. (1993) Association of the APC tumor suppressor protein with catenins Science 262:1734–7

Suzuki H, Watkins DN, Jair KW, *et al.* (2004) Epigenetic inactivation of SFRP genes allows constitutive WNT signaling in colorectal cancer Nat Genet 36:417–22

Takemaru KI and Moon RT. (2000) The transcriptional coactivator CBP interacts with beta-catenin to activate gene expression J Cell Biol 149:249–54

Tamai K, Semenov M, Kato Y, *et al.* (2000) LDL-receptor-related proteins in Wnt signal transduction Nature 407:530–5

Tetsu O and McCormick F. (1999) Beta-catenin regulates expression of cyclin D1 in colon carcinoma cells Nature 398:422–6

Thompson B, Townsley F, Rosin-Arbesfeld R, Musisi H and Bienz M. (2002) A new nuclear component of the Wnt signalling pathway Nat Cell Biol 4:367–73

Thorstensen L, Lind GE, Lovig T, *et al.* (2005) Genetic and epigenetic changes of components affecting the WNT pathway in colorectal carcinomas stratified by microsatellite instability Neoplasia 7:99–108

van den Heuvel M, Nusse R, Johnston P and Lawrence PA. (1989) Distribution of the wingless gene product in Drosophila embryos: a protein involved in cell-cell communication Cell 59:739–49

Varmus HE, Heasley S and Bishop JM. (1974) Use of DNA-DNA annealing to detect new virus-specific DNA sequences in chicken embryo fibroblasts after infection by avian sarcoma virus J Virol 14:895–903

Waterman ML, Fischer WH and Jones KA. (1991) A thymus-specific member of the HMG protein family regulates the human T cell receptor C alpha enhancer Genes Dev 5:656–69

Webster MT, Rozycka M, Sara E, *et al.* (2000) Sequence variants of the axin gene in breast, colon, and other cancers: an analysis of mutations that interfere with GSK3 binding Genes Chromosomes Cancer 28:443–53

Wehrli M, Dougan ST, Caldwell K, *et al.* (2000) arrow encodes an LDL-receptor-related protein essential for Wingless signalling Nature 407:527–30

Whitehead I, Kirk H and Kay R. (1995) Expression cloning of oncogenes by retroviral transfer of cDNA libraries Mol Cell Biol 15:704–10

Wieschaus E and Riggleman R. (1987) Autonomous requirements for the segment polarity gene armadillo during Drosophila embryogenesis Cell 49:177–84

Willert K, Brown JD, Danenberg E, *et al.* (2003) Wnt proteins are lipid-modified and can act as stem cell growth factors Nature 423:448–52

Wong HC, Bourdelas A, Krauss A, *et al.* (2003) Direct binding of the PDZ domain of Dishevelled to a conserved internal sequence in the C-terminal region of Frizzled Mol Cell 12:1251–60

Xie J, Murone M, Luoh SM, *et al.* (1998) Activating Smoothened mutations in sporadic basal-cell carcinoma Nature 391:90–2

Xing Y, Clements WK, Kimelman D and Xu W. (2003) Crystal structure of a beta-catenin/axin complex suggests a mechanism for the beta-catenin destruction complex Genes Dev 17:2753–64

Yanagawa S, Matsuda Y, Lee JS, *et al.* (2002) Casein kinase I phosphorylates the Armadillo protein and induces its degradation in Drosophila Embo J 21:1733–42

Yost C, Torres M, Miller JR, *et al.* (1996) The axis-inducing activity, stability, and subcellular distribution of beta-catenin is regulated in Xenopus embryos by glycogen synthase kinase 3 Genes Dev 10:1443–54

Zeng L, Fagotto F, Zhang T, *et al.* (1997) The mouse Fused locus encodes Axin, an inhibitor of the Wnt signaling pathway that regulates embryonic axis formation Cell 90:181–92

Zeng X, Tamai K, Doble B, *et al.* (2005) A dual-kinase mechanism for Wnt co-receptor phosphorylation and activation Nature 438:873–7

Chapter 2
Regulation of Wnt Secretion and Distribution

Xiaofang Tang, Xiaolan Fan, and Xinhua Lin

Abstract Wnts are a family of signaling glycoproteins which play essential roles in many developmental processes and adult homeostasis. Misregulated Wnt signaling has been implicated in a variety of human diseases including cancers. The tight regulation of Wnt signaling is not only reflected by the diverse responses triggered in the Wnt-receiving cells, but also, as more recent work suggested, by the complex control on Wnt processing, secretion, and subsequent distribution. The characterization of the nature and roles of posttranslational modifications of Wnt molecules and the discovery of Wntless (Wls) and the retromer complex as novel and indispensable players in Wnt release have led to closer inspection of the Wnt secretory routes. Moreover, dissection of the functions of lipoproteins and heparan sulfate proteoglycans (HSPGs) in Wnt diffusion shed new light on the mechanism of morphogen distribution. In this chapter, we will summarize the recent advances in the studies of Wnt processing, secretion, and spreading and discuss how these components are integrated into the regulating network of Wnt pathway.

Keywords Wnt processing • Wnt secretion • Wingless (Wg) • Wntless (Wls) • The retromer complex • Lipoprotein • Heparan sulfate proteoglycan (HSPG)

X. Lin (✉)
Division of Developmental Biology, Cincinnati Children's Hospital Medical Center,
and The Graduate Program in Molecular and Developmental Biology,
University of Cincinnati College of Medicine, Cincinnati, OH 45229, USA
and
State Key Laboratory of Biomembrane and Membrane Biotechnology, and Key Laboratory
of stem cell, Institute of Zoology, Chinese Academy of Sciences, Beijing, 100101, China
e-mail: xinhua.lin@cchmc.org

K.H. Goss and M. Kahn (eds.), *Targeting the Wnt Pathway in Cancer*,
DOI 10.1007/978-1-4419-8023-6_2, © Springer Science+Business Media, LLC 2011

2.1   Introduction

The Wnt family of secreted cysteine-rich glycoproteins is evolutionarily conserved in metazoans. As one of the best-studied morphogen families, Wnt molecules provide cells in the morphogenetic field with positional information and trigger cellular responses in a concentration-dependent manner. Although a great deal is known about Wnt perception and signal transduction in the Wnt-receiving cells, relatively limited information is available about the events occurring in Wnt-producing cells and the extracellular space. In this chapter, we will review the recent studies on the molecules and mechanisms involved in these events and discuss how the players interact with each other and integrate into the dedicated Wnt secretion route(s).

2.2   Wnts Are Posttranslationally Modified in the ER

As a common structural characteristic, Wnts contain several charged residues and a relatively high number of conserved cysteines (23–25 on average), which might be involved in the establishment of intra- and intermolecular disulfide bonds and thus be important for the proper folding and multimerization of Wnt proteins (Miller 2002; Coudreuse and Korswagen 2007) (Fig. 2.1). In contrast to predictions made based on their primary amino-acid sequences, Wnt proteins are more hydrophobic and insoluble. These characteristics have long hampered the isolation of active Wnts. The first successful attempt in Wnt purification was made by the Nusse group in 2003 (Willert et al. 2003). From their work, they isolated active products of mouse *Wnt3a* and *Drosophila Wnt8* genes. Moreover, they found that

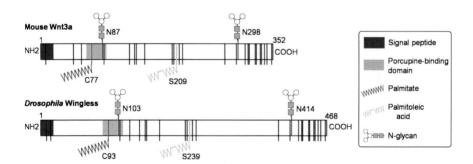

Fig. 2.1 Schematic overview of mouse Wnt3a and *Drosophila* Wingless proteins, showing the approximate positions of cysteine residues (*black vertical lines*). Both Wnts are acylated probably by Porcupine which binds Wnts at the corresponding region. Two lipids are appended to Wnts: one palmitate to the N-terminal cysteine and one palmitoleic acid to the internal serine. Wnts also harbor several potential N-glycosylation sites as indicated. The signal sequence is represented by the boxed area in the N-terminus

both molecules were palmitoylated at a conserved cysteine residue (C77 in Wnt3a) and this modification was essential for Wnt signaling activity. Subsequent work revealed that *Drosophila* Wingless (Wg), murine Wnt5a, as well as chick Wnt1 and Wnt3a are all palmitoylated at the corresponding cysteine residues (Willert et al. 2003; Miura and Treisman 2006; Galli et al. 2007; Kurayoshi et al. 2007). More recently, Takada et al. reported that mouse Wnt3a was also lipid-modified by palmitoleic acid at a conserved serine residue (S239) (Takada et al. 2006). Therefore, Wnts are potentially acylated at two conserved sites: one palmitate at an N-terminal cysteine and one palmitoleic acid at an internal serine (Fig. 2.1). The only exception so far is WntD, a recently characterized *Drosophila* Wnt family member (Ganguly et al. 2005; Gordon et al. 2005; Ching et al. 2008). WntD does not undergo lipid modification and it takes a secretion route different from other Wnts which will be discussed later (Ching et al. 2008).

Many lines of evidence suggest that lipid modifications play essential roles in Wnt secretion and signaling. In vertebrates, it is generally believed that palmitate at cysteine is required for Wnt action, whereas palmitoleic acid at serine is necessary for Wnt secretion. Point mutations of the palmitoylated cysteine in Wnt3a, Wnt1, and Wnt5a do not interfere with their secretion, but strongly decrease their signaling activity in cell-based assays (Willert et al. 2003; Galli et al. 2007; Kurayoshi et al. 2007). Takada et al. demonstrated that Wnt3a defective in serine palmitoleoylation is not secreted from cells, but is rather retained in the endoplasmic reticulum (ER) (Takada et al. 2006), suggesting a possible role of this residue in protein folding and intracellular transport. However, the recent report using *Drosophila* Wg disagreed on the exact roles of two lipid adducts (Franch-Marro et al. 2008a). In this study, it is found that removal of palmitate moiety at the conserved cysteine residue (C93) causes inefficient exit of Wg from ER in the wing imaginal discs, although this mutant can be readily secreted in cultured *Drosophila* S2 cells. On the other hand, mutation of the equivalent serine site (S209) causes no major defect in secretion and membrane association, but results in poor signaling activities. Nevertheless, all of the mutations in this work were made on Wg with an internal HA tag, so it will be important to repeat all experiments on native Wg to confirm the results. How is lipid modification involved in Wnt secretion and signaling activity? While it is still unclear on the aspect of Wnt secretion, current data argue that acylation contributes to Wnt signaling activity by facilitating its interaction with the Frizzled receptor (Willert et al. 2003; Cong et al. 2004; Komekado et al. 2007; Kurayoshi et al. 2007).

Another posttranslational modification of Wnts is N-glycosylation, in which N-linked oligosaccharide chains are attached to the peptide backbone (Fig. 2.1). Unlike lipid modification, the number and position of glycosylation sites seem to be flexible and its function is poorly understood. In the early studies, it was demonstrated that replacement of all four asparagine-linked glycosylation sites did not affect Wnt1-induced or paracrine signaling in tissue culture system, indicating that glycosylation was not essential for either secretion or signaling of Wnts (Mason et al. 1992). However, the Kikuchi group recently argued that in the case of Wnt3a and Wnt5a, glycosylation precedes lipid modification and is important for Wnt secretion, but not for their actions (Komekado et al. 2007; Kurayoshi et al. 2007). As most of the published studies were based on in vitro assays, further in vivo studies on more Wnt members are required to fully unravel the functions of Wnt posttranslational modifications.

The enzyme most likely to be responsible for Wnt lipid modification is the ER protein Porcupine (Porc). *Porc* was first identified in *Drosophila* as a segment polarity gene (van den Heuvel et al. 1993), which encodes a conserved multiple-pass transmembrane protein in the family of membrane-bound O-acyltransferases (MBOATs) (Hofmann 2000). Despite the lack of direct evidence, the role of Porc as the lipid-modifying enzyme of Wnt is supported by three lines of evidence. First, Porc controls the hydrophobicity levels of Wnts: in the absence of Porc, Wg becomes less hydrophobic (Zhai et al. 2004), while when Porc is overexpressed, Wnt1 and Wnt3a are more hydrophobic (Galli et al. 2007). Second, the Porc-binding domain in Wnt sequence contains the conserved palmitoylated cysteine residue (Fig. 2.1) (Tanaka et al. 2002). Third, Porc loss-of-function mutations phenocopy mutations of Wnt acylation and show similar disrupted secretion of Wg and Wnt3a (van den Heuvel et al. 1993; Takada et al. 2006). Although the link of Wnt acylation and Porc is well established, we cannot rule out the possibility that Porc is involved in lipid-modifying other sites besides the conserved cysteine and serine. Also, Porc may control Wnt signaling via roles more than acylation, but such roles could not be exhibited in Porc mutant due to its dominating secretion defect. Previously, Porc was also shown to be required for Wg glycosylation and its enzymatic activity correlated with the glycosylation levels of Wg (Tanaka et al. 2002). Inconsistently, the Takada group demonstrated that the glycosylation of Wnt3a was not perturbed when Porc expression was knocked down by RNAi (Takada et al. 2006). One explanation for this discrepancy is that the role of Porc in glycosylation may not be conserved among different Wnt members.

2.3 Wls and the Retromer Complex Are Involved in the Intracellular Trafficking of Wnts

In addition to Porc, Wls (also known as Evenness interrupted or Sprinter) is another key regulator for Wnt secretion (Banziger et al. 2006; Bartscherer et al. 2006; Goodman et al. 2006). The initial identification of Wls was made in *Drosophila* by three independent groups (Banziger et al. 2006; Bartscherer et al. 2006; Goodman et al. 2006). As a multipass transmembrane protein, Wls has been shown to localize in components of the secretory pathway, including the Golgi apparatus, plasma membrane, and endosomes, suggesting a role of Wls in Wnt trafficking downstream of Porc (Banziger et al. 2006; Bartscherer et al. 2006; Belenkaya et al. 2008; Franch-Marro et al. 2008b; Port et al. 2008; Yang et al. 2008). Indeed, mutations of Wls result in cell-autonomous accumulation of Wg and therefore failure in target gene activation in embryos and wing imaginal discs (Banziger et al. 2006;

Bartscherer et al. 2006; Goodman et al. 2006). Particularly, in the absence of Wls, Wg is accumulated in the Golgi and it can no longer reach the cell surface (Banziger et al. 2006). Furthermore, co-immunoprecipitation experiments confirm that Wls physically interacts with Wnt proteins (Banziger et al. 2006). All of the data lead to a model that Wls helps Wnt transport from Golgi to the plasma membrane for secretion, but the underlying mechanism is still unknown. Several possibilities have been raised: Wls could function as a modifying enzyme or chaperone which assists in the proper folding and maturation of Wnt before it is admitted to the public transportation; or, Wls could act as a cargo receptor or router which carries or sorts Wnt into the dedicated secretion track. On this point, one related question needs to be answered, i.e., whether Wls is associated with Wnt during or after the passage of Wnt to the cell surface? One intriguing hypothesis is that Wls can also function in the endocytosis and rerouting of membrane-bound Wnt molecules. As an evolutionarily conserved protein family, Wls and its homologs in *C. elegans*, planarian, mouse, and *Xenopus* have been shown to regulate the secretion of various Wnt ligands both in vitro and in vivo (Banziger et al. 2006; Adell et al. 2009; Fu et al. 2009; Kim et al. 2009). Interestingly, recent work uncovered that mouse Wls is a direct target of the canonical Wnt pathway during embryonic axis formation (Fu et al. 2009), suggesting a feedback mechanism underlying the reciprocal regulation of Wls and Wnt. As mentioned before, *Drosophila* WntD is the only lipid-unmodified Wnt member. Actually, it is also the only Wnt member which can be efficiently secreted without Wls action (Ching et al. 2008). The secretion of WntD, however, does maintain the requirement of Rab1, which is an ER-to-Golgi trafficking component (Ching et al. 2008). This observation strongly argues that the unpalmitoylated WntD takes a different secretion mode subsequent to its Golgi entrance. In other words, lipid modification renders Wnt dependent on a dedicated mechanism for secretion in which Wls is required.

First identified in yeast decades ago, the retromer was recently implicated in the same Wnt secretion pathway as Wls. The retromer is an evolutionarily conserved multisubunit complex, consisting of two smaller complexes, the cargo recognition Vps26-Vps29-Vps35 heterotrimer and a membrane-targeting SNX heterodimer or homodimer (Seaman et al. 1998; Seaman 2005; Verges 2007). It has been shown that the retromer mediates various intracellular transporting processes, including endosome-Golgi trafficking of yeast hydrolase transporter Vps10 and mammalian cation-independent mannose-6-phosphate receptor, and transcytosis of the polymeric immunoglobulin receptor (Seaman et al. 1997; Seaman et al. 1998; Verges et al. 2004; Seaman 2005).The function of the retromer complex in Wnt signaling was first uncovered in *C. elegans* by two independent groups (Coudreuse et al. 2006; Prasad and Clark 2006). In *C. elegans*, mutations in components of the retromer complex, especially Vps35, show disrupted Wnt signaling and, by epistatic assays, both groups established the role of the retromer in Wnt-producing cells (Coudreuse et al. 2006; Prasad and Clark 2006). Of note, Coudreuse and colleagues observed a much stronger impairment in long-range Wnt signaling vs. short-range Wnt signaling and more importantly a loss of Wnt gradient (Coudreuse et al. 2006), arguing a role of the retromer in packaging and/or transporting Wnt for secretion.

The similarity of Wnt signaling defects in the retromer and *wls* mutants suggests that they may act together to facilitate Wnt secretion. This hypothesis is supported by parallel studies from five independent groups. The authors of this chapter as well as others demonstrated that the retromer complex regulates Wls stability by preventing it from degradation in the lysosomes (Belenkaya et al. 2008; Franch-Marro et al. 2008b; Pan et al. 2008; Port et al. 2008; Yang et al. 2008). Wls is internalized from the plasma membrane by a clathrin-dependent endocytosis (Belenkaya et al. 2008; Pan et al. 2008; Port et al. 2008; Yang et al. 2008) and can be recycled back to the trans-Golgi network (TGN) as shown by antibody-uptake assays (Belenkaya et al. 2008; Franch-Marro et al. 2008b). Interference of AP-2, Rab5, and dynamin function causes accumulation of Wls on the cell surface, increase in total Wls levels, and reduced amount of Wls in the Golgi, indicating recycling of Wls following endocytosis from the cell surface (Belenkaya et al. 2008; Franch-Marro et al. 2008b; Pan et al. 2008; Port et al. 2008; Yang et al. 2008). An interaction between Wls and the retromer complex has been proposed based on colocalization in endocytic vesicles and co-immunoprecipitation assays (Belenkaya et al. 2008; Franch-Marro et al. 2008b; Port et al. 2008; Yang et al. 2008). By analogy with the previous reported role of the retromer in selective recycling of cargo receptors, it is proposed that the retromer supports Wnt secretion by retrieving Wls from endosomes to the Golgi after its clathrin-mediated endocytosis. So far, the function of the retromer in Wls recycling is shown to be conserved in *C. elegans* (Pan et al. 2008; Yang et al. 2008), *Drosophila* (Belenkaya et al. 2008; Franch-Marro et al. 2008b; Port et al. 2008), *Xenopus* (Kim et al. 2009), and mammalian cells (Belenkaya et al. 2008; Franch-Marro et al. 2008b; Port et al. 2008).

2.4 Wnts Associate with Lipoproteins in the Dedicated Secretory Route

As mentioned before, Wnt proteins are hydrophobic due to attachment of lipid moieties. In vitro purified Wnt proteins are poorly diffusible and insoluble, which seems inconsistent with the in vivo role of Wnt in tissue patterning. During development, Wnt molecules act both as a short-range inducer and a long-range morphogen which spreads in long distances to activate expression of different target genes at different threshold levels. Therefore, it has been speculated that a dedicated secretion route exists in addition to the unregulated bulk flow pathway. While the later releases poorly mobile molecules close to the source of production, the former produces specifically packed morphogens for efficient spreading and long-range signaling. The existence of such a dedicated pathway has been implicated in the secretion of Hedgehog (Hh) (Gallet et al. 2003). In this study, they found that in the *Drosophila* embryonic epithelium, Hh forms large punctate structures and the movement of these puncta segregates away from a secreted form of GFP. As the morphogen family of Hh shares significant structural (both are lipid-modified) and functional similarities with Wnt (Nusse 2003). Wnt may take a similar route in secretion. Moreover, the discovery of Wls as a specific player in Wnt-producing cells hints again at specific cellular machinery dedicated to controlling Wnt release. Interestingly, the functional equivalent of Wls in Hh secretion is the multipass transmembrane protein Dispatched, which contains a sterol-sensing domain potentially interacting with the cholesterol modification of Hh (Burke et al. 1999). The last evidence resides in the association of Wnt with lipid rafts (Zhai et al. 2004). Lipid rafts are specialized detergent-resistant membrane microdomains which are shown to act as platforms for the sorting and trafficking of particular subgroups of proteins (Rietveld et al. 1999; Schmidt et al. 2001; Le Roy and Wrana 2005). Importantly, the Basler group recently reported that in *Drosophila*, a major component of membrane micro-domains, Reggie-1/Flotillin-2, promotes the secretion and spreading of Wnt and Hh especially for long-range signaling (Katanaev et al. 2008). This result consistently supports the view that targeting to lipid rafts may direct Wnt to specialized sorting and secretion routes.

How could Wnt overcome its hydrophobic nature and achieve effective secretion and diffusion in vivo? Generally, two models have been proposed. In the first model, acylated Wnts may form micelle-like multimers with the lipid chains facing the interior. This multimeric complex has recently been suggested by the sucrose-density gradient experiments with secreted Wnts from tissue-cultured cells (Katanaev et al. 2008). Although Wnt oligomerization is ambiguous, the formation of Hh oligomers has been much better demonstrated. In addition to previous bio-chemical evidence (Zeng et al. 2001; Chen et al. 2004; Gallet et al. 2006), Neha Vyas and colleagues predicted, based on FRET microscopy, that Hh forms nano-scale oligomers which require the electrostatic interaction between Hh molecules (Vyas et al. 2008). Another model for the movement of lipid-modified morphogens involves the association of Wnt with the lipoprotein particles (LPPs), which were demonstrated in *Drosophila* and originally termed "argosomes" (Greco et al. 2001; Panakova et al. 2005). LPPs consist of a hydrophobic core of lipids, surrounded by a hydrophilic monolayer harboring specific apolipoproteins (Rodenburg and Van der Horst 2005). In *Drosophila*, LPPs are derived from fat body and are found in endocytic compartments in the secreting cell and in the extracellular space of wing imaginal discs (Kutty et al. 1996; Panakova et al. 2005). Both Wnt and Hh are shown to associate with LPPs and this association is important for morphogen spreading and activation of long-range signaling. In the *Drosophila* wing epithe-lium, loss of lipoproteins reduces the range of spreading and signaling of Wg and Hh (Panakova et al. 2005). In the mammalian tissue culture system, it was recently shown that Wnt3a is released on high-density LPPs (Neumann et al. 2009). However, it remains unclear by which manner Wnt proteins distribute on LPPs. One possibility is that cell surface Wnt is "brushed off" by the LPPs in the extracel-lular space. Alternatively, a more attractive model would be that Wnts are loaded onto LPPs in endocytic compartments of Wnt-producing cells in which process Wls may play a role.

2.5 HSPGs Regulate Extracellular Diffusion and Gradient Formation of Wnts

Heparan sulfate proteoglycan (HSPGs) are cell-surface and extracellular matrix (ECM) macromolecules consisting of a protein core attached by heparin sulfate (HS) glycosaminoglycan (GAG) chains (Bernfield et al. 1999; Esko and Selleck 2002). Over the past decades, studies in *Drosophila* and vertebrates have demonstrated that HSPGs are involved in several signaling pathways, including Wnt, Hh, transforming growth factor-β (TGFβ), and fibroblast growth factor (FGF).

Based on the structure of the core protein, HSPGs are classified into three major families. Glypicans and syndecans are cell-surface HSPGs and are linked to the plasma membrane by a glycosylphosphatidylinositol (GPI) linkage or a transmembrane domain, respectively. Perlecans are secreted HSPGs mainly distributed in the ECM. Besides HS chains, syndecans are decorated with chondroitin sulfate. All three HSPG families are evolutionarily conserved from *C. elegans*, *Drosophila* to vertebrates (Esko and Selleck 2002; Nybakken and Perrimon 2002). HS chain biosynthesis is initiated at the GAG attachment site(s) of the core proteins and involves various glycosyltransferases and modification enzymes which are also evolutionarily conserved (Bernfield et al. 1999; Lin and Perrimon 2002; Nybakken and Perrimon 2002). The function of HSPGs in Wnt signaling was first revealed by the characterization of sugarless (sgl) (Binari et al. 1997; Hacker et al. 1997; Haerry et al. 1997) and sulfateless (sfl) (Lin and Perrimon 1999), both of which are important enzymes involved in HS biosynthesis. *sgl* and *sfl* mutants develop Wg-dependent embryonic defects (Hacker et al. 1997; Lin and Perrimon 1999) and loss of Sfl activity results in reduced Wg target gene expression and extracellular Wg levels (Lin and Perrimon 1999; Baeg et al. 2001). In subsequent research, other enzymes, such as the EXT proteins, are also shown to be involved in Wg/Wnt signaling and distribution (Lin 2004). To date, various studies support the idea that HSPGs regulate Wnt signaling and its gradient formation via their attached HS GAG chains.

Existing evidence, especially those from *Drosophila,* suggests that glypican core proteins also play important roles in regulating the gradient formation of morphogens, including Wnt and Hh. The *Drosophila* genome encodes two glypicans (division abnormally delayed [Dally] and Dally-like [Dlp]) (Nakato et al. 1995; Khare and Baumgartner 2000; Baeg et al. 2001). It has been shown that Dally and Dlp play cooperative and distinct roles in regulating Wg signaling and distribution. First, Dally-Dlp double mutants exhibit stronger reduction in Wg signaling and extracellular deposition in the embryos and wing discs than in either alone (Baeg et al. 2001; Han et al. 2005). Second, as opposed to the positive role of Dally in Wg signaling (Lin and Perrimon 1999), Dlp shows biphasic activities, functioning to repress short-range Wg signaling but activate long-range Wg signaling (Baeg et al. 2004; Kirkpatrick et al. 2004; Franch-Marro et al. 2005). One explanation for it resides in the fact that Dlp has stronger affinity for Wg. Both Dally and Dlp can bind Wg in cell culture, but only overexpression of Dlp causes Wg accumulation in the imaginal discs (Baeg et al. 2001; Franch-Marro et al. 2005). Therefore, while

Dally helps present Wg to the signaling receptor dFz2 as a coreceptor (Lin and Perrimon 1999; Franch-Marro et al. 2005), Dlp retains Wg on the cell surface to either compete with dFz2 or facilitate its binding with Wg depending on the ratio of Wg, dFz2, and Dlp (Yan et al. 2009). Concerning the distinct functions of Dally and Dlp, HSPG core proteins may contribute to Wnt signaling much more than being a carrier for HS GAG chains. Indeed, HSPG core proteins can affect the modifications of HS GAG chains (Esko and Zhang 1996; Chen and Lander 2001). Moreover, several studies indicate that HSPG core proteins can be directly involved in Wnt signaling. In vertebrate cells, the nonglycanated glypican-3 (GPC3) core protein can form complexes with Wnts and stimulate Wnt signaling (Capurro et al. 2005). In *Drosophila* wing discs, it was recently demonstrated that Dlp core protein has similar biphasic activity as wild-type Dlp (Yan et al. 2009; Hufnagel et al. 2006).

The functions of vertebrate HSPGs are not well characterized, but accumulating data suggest that HSPGs are also involved in Wnt signaling during development. Examples include the *zebrafish* glypican knypek in Wnt11 signaling (Topczewski et al. 2001), *Xenopus* EXT1 in Wnt11 signaling and distribution (Tao et al. 2005), as well as mammalian GPC3 in Wnt signaling in cancer cells (Filmus and Capurro 2008; Stigliano et al. 2009). As major regulators in morphogen molecules, HSPGs are under a hierarchical regulation during development. First, the expression of HSPGs and the related enzymes is tightly controlled. Both *Dally* and *Dlp* are transcriptionally regulated by Wg and Hh signaling, forming a feedback loop (Fujise et al. 2001; Han et al. 2005; Gallet et al. 2008). The translation of Ttv (one Drosophila EXT protein) and Sfl is controlled by internal ribosome entry sites (Bornemann et al. 2008). Interestingly, the Hippo pathway that modulates multiple morphogen signaling pathways also regulates the transcriptional control of *Dally* and *Dlp* (Baena-Lopez et al. 2008). Second, the intracellular trafficking of HSPGs is a regulated process. Several studies demonstrated that HSPGs are transported to specific membrane domains after synthesis and are actively endocytosed (Bernfield et al. 1999; Kramer and Yost 2003; Bishop et al. 2007). In a recent study, Dlp, which is apically targeted by the GPI anchor, undergoes internalization and redistribution to the basolateral compartment, and this so-called "transcytosis" of Dlp is required for Wg basolateral spreading (Gallet et al. 2008). Finally, HSPGs can be regulated by various shedding mechanisms. The membrane-tethered sydecans and glypicans can be shed into the ECM by proteolytic cleavage (Kato et al. 1998) and GPI cleavage, respectively. Notum, an extracellular lipase, was shown to be involved in the release of glypicans from the cell surface (Gerlitz and Basler 2002; Giraldez et al. 2002; Kreuger et al. 2004; Traister et al. 2008). Alternatively, the HS GAG chains can be cleaved by extracellular heparanase (Sanderson et al. 2004). Although shedding is proposed to regulate cell surface HSPG levels and affect its activities, the in vivo roles await further investigation.

How do HSPGs modulate Wnt distribution? Current data support roles of HSPGs in controlling the spreading of morphogens along the epithelial cell surface through a "restricted diffusion mechanism" in which the secreted morphogen molecules move while interacting with their receptors and other ECM proteins especially HSPGs (Strigini and Cohen 2000; Baeg et al. 2004; Lin 2004;

Han et al. 2005; Hufnagel et al. 2006). In restricted diffusion, HSPGs may play two roles in regulating Wnt movement. First, Wnt movement may be mediated by transferring between HSPGs, especially HS GAG chains. Alternatively, HSPGs control Wnt stability to ensure it moves across a field of cells without being degraded. The two mechanisms may be coupled in Wnt gradient formation. Particularly, it was recently reported that membrane-associated glypicans recruit LPPs in the wing disc cells (Eugster et al. 2007), adding another level of complexity to Wnt gradient formation. In addition to a role in Wnt planar transportation, HSPGs can also regulate Wnt apical/basolateral distribution in epithelial cells. As mentioned before, the apicobasal trafficking of Dlp was recently shown to be involved in the basolateral redistribution of apically secreted Wg in polarized wing disc cells (Gallet et al. 2008).

2.6   Concluding Remarks

Left aside for a long period, the process of Wnt maturation, sorting, and secretion is attracting the interest of more and more researchers in the Wnt field. Especially in the past decade, many important discoveries have been made, including the characterization of Wnt posttranslational modifications, the involvement of LPPs in Wnt trafficking, and the discovery of Wls and the retromer complex in Wnt secretion (as summarized in Fig. 2.2). However, many questions remain to be answered. Regarding Wnt processing and maturation, systematic analysis is needed to verify the results from cell-based assays and to resolve the inconsistence between published data. Particularly, the role of lipid and glycosyl group in Wnt gradient formation as well as short-range vs. long-range signaling has not been examined yet. Recently, the Nusse group identified WntD, the Wnt member which is not lipid-modified and not dependent on Wls for secretion. This exceptional case links Wnt acylation with the need of specialized accessory proteins. It seems that as acylation renders Wnt hydrophobic, certain dedicated secretion mechanisms are required to enable long-range movement and signaling and Wls as well as LPPs may be part of it. In this dedicated pathway, several molecular mechanisms are still elusive. First, how lipid modification affects Wnt-Wls interaction is unknown. Second, the mode of Wls action in Wnt secretion is not fully understood. Third, mechanisms of Wnt apical/basolateral distribution are unclear. Finally, both working in Wnt secretion, the cooperation of Wls and LPPs has not been characterized.

While intensive studies have illustrated the major functions of HSPGs in Wnt gradient formation (Fig. 2.2), the molecular nature of Wnt-HS GAG or Wnt-HSPG core protein interaction waits to be resolved, which may need combined approaches and advanced technology. Clearly, the characterization of HSPG-binding partners, the investigation of HSPG function in vertebrates, as well as lessons from other morphogenic fields will make important contributions to our understanding of the mechanisms by which HSPGs regulate Wnt distribution.

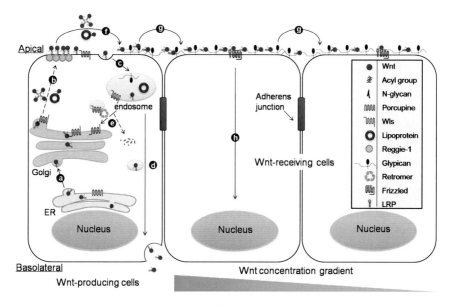

Fig. 2.2 Models of Wnt secretion and distribution. (**a**) Wnt synthesized in the endoplasmic reticulum undergoes N-glycosylation and acylation by the ER enzyme Porcupine. (**b**) In the Golgi apparatus, Wls binds Wnt and helps its delivery to the cell surface by an unknown mechanism. The efficient secretion of Wnt may involve Wnt oligomerization and its association with lipoprotein particles. (**c**) Secreted Wnt is enriched in Reggie-1/Flotillin-2 containing lipid rafts and can be internalized into endocytic vesicles dependent or independent from the endocytosis of Wls, glypican, and lipoprotein. (**d**) Internalized Wnt may be rerouted for basolateral secretion. (**e**) After dissociation with Wnt, Wls, otherwise degraded in the lysosome, is recycled by the retromer complex to the trans-Golgi network. (**f**) Wnt after secretion moves in the extracellular space possibly in the form of Wnt oligomers and/or Wnt–lipoprotein complex. (**g**) The cell surface glypicans facilitate the restricted diffusion and gradient formation of Wnt across a field of cells. (**h**) When captured by Frizzled and the coreceptor LRP, Wnt induces a series of signaling events in the receiving cells in a concentration-dependent manner

Acknowledgments We thank Lin lab members for discussions and critical reading of the manuscript. We apologize to our colleagues whose work could not be cited because of space constraints. Studies of Wnt signaling in the Lin lab were funded by NIH grants (2R01 GM063891 and RO1 GM087517) and American Cancer Society (RSG-07-051), and the grants from Chinese Academy of Sciences (KSCX2-YW-R-263 and KSCX2-YW-R-240).

References

Adell T, Salo E, Boutros M et al (2009) Smed-Evi/Wntless is required for beta-catenin-dependent and -independent processes during planarian regeneration. Development 136(6):905–910

Baeg GH, Lin X, Khare N et al (2001) Heparan sulfate proteoglycans are critical for the organization of the extracellular distribution of Wingless. Development 128(1):87–94

Baeg GH, Selva EM, Goodman RM et al (2004) The Wingless morphogen gradient is established by the cooperative action of Frizzled and Heparan Sulfate Proteoglycan receptors. Dev Biol 276(1):89–100

Baena-Lopez LA, Rodriguez I, Baonza A (2008) The tumor suppressor genes dachsous and fat modulate different signalling pathways by regulating dally and dally-like. Proc Natl Acad Sci U S A 105(28):9645–9650

Banziger C, Soldini D, Schutt C et al (2006) Wntless, a conserved membrane protein dedicated to the secretion of Wnt proteins from signaling cells. Cell 125(3):509–522

Bartscherer K, Pelte N, Ingelfinger D et al (2006) Secretion of Wnt ligands requires Evi, a conserved transmembrane protein. Cell 125(3):523–533

Belenkaya TY, Wu Y, Tang X et al (2008) The retromer complex influences Wnt secretion by recycling wntless from endosomes to the trans-Golgi network. Dev Cell 14(1):120–131

Bernfield M, Gotte M, Park PW et al (1999) Functions of cell surface heparan sulfate proteoglycans. Annu Rev Biochem 68:729–777

Binari RC, Staveley BE, Johnson WA et al (1997) Genetic evidence that heparin-like glycosaminoglycans are involved in wingless signaling. Development 124(13):2623–2632

Bishop JR, Schuksz M, Esko JD (2007) Heparan sulphate proteoglycans fine-tune mammalian physiology. Nature 446(7139):1030–1037

Bornemann DJ, Park S, Phin S et al (2008) A translational block to HSPG synthesis permits BMP signaling in the early Drosophila embryo. Development 135(6):1039–1047

Burke R, Nellen D, Bellotto M et al (1999) Dispatched, a novel sterol-sensing domain protein dedicated to the release of cholesterol-modified hedgehog from signaling cells. Cell 99(7): 803–815

Capurro MI, Xiang YY, Lobe C et al (2005) Glypican-3 promotes the growth of hepatocellular carcinoma by stimulating canonical Wnt signaling. Cancer Res 65(14):6245–6254

Chen MH, Li YJ, Kawakami T et al (2004) Palmitoylation is required for the production of a soluble multimeric Hedgehog protein complex and long-range signaling in vertebrates. Genes Dev 18(6):641–659

Chen RL, Lander AD (2001) Mechanisms underlying preferential assembly of heparan sulfate on glypican-1. J Biol Chem 276(10):7507–7517

Ching W, Hang HC, Nusse R (2008) Lipid-independent secretion of a Drosophila Wnt protein. J Biol Chem 283(25):17092–17098

Cong F, Schweizer L, Varmus H (2004) Wnt signals across the plasma membrane to activate the beta-catenin pathway by forming oligomers containing its receptors, Frizzled and LRP. Development 131(20):5103–5115

Coudreuse D, Korswagen HC (2007) The making of Wnt: new insights into Wnt maturation, sorting and secretion. Development 134(1):3–12

Coudreuse DY, Roel G, Betist MC et al (2006) Wnt gradient formation requires retromer function in Wnt-producing cells. Science 312(5775):921–924

Esko JD, Selleck SB (2002) Order out of chaos: assembly of ligand binding sites in heparan sulfate. Annu Rev Biochem 71:435–471

Esko JD, Zhang L (1996) Influence of core protein sequence on glycosaminoglycan assembly. Curr Opin Struct Biol 6(5):663–670

Eugster C, Panakova D, Mahmoud A et al (2007) Lipoprotein-heparan sulfate interactions in the Hh pathway. Dev Cell 13(1):57–71

Filmus J, Capurro M (2008) The role of glypican-3 in the regulation of body size and cancer. Cell Cycle 7(18):2787–2790

Franch-Marro X, Marchand O, Piddini E et al (2005) Glypicans shunt the Wingless signal between local signalling and further transport. Development 132(4):659–666

Franch-Marro X, Wendler F, Griffith J et al (2008a) In vivo role of lipid adducts on Wingless. J Cell Sci 121(Pt 10):1587–1592

Franch-Marro X, Wendler F, Guidato S et al (2008b) Wingless secretion requires endosome-to-Golgi retrieval of Wntless/Evi/Sprinter by the retromer complex. Nat Cell Biol 10(2):170–177

Fu J, Jiang M, Mirando AJ et al (2009) Reciprocal regulation of Wnt and Gpr177/mouse Wntless is required for embryonic axis formation. Proc Natl Acad Sci U S A 106(44):18598–18603

Fujise M, Izumi S, Selleck SB et al (2001) Regulation of dally, an integral membrane proteoglycan, and its function during adult sensory organ formation of Drosophila. Dev Biol 235(2):433–448

Gallet A, Rodriguez R, Ruel L et al (2003) Cholesterol modification of hedgehog is required for trafficking and movement, revealing an asymmetric cellular response to hedgehog. Dev Cell 4(2):191–204

Gallet A, Ruel L, Staccini-Lavenant L et al (2006) Cholesterol modification is necessary for controlled planar long-range activity of Hedgehog in Drosophila epithelia. Development 133(3):407–418

Gallet A, Staccini-Lavenant L, Therond PP (2008) Cellular trafficking of the glypican Dally-like is required for full-strength Hedgehog signaling and wingless transcytosis. Dev Cell 14(5):712–725

Galli LM, Barnes TL, Secrest SS et al (2007) Porcupine-mediated lipid-modification regulates the activity and distribution of Wnt proteins in the chick neural tube. Development 134(18):3339–3348

Ganguly A, Jiang J, Ip YT (2005) Drosophila WntD is a target and an inhibitor of the Dorsal/Twist/Snail network in the gastrulating embryo. Development 132(15):3419–3429

Gerlitz O, Basler K (2002) Wingful, an extracellular feedback inhibitor of Wingless. Genes Dev 16(9):1055–1059

Giraldez AJ, Copley RR, Cohen SM (2002) HSPG modification by the secreted enzyme Notum shapes the Wingless morphogen gradient. Dev Cell 2(5):667–676

Goodman RM, Thombre S, Firtina Z et al (2006) Sprinter: a novel transmembrane protein required for Wg secretion and signaling. Development 133(24):4901–4911

Gordon MD, Dionne MS, Schneider DS et al (2005) WntD is a feedback inhibitor of Dorsal/NF-kappaB in Drosophila development and immunity. Nature 437(7059):746–749

Greco V, Hannus M, Eaton S (2001) Argosomes: a potential vehicle for the spread of morphogens through epithelia. Cell 106(5):633–645

Hacker U, Lin X, Perrimon N (1997) The Drosophila sugarless gene modulates Wingless signaling and encodes an enzyme involved in polysaccharide biosynthesis. Development 124(18):3565–3573

Haerry TE, Heslip TR, Marsh JL et al (1997) Defects in glucuronate biosynthesis disrupt Wingless signaling in Drosophila. Development 124(16):3055–3064

Han C, Yan D, Belenkaya TY et al (2005) Drosophila glypicans Dally and Dally-like shape the extracellular Wingless morphogen gradient in the wing disc. Development 132(4):667–679

Hofmann K (2000) A superfamily of membrane-bound O-acyltransferases with implications for wnt signaling. Trends Biochem Sci 25(3):111–112

Hufnagel L, Kreuger J, Cohen SM et al (2006) On the role of glypicans in the process of morphogen gradient formation. Dev Biol 300(2):512–522

Katanaev VL, Solis GP, Hausmann G et al (2008) Reggie-1/flotillin-2 promotes secretion of the long-range signalling forms of Wingless and Hedgehog in Drosophila. Embo J 27(3):509–521

Kato M, Wang H, Kainulainen V et al (1998) Physiological degradation converts the soluble syndecan-1 ectodomain from an inhibitor to a potent activator of FGF-2. Nat Med 4(6):691–697

Khare N, Baumgartner S (2000) Dally-like protein, a new Drosophila glypican with expression overlapping with wingless. Mech Dev 99(1–2):199–202

Kim H, Cheong SM, Ryu J et al (2009) Xenopus Wntless and the retromer complex cooperate to regulate XWnt4 secretion. Mol Cell Biol 29(8):2118–2128

Kirkpatrick CA, Dimitroff BD, Rawson JM et al (2004) Spatial regulation of Wingless morphogen distribution and signaling by Dally-like protein. Dev Cell 7(4):513–523

Komekado H, Yamamoto H, Chiba T et al (2007) Glycosylation and palmitoylation of Wnt-3a are coupled to produce an active form of Wnt-3a. Genes Cells 12(4):521–534

Kramer KL, Yost HJ (2003) Heparan sulfate core proteins in cell-cell signaling. Annu Rev Genet 37:461–484

Kreuger J, Perez L, Giraldez AJ et al (2004) Opposing activities of Dally-like glypican at high and low levels of Wingless morphogen activity. Dev Cell 7(4):503–512

Kurayoshi M, Yamamoto H, Izumi S et al (2007) Post-translational palmitoylation and glycosylation of Wnt-5a are necessary for its signalling. Biochem J 402(3):515–523

Kutty RK, Kutty G, Kambadur R et al (1996) Molecular characterization and developmental expression of a retinoid- and fatty acid-binding glycoprotein from Drosophila. A putative lipophorin. J Biol Chem 271(34):20641–20649

Le Roy C, Wrana JL (2005) Clathrin- and non-clathrin-mediated endocytic regulation of cell signalling. Nat Rev Mol Cell Biol 6(2):112–126

Lin X (2004) Functions of heparan sulfate proteoglycans in cell signaling during development. Development 131(24):6009–6021

Lin X, Perrimon N (1999) Dally cooperates with Drosophila Frizzled 2 to transduce Wingless signalling. Nature 400(6741):281–284

Lin X, Perrimon N (2002) Developmental roles of heparan sulfate proteoglycans in Drosophila. Glycoconj J 19(4–5):363–368

Mason JO, Kitajewski J, Varmus HE (1992) Mutational analysis of mouse Wnt-1 identifies two temperature-sensitive alleles and attributes of Wnt-1 protein essential for transformation of a mammary cell line. Mol Biol Cell 3(5):521–533

Miller JR (2002) The Wnts. Genome Biol 3(1):REVIEWS3001

Miura GI, Treisman JE (2006) Lipid modification of secreted signaling proteins. Cell Cycle 5(11):1184–1188

Nakato H, Futch TA, Selleck SB (1995) The division abnormally delayed (dally) gene: a putative integral membrane proteoglycan required for cell division patterning during postembryonic development of the nervous system in Drosophila. Development 121(11):3687–3702

Neumann S, Coudreuse DY, van der Westhuyzen DR et al (2009) Mammalian Wnt3a is released on lipoprotein particles. Traffic 10(3):334–343

Nusse R (2003) Wnts and Hedgehogs: lipid-modified proteins and similarities in signaling mechanisms at the cell surface. Development 130(22):5297–5305

Nybakken K, Perrimon N (2002) Heparan sulfate proteoglycan modulation of developmental signaling in Drosophila. Biochim Biophys Acta 1573(3):280–291

Pan CL, Baum PD, Gu M et al (2008) C. elegans AP-2 and retromer control Wnt signaling by regulating mig-14/Wntless. Dev Cell 14(1):132–139

Panakova D, Sprong H, Marois E et al (2005) Lipoprotein particles are required for Hedgehog and Wingless signalling. Nature 435(7038):58–65

Port F, Kuster M, Herr P et al (2008) Wingless secretion promotes and requires retromer-dependent cycling of Wntless. Nat Cell Biol 10(2):178–185

Prasad BC, Clark SG (2006) Wnt signaling establishes anteroposterior neuronal polarity and requires retromer in C. elegans. Development 133(9):1757–1766

Rietveld A, Neutz S, Simons K et al (1999) Association of sterol- and glycosylphosphatidylinositol-linked proteins with Drosophila raft lipid microdomains. J Biol Chem 274(17):12049–12054

Rodenburg KW, Van der Horst DJ (2005) Lipoprotein-mediated lipid transport in insects: analogy to the mammalian lipid carrier system and novel concepts for the functioning of LDL receptor family members. Biochim Biophys Acta 1736(1):10–29

Sanderson RD, Yang Y, Suva LJ et al (2004) Heparan sulfate proteoglycans and heparanase–partners in osteolytic tumor growth and metastasis. Matrix Biol 23(6):341–352

Schmidt K, Schrader M, Kern HF et al (2001) Regulated apical secretion of zymogens in rat pancreas. Involvement of the glycosylphosphatidylinositol-anchored glycoprotein GP-2, the lectin ZG16p, and cholesterol-glycosphingolipid-enriched microdomains. J Biol Chem 276(17):14315–14323

Seaman MN (2005) Recycle your receptors with retromer. Trends Cell Biol 15(2):68–75

Seaman MN, Marcusson EG, Cereghino JL et al (1997) Endosome to Golgi retrieval of the vacuolar protein sorting receptor, Vps10p, requires the function of the VPS29, VPS30, and VPS35 gene products. J Cell Biol 137(1):79–92

Seaman MN, McCaffery JM, Emr SD (1998) A membrane coat complex essential for endosome-to-Golgi retrograde transport in yeast. J Cell Biol 142(3):665–681

Stigliano I, Puricelli L, Filmus J et al (2009) Glypican-3 regulates migration, adhesion and actin cytoskeleton organization in mammary tumor cells through Wnt signaling modulation. Breast Cancer Res Treat 114(2):251–262

Strigini M, Cohen SM (2000) Wingless gradient formation in the Drosophila wing. Curr Biol 10(6):293–300

Takada R, Satomi Y, Kurata T et al (2006) Monounsaturated fatty acid modification of Wnt protein: its role in Wnt secretion. Dev Cell 11(6):791–801

Tanaka K, Kitagawa Y, Kadowaki T (2002) Drosophila segment polarity gene product porcupine stimulates the posttranslational N-glycosylation of wingless in the endoplasmic reticulum. J Biol Chem 277(15):12816–12823

Tao Q, Yokota C, Puck H et al (2005) Maternal wnt11 activates the canonical wnt signaling pathway required for axis formation in Xenopus embryos. Cell 120(6):857–871

Topczewski J, Sepich DS, Myers DC et al (2001) The zebrafish glypican knypek controls cell polarity during gastrulation movements of convergent extension. Dev Cell 1(2):251–264

Traister A, Shi W, Filmus J (2008) Mammalian Notum induces the release of glypicans and other GPI-anchored proteins from the cell surface. Biochem J 410(3):503–511

van den Heuvel M, Harryman-Samos C, Klingensmith J et al (1993) Mutations in the segment polarity genes wingless and porcupine impair secretion of the wingless protein. Embo J 12(13):5293–5302

Verges M (2007) Retromer and sorting nexins in development. Front Biosci 12:3825–3851

Verges M, Luton F, Gruber C et al (2004) The mammalian retromer regulates transcytosis of the polymeric immunoglobulin receptor. Nat Cell Biol 6(8):763–769

Vyas N, Goswami D, Manonmani A et al (2008) Nanoscale organization of hedgehog is essential for long-range signaling. Cell 133(7):1214–1227

Willert K, Brown JD, Danenberg E et al (2003) Wnt proteins are lipid-modified and can act as stem cell growth factors. Nature 423(6938):448–452

Yan D, Wu Y, Feng Y et al (2009) The core protein of glypican Dally-like determines its biphasic activity in wingless morphogen signaling. Dev Cell 17(4):470–481

Yang PT, Lorenowicz MJ, Silhankova M et al (2008) Wnt signaling requires retromer-dependent recycling of MIG-14/Wntless in Wnt-producing cells. Dev Cell 14(1):140–147

Zeng X, Goetz JA, Suber LM et al (2001) A freely diffusible form of Sonic hedgehog mediates long-range signalling. Nature 411(6838):716–720

Zhai L, Chaturvedi D, Cumberledge S (2004) Drosophila wnt-1 undergoes a hydrophobic modification and is targeted to lipid rafts, a process that requires porcupine. J Biol Chem 279(32):33220–33227

Chapter 3
Wnt Signaling in Stem Cells

Philipp C. Manegold, Jia-Ling Teo, and Michael Kahn

Abstract Wnt signaling pathways play divergent roles during development, normal homeostasis and disease. Wnt signaling is also critically important in stem cell biology. It has been demonstrated to be involved in both the proliferation and differentiation of stem and progenitor populations. Wnt/β-catenin signaling also plays a critical role in lineage decision/commitment. These dramatically different outcomes upon activation of the Wnt signaling cascade has fueled enormous controversy concerning the role of Wnt signaling in maintenance of potency and induction of differentiation. Tight regulation and controlled coordination of the Wnt signaling cascade is required to maintain the balance between proliferation and differentiation. The diverse and titrated responses that result from the activation of the Wnt signaling pathway however begs the question of how the Wnt signaling network integrates the various inputs that a cell receives to elicit the correct and coordinated responses.

Until recently, a rationale for the dichotomous behavior of Wnt/beta-catenin signaling in controlling both proliferation and differentiation has been unclear. Using a selective antagonist of the CBP/beta-catenin interaction that we identified using a chemical genomic approach, we have developed a model to explain the divergent activities of Wnt/beta-catenin signaling. Our model highlights the distinct and non-redundant roles of the coactivators CBP and p300 in the Wnt/beta-catenin signaling cascade. The critical feature of the model is that CBP/catenin mediated transcription is critical for proliferation and stem cell/progenitor cell maintenance; whereas p300/catenin mediated transcription leads to the differentiation program.

M. Kahn (✉)
Eli and Edythe Broad Center for Regenerative Medicine and Stem Cell Research at USC,
University of Southern California, 1425 San Pablo Street, Los Angeles, CA 90033, USA
and
Department of Biochemistry and Molecular Biology Keck School of Medicine,
University of Southern California, 1425 San Pablo Street, Los Angeles, CA 90033, USA
and
Department of Molecular Pharmacology and Toxicology, University of Southern California,
1425 San Pablo Street, Los Angeles, CA 90033, USA
e-mail: kahnm@usc.edu

K.H. Goss and M. Kahn (eds.), *Targeting the Wnt Pathway in Cancer*,
DOI 10.1007/978-1-4419-8023-6_3, © Springer Science+Business Media, LLC 2011

The 'decision' to partner with either CBP or p300 is the first key decision point to initiate either a proliferative or a differentiative program, respectively. This initiation of proliferation or differentiation is followed by additional epigenetic modifications as well as the recruitment of additional transcription factors for both subsequent expansion of transient amplifying populations and/or lineage commitment.

The ultimate decision for a cell to either initiate differentiation, or not, must be integrated and funneled down into a decision point. We propose that essentially all cellular information – i.e. from other signaling pathways, nutrient levels, etc. – is funneled down into a choice of coactivators usage, either CBP or p300, by their interacting partner beta-catenin (or catenin-like molecules in the absence of beta-catenin) to make the critical decision to either remain quiescent, or once entering cycle to proliferate without differentiation or to initiate the differentiation process.

Keywords Role of coactivators CBP and p300 • Wnt signaling • Stem cells • Potency

3.1 Introduction

3.1.1 Stem Cells

Embryonic stem cells (ESCs) are undifferentiated cells that can develop into any of the more than 200 different cell types that make up the adult human body. Apart from the political and ethical controversies that surround them, few argue over predictions of the unlimited potential that stem cell research holds. In many tissues, somatic stem cells (SSCs) serve as a reservoir for internal repair and maintenance through their ability to essentially divide without limit, to replenish and replace cells, as long as the organism is alive. What is a stem cell? A stem cell is distinguished from other cell types by two traits (1) capacity to self-renew, i.e., to make at least one identical copy of itself at each division; (2) the capacity to differentiate into more mature and differentiated (thus less potent) specialized cells.

The term stem cell covers an extremely diverse array of cell types. Stem cells can be embryonic, if derived from an embryo, or adult/somatic if derived from tissue. ESCs possess the unique property of pluripotency – they possess the rare and precious capacity to generate all the cell types found in embryos, as well as adult developed organisms. This unique property has been lost or at least silenced in other SSCs. SSCs are therefore described as being multipotent, i.e., capable of generating multiple differentiated cell types but generally restricted to that of a particular tissue, organ, or physiological system (e.g., hematopoietic stem cells, neural stem cells, etc.) in which they reside, as opposed to being pluripotent.

Today, the basic molecular pharmacology and signaling networks in ESCs are coming into focus. Considerable effort has been devoted to understanding the maintenance of the pluripotent state. It is believed to rely heavily on the expression of a relatively few factors, such as Oct4 and Nanog. Oct4 appears to be the most specific and critical gene for the maintenance of pluripotency, as its expression is mandatory for this purpose and also for the generation of induced pluripotent cells (iPS) (Nichols et al. 1998; Hay et al. 2004). However, expanding our knowledge of the biology of ES cell pluripotency, SSC multipotency and the differentiation programs implemented during development are critical. Furthermore, these same pathways appear to be corrupted in cancer (and in particular cancer stem cells/tumor-initiating cells) to drive malignancies. Aberrant regulation of these same pathways leads to neoplastic proliferation in the same tissues. Understanding how to correct these aberrantly utilized pathways in cancer stem cells (CSCs) will be critical to the effective treatment of malignancies.

Stem cell research is one of the most fascinating areas of contemporary biology, but as with many areas of expanding scientific inquiry, stem cell research raises scientific questions as rapidly as it generates new discoveries. We will briefly discuss the role of the Wnt signaling cascade in stem cells – ES, iPS, SSC, and CSC – in the maintenance of potency and in driving differentiation.

3.1.2 Human Embryonic Stem Cells

Since the first human embryonic stem cells (hESCs) were generated and described, a number of additional lines have been generated (Thomson et al. 1998). These lines, which are derived from the inner cell mass (ICM) of blastocyst-stage embryos, can be cultured on feeder layers of mouse embryonic fibroblasts (MEFs) in the presence of serum and/or basic fibroblast growth factors (bFGF), where they maintain self-renewal and pluripotency. Protocols for directed differentiation of hESCs into various specific cell types have been established (Odorico et al. 2001). However, there is still significant room for improvement. A deeper understanding of the molecular players and signaling pathways governing lineage commitment is needed to achieve homogeneous enrichment for cell types of interest. Interestingly, in ES cells, the transcription factor T-cell factor-3 (Tcf3), a key component of the Wnt signaling cascade, co-occupies promoters throughout the genome in association with the pluripotency regulators Oct4 and Nanog.

3.1.3 Induced Pluripotent Stem Cells (iPSCs)

As science and technology continue to advance, so also do ethical and technical issues surrounding these advancements. The generation of iPSCs represents a way to circumvent some of the ethical and technical issues associated with the use of hESCs. iPSCs are adult cells that have been genetically reprogrammed to an ES-like state directly from somatic cells, by the forced expression of genes and factors that are required for maintaining pluripotency that define an ES cell. Several years ago, Yamanaka and colleagues screened for combinations of factors that could induce the reprogramming of somatic cells and demonstrated that the forced expression of only four transcription factors – Oct4, Sox2, Klf4, and c-Myc – is sufficient to dedifferentiate mouse embryonic and adult fibroblasts into pluripotent stem-like cells (Yamanaka 2009). Oct4 and Sox2 are known to be key representatives of the core transcriptional apparatus, which synergistically upregulate "stemness genes" while repressing differentiation pathways. However, Oct4 and Sox2 appear to operate only in an environment that is not provided in differentiated cells such as fibroblasts, but is created by epigenetic modifications by the transcription factors Klf4 and c-Myc, or Nanog and the RNA binding protein Lin28.

The overexpression of c-Myc, a well-known Wnt-regulated proto-oncogene raised concerns for increased risk of tumorigenicity with early iPS protocols. Alternative methods have already been developed, using nonintegrating adenovirus, repeated transfection of plasmids, nonintegrating episomal vectors or protein expression, providing integration-free, and/or xeno-free conditions. The absence of c-Myc can also be compensated for by Wnt3a addition (Marson et al. 2008).

3.1.4   Somatic Stem Cells

Research on SSCs or tissue stem cells has generated a great deal of excitement. SSCs have been identified and isolated from bone marrow, the eye, and many other tissues and organs that were once thought impossible, like the skeletal muscle and brain. These cells reside in specialized niches within the body, and their main function is to replenish and replace cells that are continually lost through depletion or damage. Therefore, SSCs are critical in normal tissue homeostasis and repair. Unlike ESCs, which are defined by their origin (the ICM of the blastocyst), the origin of adult stem cells in some mature tissues is still under investigation.

The first type of SSC to be isolated and utilized therapeutically was the hematopoietic stem cell (HSC) in the form of bone marrow for transplantation therapy. In the 1950s, scientists discovered that the bone marrow contains at least two kinds of stem cells. One population, called HSCs, forms all the types of blood cells in the body. The second population, called bone marrow stromal stem cells (also called mesenchymal stem cells or skeletal stem cells by some), was discovered a few years later. These nonHSCs make up a small proportion of the stromal cell population in the bone marrow, and can generate bone, cartilage, and fat, cells that support the formation of blood, and fibrous connective tissue. More than half a century later, their self-renewal and multilineage differentiation capacity has been fully demonstrated.

In the 1960s, two regions of fully mature rat brains were discovered to have dividing cells that ultimately could become nerve cells. Despite these findings, most scientists believed that the adult brain could not generate new nerve cells. It was not until the 1990s that the scientific community came to a consensus that the adult brain does contain stem cells that are able to generate the brain's three major cell types – astrocytes and oligodendrocytes, which are nonneuronal cells, and neurons or nerve cells.

Adult SSCs, although frequently present in only limited numbers, are the source for naturally occurring tissue regeneration and repair in adult tissues, as already demonstrated in the lung, in the heart after myocardial infarction or in the adult central nervous system.

3.1.5 Cancer Stem Cells

The presence of CSC or tumor initiating cells (TICs) had been hypothesized for many decades, but it was not until 1997 that these cells were first isolated from acute myeloid leukemia (AML). The term CSC/TIC refers to cells that propagate the tumor phenotype, hence their name. Like their normal counterpart SSCs, CSCs exhibit self-renewal capacity and differentiation potential, albeit an aberrant and incomplete differentiation potential (Reya et al. 2001). Since the initial isolation of CSCs in AML, their existence in a wide variety of other cancers has been successfully demonstrated. It is worth noting that the term CSCs does not necessarily imply that these cells were directly derived from mutations to normal tissue SSCs. Alternatively, CSC/TIC may be derived from progenitor populations that have acquired mutations that have essentially reprogrammed the cell to a "stem-like" status (Krivtsov et al. 2006). Therefore, the term TIC may be generically more appropriate. CSCs are similar to ESCs in that they have the ability, and in fact may be biased toward self-renewing cell divisions.

Signaling cascades including the Wnt, Shh, and Notch pathways, all associated with normal stem cell development, are also active in CSCs and play critical roles in cancer development. The presence of ATP-binding (multidrug resistance) cassette transporters, which actively remove drugs/xenobiotics from the cell, is notable in ESCs. CSCs retain this characteristic that partially accounts for the ineffectiveness of current therapies to eliminate these cells. Normal SSCs are under tight metabolic control and divide only under specific conditions, for example after tissue injury. CSCs appear to have lost some of these tight controls.

CSCs are generally present in small numbers in tumors. Current therapies, targeting rapidly proliferating cell populations, often with cytotoxic agents, may kill the bulk of the tumor, yet are inefficient at targeting the CSC/TICs. For this reason, alternative therapies, which directly target CSCs, are needed to complement classic approaches. A significant caveat to this approach is that given the similarities between endogenous SSC and CSC/TIC, the potential to damage the endogenous normal population is ever present. To successfully accomplish this approach, we will need to improve our understanding of stem cell biology; understanding the molecular pathways that regulate normal SSC vs. CSC activation vs. quiescence in tissues. This may be the key to successful cancer chemotherapy, as most cancers probably originate from an inappropriate perturbation of the finely tuned balance of stem cell quiescence vs. activation and subsequent terminal differentiation.

3.1.6   Wnt Signaling

The Wnt signaling cascade is an extremely complex signal transduction system involving 19 extracellular mammalian glycoprotein Wnt ligands, 10 Fzd family 7-TM spanning receptors, and the coreceptors LRP 5, 6 as well as additional nonclassical Wnt receptors (e.g., Ryk, Ror). Wnt ligands trigger a variety of intracellular responses, broadly associated with canonical (increase in nuclear β-catenin) and noncanonical (planar cell polarity, Ca^{++}/PKC activation) signaling (Komiya and Habas 2008). In a gross oversimplification, the former is often associated with proliferation and lack of differentiation (e.g., as a hallmark of dysregulated Wnt signaling in cancer), whereas the latter is often associated with cell and organismal differentiation. Beyond the classical Wnt-activated translocation of β-catenin to the nucleus, a number of other factors (growth factors, prostaglandins, etc.) can induce the nuclear localization of β-catenin.

Beta-catenin plays a key role in both aspects of the Wnt signaling cascade (canonical and noncanonical) through both its nuclear functions and cytoskeletal/cytoplasmic membrane interactions. Nuclear β-catenin drives the expression of a Wnt/catenin regulated-cassette of genes, whereas outside of the nucleus, β-catenin plays a critical role in cell–cell interactions and cellular polarization. Rather than being thought of as distinct signal transduction systems, we believe that the balance and coordination between nuclear/transcriptionally active β-catenin and cytoplasmic/cytoskeletal β-catenin couple canonical with noncanonical Wnt signaling. A number of excellent reviews on both the canonical and noncanonical Wnt signaling cascades have recently been published.

3.1.7   Wnt Signaling in Stem Cells

Wnt signaling plays important roles throughout development and also in day-to-day processes including maintenance of intestinal homeostasis, regulation of hematopoietic stem/progenitors, and in addition, lineage commitment of progenitors during hematopoiesis. Erythrocytes only live for about 120–130 days, at which point they become inefficient in the transport of oxygen and have to be replaced. This task is taken over by the HSCs found in the bone marrow. Expression of *survivin*, which we have demonstrated is a Wnt/CBP/β-catenin regulated gene, is important during hematopoeisis, and it is prominently upregulated in CD34[+] hematopoietic stem/progenitor cells upon growth factor treatment (Fukuda et al. 2002; Ma et al. 2005). *Survivin*-deficient hematopoietic progenitors show defects in erythroid and megakaryocytic formation. However, it is worth noting that β-catenin-deficient, and even beta-, gamma-double-deficient mice maintain apparently normal hematopoiesis through the Wnt signaling cascade, pointing to yet uncharacterized catenin-like molecule(s) that can compensate for the loss of both beta- and gamma-catenin (Jeannet et al. 2008). The role of Wnt signaling in SSCs is not restricted to HSCs. Other somatic cell replacement activities that occur in the human body, like liver and intestinal epithelial cell turnover, involve Wnt signal transduction (Radtke and Clevers 2005).

Although most would agree that Wnt signaling is important in stem cell biology, there is no consensus as to whether Wnt signaling is important for proliferation and maintenance of pluri- or multipotency, or differentiation of stem/progenitor cells (Sato et al. 2004). Wnt/β-catenin signaling has been demonstrated to maintain pluripotency in ESCs and is critical for the expansion of neural progenitors thereby increasing brain size (Chenn and Walsh 2002). However, Wnt/β-catenin signaling is also required for neural differentiation of ES cells, fate decision in neural crest stem cells and Wnt3a has been reported to promote differentiation into the neural and astrocytic lineages by inhibiting neural stem cell maintenance (Otero et al. 2004). Clearly, Wnt/β-catenin signaling also plays a critical role in lineage decision/commitment. These dramatically different outcomes upon activation of the Wnt signaling cascade have fueled enormous controversy concerning the role of Wnt signaling in maintenance of potency and induction of differentiation.

The rationale for the dichotomous behavior of Wnt/β-catenin signaling in controlling both proliferation and differentiation has been unclear. Recently, using a selective antagonist of the CBP/β-catenin interaction ICG-001 that we identified utilizing a chemical genomic approach, we have developed a model to explain the divergent activities of Wnt/β-catenin signaling (Fig. 3.1) (Emami et al. 2004). Our model highlights the distinct roles of the coactivators CBP and p300 in the Wnt/β-catenin signaling cascade. The critical feature of the model is that CBP/β-catenin-mediated transcription is critical for stem cell/progenitor cell maintenance and proliferation, whereas a switch to p300/β-catenin-mediated transcription is the initial critical step to initiate differentiation and a decrease in cellular potency (McMillan and Kahn 2005; Teo et al. 2005; Miyabayashi et al. 2007; McKinnon et al. 2009). Again, this represents an oversimplification. In reality, although a subset of the gene expression cassette that is regulated by the CBP/β-catenin arm is critical for the maintenance of potency and proliferation (e.g., Oct4, survivin, etc.), other genes that are regulated in this manner (e.g., hNkd and axin2) are in fact negative regulators of the CBP/β-catenin arm of the cascade (Fig. 3.2). Assuming potency and activation of the CBP/β-catenin arm is the default pathway, at some point, in order for development to proceed, one must stop proliferation, exit cell cycle, and initiate the process of differentiation (Fig. 3.2).

The recent identification of the small molecule IQ-1 that allows for the Wnt/β-catenin-driven long-term expansion of mouse ES cells by blocking the p300/β-catenin interaction, and thereby preventing spontaneous differentiation in the absence of LIF, is consistent and lends further credence to our model. This study demonstrated that IQ-1, in combination with Wnt3a to stimulate nuclear translocation of β-catenin, is sufficient to maintain long-term pluripotency (Miyabayashi et al. 2007). This is achieved by decreasing the interaction of β-catenin with p300 and consequently increasing its interaction with CBP. Removal of IQ-1 from the mES cultures rapidly leads to loss of pluripotency, even in the presence of Wnt3a. The switch to p300/β-catenin-mediated transcription, whether induced pharmacologically, by removal of IQ-1, or addition of ICG-001 (Fig. 3.2), or naturally, for

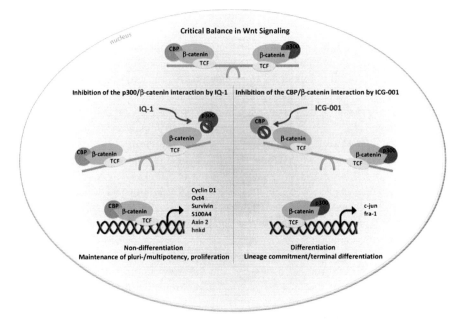

Fig. 3.1 Wnt signaling is a complex pathway, believed to be involved in the regulation of divergent processes, including the maintenance of pluripotency and commitment to differentiation. To resolve these divergent responses to activation of Wnt/β-catenin signaling, we have developed a model in which β-catenin/CBP-mediated transcription is critical for the maintenance of potency, whereas a switch to β-catenin/p300-mediated transcription is the first critical step to initiate differentiation. Hence the balance between CBP and p300-mediated β-catenin transcription regulates the balance between maintenance of potency and the initiation of commitment to differentiate. The interaction of β-catenin with either CBP or p300 can be modulated by two small molecules, respectively ICG-001 and IQ-1, identified in our laboratory. As a consequence, these small molecules regulate Wnt signaling pathway outcomes

example, LIF withdrawal, is critical to initiate a differentiative program with a more limited proliferative capacity. More recently, we identified the small molecule ID-8, which via a similar mechanism (i.e., blocking the p300/β-catenin interaction thereby enhancing the CBP/β-catenin interaction) allows for long-term Wnt-mediated maintenance of pluripotency in human ES cells (Hasegawa et al. 2009). We have also demonstrated that this β-catenin coactivator switching mechanism is also critical in the maintenance of both mouse and human SSC populations (McKinnon et al. 2009).

3.1.8 Wnt Signaling in Cancer Stem Cells

As discussed previously, the similarities between normal SSCs and CSCs suggest that the signaling pathways Wnt, Hedgehog, and Notch, which are involved in maintenance of ESCs and SSCs, are also involved in the regulation of CSCs.

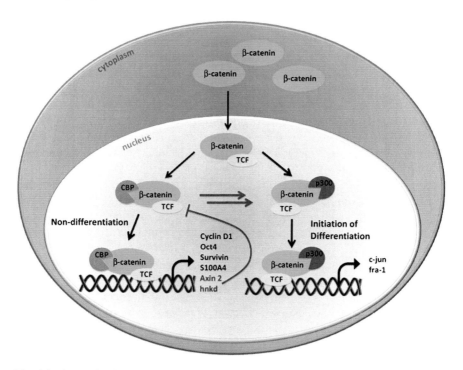

Fig. 3.2 A negative feedback normally turns off the CBP/β-catenin arm of the pathway and initiates differentiation via the p300/β-catenin arm

Aberrant regulation of these same pathways leads to neoplastic proliferation in the same tissues. Interestingly, progression of chronic myelogenous leukemia from chronic phase to blast crisis, which is associated with imatinib resistance, was correlated with increased nuclear β-catenin levels, a hallmark of increased Wnt/TCF/β-catenin transcription. Recent studies have revealed that multidrug resistance genes, including *MDR-1*, *ABCG2*, *ABCA3*, and *BRCP1*, are also intrinsically expressed in stem/progenitor cells from multiple adult tissues and that they may contribute to the side population (SP) phenotype of malignant cells (Hirschmann-Jax et al. 2005). Wnt/β-catenin signaling appears to play an important role in *ABCB1/MDR-1* expression via Wnt/TCF/β-catenin-mediated transcription. This observation was initially based upon the increased expression of *MDR-1* associated with intestinal crypt cells, which carry a defective *APC* tumor suppressor gene in both the Min mouse and FAP patients. Putative TCF binding elements were also identified in the *ABCB1* promoter (−1813 to −275 bp) (Yamada et al. 2000; Yamada et al. 2003). Interestingly, many of the cell surface markers, including LGR5/GPR49, CD44, CD24, and Epcam that have been utilized to identify and isolate putative tumor stem cell populations in a variety of tissues, are direct Wnt targets.

The role of the Wnt signaling cascade, particularly in CSC and in other malignancies, which do not carry classical activating mutations in the Wnt pathway, is becoming more apparent. For example, multiple myeloma (MM) is quite responsive to a wide array of therapeutic protocols including conventional cytotoxics, corticosterioids, radiation therapy, and an increasing number of targeted chemotherapeutic agents, e.g., the proteasome inhibitor Bortezomib. Despite this, few, if any, patients are "cured" utilizing these approaches and relapse remains a critical issue. The majority of MM infiltrates phenotypically resemble normal terminally differentiated plasma cells with the ability to produce monoclonal immunoglobin. That the majority of myeloma plasma cells are quiescent, particularly at diagnosis, led to the investigation of a restricted "stem cell" population critical for tumor growth. Thirty years ago, Hamburger and Salmon (1980) demonstrated the ability of ~90% of tumor samples from MM patients to form colonies and that clonogenic growth occurred at a frequency of between 1 in 100 and 100,000 cells. Importantly, as with other CSC populations, multiple myeloma CSC have been found to be relatively resistant to existing chemotherapies. Moreover, MM stem cells display high expression of multidrug resistance transporters, intracellular detoxification enzymes, and relative quiescence, similar to both other CSC populations as well as normal stem cell populations.

Despite a lack of mutations in the classical Wnt signaling genes *adenomatous polyposis coli* (*APC*) or *β-catenin* (CTNNB1), MM cells exhibit hallmarks of active Wnt signaling. As in most cases, the exact effects of Wnt signaling activation on MM cells, e.g., cell proliferation vs. migration and invasion appear dependent on the particular assay conditions. However, in contemplating antagonizing the Wnt signaling cascade as a therapeutic strategy for MM, it must be taken into account that Wnt signaling also plays a critical role in normal stem cell maintenance and differentiation. In the case of MM particularly, the anabolic effects of Wnt signaling on bone development also has to be considered. In this regard, a recent paper by Yaccoby and colleagues demonstrated that increasing Wnt signaling within the myeloma bone microenvironment inhibits myeloma bone disease and consequently decreases tumor burden.

Interestingly, cancer-specific overexpression of survivin in myeloma cells and a significant correlation between survivin expression at the protein level and clinical course of MM have been demonstrated. Moreover, survivin knockdown by RNA interference led to growth rate inhibition of myeloma cells related to apoptosis induction and cell-cycle disruption. Bortezomib activates and upregulates β-catenin, both by activating Akt and inhibiting proteasomal degradation of β-catenin, thereby upregulating survivin expression. Finally, survivin knockdown sensitized myeloma cells to conventional antimyeloma agents and Bortezomib. Therefore, targeting survivin expression by blocking Wnt/CBP/β-catenin-driven gene expression, in conjunction with standard chemotherapies, would appear to be a very attractive approach to maximize effectiveness in treating MM without increasing toxicity.

Although our knowledge concerning the role of Wnt signaling in breast cancer is far from complete, its importance and significance has been the subject of numerous reports during the past 5 years. In human breast cancer, there are many reports of inactivation of negative regulators of the Wnt signaling pathway. Similarly, there are numerous studies that have documented the amplification or overexpression of positive regulators of components of this pathway. Disheveled

(Dsh), a downstream activator, is amplified and upregulated in 50% of ductal breast cancers. Frizzled-related protein 1 (*FRP1/FRZB*), a secreted Wnt inhibitor, located within chromosomal locus 8p11-21, is frequently deleted in human breast cancers. In approximately 80% of malignant breast carcinomas, Frp1 expression is either repressed or absent, making it one of the most frequent alterations in breast cancer. Axin is downregulated in a small percentage of breast cancers. *AXIN2*, on chromosome 17q23-q24, exhibits frequent loss of heterozygosity (LOH) in breast cancers. Both are negative regulators of the canonical Wnt signaling pathway. Collectively, LOH (23–40%), mutation (6–18%), and hypermethylation of the *APC* gene, has been shown to result in loss of expression in approximately 36–50% of breast tumors. In mice, it has long been known that misexpression of Wnt-1, -3, or -10 induces mammary adenocarcinomas. The APC[Min] mouse has also been shown to exhibit an enhanced incidence (~10%) of spontaneous mammary cancer and a greatly increased susceptibility (90%) to carcinogen-induced mammary cancer (Zhang and Rosen 2006).

With the use of a small selective molecule CBP/β-catenin antagonistic ICG-001, we have found that while the expression of the Wnt target gene survivin is downregulated, the Wnt targets E-cadherin and connexin 43 are consistently upregulated in breast cancer cell lines. The increased expression of these genes is effected by differential coactivator usage (i.e., p300 rather than CBP) in the Wnt signaling cascade, and is associated with a more epithelial phenotype and a decrease in invasiveness and metastatic ability. MDA-MB-231 ER- breast cancer cells have low expression of the Wnt-regulated cell surface marker CD24, yet relatively high expression of another Wnt-regulated gene CD44. This phenotype CD44hi, CD24lo has been associated with a subpopulation of cells that behave like a breast CSC/TIC population. Interestingly, treatment with the ICG-001 significantly increased the expression of cell surface CD24 at 24 h, while decreasing CD44 expression.

Pancreatic cancers are one of the most difficult cancers to treat with a 5-year life expectancy of less than 5%. Pancreatic ductal adenocarcinoma (PDAC) is the most common pancreatic neoplasm. There are approximately 33,000 new cases of PDAC annually in the United States with approximately the same number of deaths. To date, surgery represents the only opportunity for cure, but this is restricted to early stage pancreatic cancer. With only two FDA-approved drugs for the treatment of pancreatic cancer, there exists a significant need to develop more effective therapies, attacking pancreatic cancer and in particular pancreatic CSC, the root cause of the disease. Almost all PDACs involve mutations in the K-Ras oncogene. Thus, it is believed that activating K-Ras mutations is critical for initiation of pancreatic ductal carcinogenesis. Again, although PDAC do not generally carry mutations in classic Wnt regulators (such as APC), recent in vitro and in vivo functional studies demonstrate that canonical Wnt signaling promotes tumorigenesis in PDAC, and a majority of PDAC tumors demonstrate an activated Wnt/β-catenin transcriptional signature. Synchronous activation of the Wnt and Ras signaling cascades has been observed in a number of transgenic mouse tumor models, including colon, intestine, and liver. The convergence of these signaling pathways upregulates the expression of a number of genes (i.e., Cox2, C-myc, and Interleukin-8) that promote tumorigenesis. Interestingly, monoallelic expression of an activating K-Ras mutation in the mouse intestine has no phenotype, but can promote tumorigenesis in APC-deficient mice. Furthermore, the Wnt/β-catenin-driven maintenance of CSCs/TICs within the pancreatic tumor may be closely associated with chemotherapy resistance.

Given the fact that multiple mutations can lead to the aberrant activation of nuclear β-catenin signaling, there is a clear need for drugs that attenuate the nuclear functions of β-catenin. The small molecule antagonist that our laboratory developed, ICG-001, by binding to the coactivator CBP and not to its highly homologous relative p300, specifically downregulates a subset of Wnt/β-catenin-driven genes including *S100A4* and *survivin* the number 1 and 4 transcriptomes upregulated in cancer. Recently, it has also been demonstrated that continued expression of *survivin* is associated with teratoma formation by hES cells (Blum et al. 2009). Importantly, specific inhibition of Wnt/CBP/β-catenin expression appears quite safe in a number of preclinical studies.

3.1.9 Concluding Thoughts

Even from the brief discussion above, certain characteristics about "stemness" in a variety of systems, i.e., ESCs, iPSCs, SSCs, and CSC, appear to be conserved. For example, there are a number of critical pathways that are involved in the maintenance or loss of potency in all of these cell types (i.e., Wnt, Notch, Hedeghog, TGFβ/BMP, JAK/Stat, FGF/MAPK/PI3K). A second conclusion that one can draw from published studies is that there are many potential points of intersection, or crosstalk along these critical signaling networks that modulate "stemness" as well as the maintenance or loss of potency (initiation of differentiation) (Xu and Ding 2008). In the end, the ultimate decision for a cell to retain potency or initiate differentiation, although enormously complex, taking in hundreds if not thousands of inputs (e.g., concentrations of different growth factors, cytokines and hormones, and the subsequent activation of different signal transduction complexes and kinase cascades, ionic concentrations [e.g., Ca++], nutrient levels, oxygen levels, genetic mutations, adhesion to substratum, etc.), must be integrated and funneled down into a simple decision point, a binary decision, a yes or no answer (Fig. 3.3). In other words, after integrating all of these inputs, the cell must decide either to maintain its level of potency (be that ES, SSC, or CSC) or to go on to differentiate and shed a level of potency. More recently, it has become clear that this decision process or decision point is also reversible under certain circumstances; iPS cells demonstrating this most clearly, as well as much earlier work on transformation and immortalization of cells.

Based upon our own investigations, we propose that this simple decision point that all of this information is funneled down into involves (1) a change in coactivators

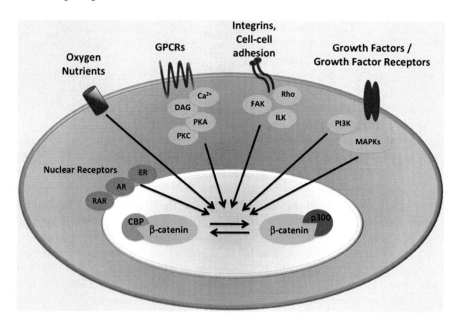

Fig. 3.3 The ultimate decision for a cell to retain potency or initiate differentiation is dependent upon numerous inputs, some of which are presented here: e.g., concentration of different growth factors, cytokines and hormones and the subsequent activation of different signal transduction complexes and kinase cascades, ionic concentrations (e.g., Ca++), nutrient levels, oxygen levels, genetic mutations, and adhesion to substratum. In the end, those multiple pathways must be integrated and funneled down into a simple decision point, i.e., a yes/no binary decision. We believe that Wnt signaling and the equilibrium between CBP-mediated and p300-mediated transcription play a central role in integrating these signals

(CBP vs. p300) interacting with β-catenin (or catenin-like molecules in the absence of β-catenin) and (2) more generally, the basal transcriptional apparatus. A model incorporating and summarizing this concept is depicted in Fig. 3.3. We have specifically not specified the transcription factor TCF as the binding partner for β-catenin in this model. Although in classical Wnt signaling (e.g., in intestinal stem cells), partnering with the TCF family of transcription factors is critical. In reality, this may represent only a fraction of the roles played by nuclear β-catenin in transcription, as β-catenin is known to interact with a much broader array of potential transcription partners, including the orphan nuclear receptors LRH-1 and Nurr1; nuclear receptors ER, AR, RAR, and VDR; Sox and Smad family members; and Oct4 itself to list but a few (Le et al. 2008).

We believe that this is an extremely fundamental switching mechanism that is present in mouse and human ES cells and that is conserved throughout essentially all stem/progenitor cell lineages. As a case in point, we have found that the earliest and perhaps most critical cellular decision point, at the embryonic 8 cell stage, is governed by the use of differential coactivator by catenin. CBP/catenin is required for the maintenance of ICM and expression of Oct4, whereas a switch to p300/catenin initiates the formation of cdx2 positive trophectoderm. Additionally, this switching mechanism appears to be important in a wide variety of somatic stem/progenitors (neural, cardiac, myogenic, hematopoietic etc.) as well as transformed somatic stem/progenitors (e.g., leukemic stem cells) (Zechner et al. 2003; Taupin et al. 2006; Warburton et al. 2008). It is also clear that there are numerous ways to perturb/modulate this coactivator decision process. In a siRNA screen of the whole human kinome in HEK293 cells, we found that almost 25% of the kinases screened had significant effects on Wnt signaling. The ability to switch coactivators within the Wnt/catenin signaling cascade, thereby, changes a gene expression cassette, including a change in micro-RNA expression. We believe that this "regulation of expression cassettes" is critical to the proper control, maintenance, and initiation of differentiation of both embryonic and SSCs. This implies that the inability to properly initiate differentiation of SSCs may be the underlying malfunction in essentially all cancers. Therefore, we would propose that cancer, rather than being an array of different diseases (breast cancer is different from colon, is different from leukemia), is a disease in which a multitude of different mutations, some of which are tissue specific (e.g., bcr/abl, K-Ras, Her2, etc.), can lead to aberrant regulation of the underlying equilibrium between CBP/catenin and p300/catenin, between proliferation and maintenance of potency, and the initiation of differentiation thereby aberrantly increasing the CBP/catenin interaction at the expense of the p300/catenin interaction (Fig. 3.3).

A big part of research is a tough slog for small reward. However, ever so often, a finding revolutionizes the field and makes us reconsider some of our fundamental beliefs. "It's not only what we have inherited from our father and mother that haunts us. It's all sorts of dead ideas, and lifeless old beliefs, and so forth. They have no vitality, but they cling to us all the same, and we can't get rid of them" Henrik Ibsen.

References

Blum B, Bar-Nur O, Golan-Lev T, Benvenisty N (2009) The anti-apoptotic gene survivin contributes to teratoma formation by human embryonic stem cells. Nat Biotechnol 27: 281–287

Chenn A, Walsh CA (2002) Regulation of cerebral cortical size by control of cell cycle exit in neural precursors. Science 297:365–369

Emami KH, Nguyen C, Ma H, Kim DH, Jeong KW, Eguchi M, Moon RT, Teo JL, Kim HY, Moon SH, Ha JR, Kahn M (2004) A small molecule inhibitor of beta-catenin/CREB-binding protein transcription [corrected]. Proc Natl Acad Sci U S A 101:12682–12687

Fukuda S, Foster RG, Porter SB, Pelus LM (2002) The antiapoptosis protein survivin is associated with cell cycle entry of normal umbilical cord blood CD34(+) cells and modulates cell cycle and proliferation of mouse hematopoietic progenitor cells. Blood 100:2463–2471

Hamburger AW, Salmon SE (1980) Development of a bioassay for human myeloma colony-forming cells. Prog Clin Biol Res 48:23–41.

Hasegawa K, Teo J.-T, Suemori H, Nakatsuji N, Pera M, Kahn M (2009) Development of a novel xeno-free human embryonic stem cell culture system using small molecules. In ISSCR 7th Annual Meeting, July 8–11, 2009, Barcelona, Spain

Hay DC, Sutherland L, Clark J, Burdon T (2004) Oct-4 knockdown induces similar patterns of endoderm and trophoblast differentiation markers in human and mouse embryonic stem cells. Stem Cells 22:225–235

Hirschmann-Jax C, Foster AE, Wulf GG, Goodell MA, Brenner MK (2005) A distinct "side population" of cells in human tumor cells: implications for tumor biology and therapy. Cell Cycle 4:203–205

Jeannet G, Scheller M, Scarpellino L, Duboux S, Gardiol N, Back J, Kuttler F, Malanchi I, Birchmeier W, Leutz A, Huelsken J, Held W (2008) Long-term, multilineage hematopoiesis occurs in the combined absence of beta-catenin and gamma-catenin. Blood 111:142–149

Komiya Y, Habas R (2008) Wnt signal transduction pathways. Organogenesis 4:68–75

Krivtsov AV, Twomey D, Feng Z, Stubbs MC, Wang Y, Faber J, Levine JE, Wang J, Hahn WC, Gilliland DG, Golub TR, Armstrong SA (2006) Transformation from committed progenitor to leukaemia stem cell initiated by MLL-AF9. Nature 442:818–822

Le NH, Franken P, Fodde R (2008) Tumour-stroma interactions in colorectal cancer: converging on beta-catenin activation and cancer stemness. Br J Cancer 98:1886–1893

Ma H, Nguyen C, Lee KS, Kahn M (2005) Differential roles for the coactivators CBP and p300 on TCF/beta-catenin-mediated survivin gene expression. Oncogene 24:3619–3631

Marson A, Foreman R, Chevalier B, Bilodeau S, Kahn M, Young RA, Jaenisch R (2008) Wnt signaling promotes reprogramming of somatic cells to pluripotency. Cell Stem Cell 3:132–135

McKinnon T, Ma H, Hasegawa K, Kahn M (2009) Trophectoderm differentiation in mouse pre-implantation embryos involves Wnt signaling and a switch to the transcriptional coactivator p300. In ISSCR Annual Meeting, Barcelona, Spain

McMillan M, Kahn M (2005) Investigating Wnt signaling: a chemogenomic safari. Drug Discov Today 10:1467–1474

Miyabayashi T, Teo JL, Yamamoto M, McMillan M, Nguyen C, Kahn M (2007) Wnt/beta-catenin/CBP signaling maintains long-term murine embryonic stem cell pluripotency. Proc Natl Acad Sci U S A 104:5668–5673

Nichols J, Zevnik B, Anastassiadis K, Niwa H, Klewe-Nebenius D, Chambers I, Scholer H, Smith A (1998) Formation of pluripotent stem cells in the mammalian embryo depends on the POU transcription factor Oct 4. Cell 95:379–391

Odorico JS, Kaufman DS, Thomson JA (2001) Multilineage differentiation from human embryonic stem cell lines. Stem Cells 19:193–204

Otero JJ, Fu W, Kan L, Cuadra AE, Kessler JA (2004) Beta-catenin signaling is required for neural differentiation of embryonic stem cells. Development 131:3545–3557

Radtke F, Clevers H (2005) Self-renewal and cancer of the gut: two sides of a coin. Science 307:1904–1909

Reya T, Morrison SJ, Clarke MF, Weissman IL (2001) Stem cells, cancer, and cancer stem cells. Nature 414:105–111

Sato N, Meijer L, Skaltsounis L, Greengard P, Brivanlou AH (2004) Maintenance of pluripotency in human and mouse embryonic stem cells through activation of Wnt signaling by a pharmacological GSK-3-specific inhibitor. Nat Med 10:55–63

Taupin P (2006) Stroke-induced neurogenesis: physiopathology and mechanisms. Curr Neurovasc Res 3:67–72

Teo JL, Ma H, Nguyen C, Lam C, Kahn M (2005) Specific inhibition of CBP/beta-catenin interaction rescues defects in neuronal differentiation caused by a presenilin-1 mutation. Proc Natl Acad Sci U S A 102:12171–12176

Thomson JA, Itskovitz-Eldor J, Shapiro SS, Waknitz MA, Swiergiel JJ, Marshall VS, Jones JM (1998) Embryonic stem cell lines derived from human blastocysts. Science 282:1145–1147

Warburton D, Perin L, Defilippo R, Bellusci S, Shi W, Driscoll B (2008) Stem/progenitor cells in lung development, injury repair, and regeneration. Proc Am Thorac Soc 5:703–706

Xu Y, Shi Y, Ding S (2008) A chemical approach to stem-cell biology and regenerative medicine. Nature 453:338–344

Yamada T, Takaoka AS, Naishiro Y, Hayashi R, Maruyama K, Maesawa C, Ochiai A, Hirohashi S
(2000) Transactivation of the multidrug resistance 1 gene by T-cell factor 4/beta-catenin
complex in early colorectal carcinogenesis. Cancer Res 60:4761–4766

Yamada T, Mori Y, Hayashi R, Takada M, Ino Y, Naishiro Y, Kondo T, Hirohashi S (2003)
Suppression of intestinal polyposis in Mdr1-deficient ApcMin/+ mice. Cancer Res
63:895–901

Yamanaka S (2009) A fresh look at iPS cells. Cell 137:13–17

Zechner D, Fujita Y, Hulsken J, Muller T, Walther I, Taketo MM, Crenshaw EB III, Birchmeier W,
Birchmeier C (2003) beta-Catenin signals regulate cell growth and the balance between progenitor cell expansion and differentiation in the nervous system. Dev Biol 258:406–418

Zhang M, Rosen JM (2006) Stem cells in the etiology and treatment of cancer. Curr Opin Genet
Dev 16:60–64

Chapter 4
Crosstalk of the Wnt Signaling Pathway

Michael Thompson, Kari Nejak-Bowen, and Satdarshan P.S. Monga

Abstract While it is very clear that activation of β-catenin through the canonical Wnt pathway plays a role in a multitude of human cancers, it has also been noted time and time again that activation of β-catenin is observed in tumors without any clear mutation in any of the major components of the pathway or any increase in Wnt signaling. This suggests that other factors maybe capable of inducing activation and downstream signaling via β-catenin. Indeed, multiple growth factor and developmental signaling pathways have been found to transactivate β-catenin. It is also reasonable to consider the converse: that the Wnt pathway is capable of transactivating other signaling pathways. In fact, multiple studies have outlined the capability of Wnt signaling to activate other pathways in various types of cancer. Such association has led to the initiative to develop approaches to therapy that are capable of targeting both the Wnt pathway and the pathways it crosstalks with simultaneously. The crosstalk that occurs between Wnt and other signaling pathways will be explored in this chapter with a primary focus on how these pathways interact in the development and progression of cancer.

Keywords Crosstalk • Cancer • Signaling • Wnt • Notch • Hedgehog • Growth factor • Receptor tyrosine kinase • Ras • PI3K • mTOR • Cox-2 • Growth • Metastasis • Proliferation • Development • Suppression • Transactivation

4.1 Growth Factor Signaling

Crosstalk between the Wnt pathway and growth factor signaling pathways is fairly prevalent in the development and progression of cancer. Some of these pathways involve β-catenin as a downstream effector of the pathway, including hepatocyte

S.P.S. Monga (✉)

Division of Experimental Pathology (EP), University of Pittsburgh School of Medicine, 200 Lothrop Street S-421 BST, Pittsburgh, PA 15261, USA

e-mail: smonga@pitt.edu

K.H. Goss and M. Kahn (eds.), *Targeting the Wnt Pathway in Cancer*, DOI 10.1007/978-1-4419-8023-6_4, © Springer Science+Business Media, LLC 2011 growth factor (HGF) and epidermal growth factor (EGF), while others seem to interact with the Wnt pathway at multiple levels, such as transforming growth factor beta (TGFβ). Association with other growth factors, such as insulin/IGF and vascular endothelial growth factor (VEGF), has been observed, but the mechanism for these crosstalks has yet to be fully elucidated (Fig. 4.1).

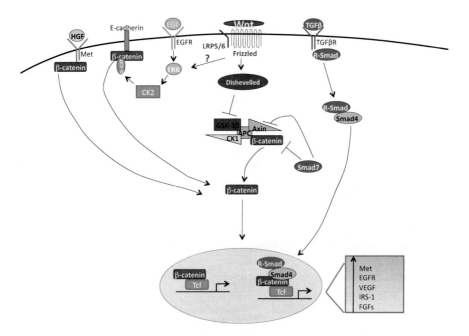

Fig. 4.1 Canonical Wnt signaling occurs when a Wnt ligand binds to one of the Frizzled receptors. This leads to phosphorylation of Disheveled, which phosphorylates and inactivates GSK3β. Inactivation of GSK3β allows for the buildup of free cytoplasmic β-catenin, which can then translocate to the nucleus bound to Tcf and induce/repress expression of downstream targets. EGF pathway activation can lead to an increase in free cytoplasmic β-catenin by inducing dissociation from α-catenin. Activated ERK phosphorylates CK2 on its α-subunit, and phosphorylated CK2 then phosphorylates α-catenin. Phosphorylation of α-catenin allows for the release of β-catenin into the cytoplasm. Wnt signaling also seems to activate ERK, although the mechanism is not yet known. The HGF pathway also can increase free cytoplasmic β-catenin. β-catenin associates with the receptor Met at the cell membrane. Upon binding of HGF, Met induces tyrosine phosphorylation of β-catenin and releases β-catenin into the cytoplasm. The TGFβ pathway can affect β-catenin's activity in the nucleus. The complex of Smad4 and a receptor Smad (R-Smad) can bind to β-catenin in the nucleus and affect target gene expression. Smad7 seems to play a dual role as it can induce degradation of β-catenin or it can inhibit Axin allowing for a buildup of free cytoplasmic β-catenin. The Wnt pathway also crosstalks with other growth factor signaling pathways, Insulin/IGF, VEGF, and FGF, by increasing expression of important players in each pathway, IRS-1, VEGF, and FGFs. No direct interaction between components of these other pathways has been observed though

4.1.1   EGF

EGF is the ligand for the epidermal growth factor receptor (EGFR) and part of a tyrosine kinase signaling cascade, which plays multiple roles in the cell including motility, growth, proliferation, and differentiation. While EGF is the primary ligand for EGFR, multiple other ligands are capable of binding agonistically to EGFR including TGFα, amphiregulin, epiregulin, epigen, heparin-binding EGF-like growth factor, and β-cellulin. Upon binding of ligand to EGFR, the receptor is induced to homo- or hetero-dimerize with another member of the EGFR family followed by tyrosine phosphorylation of various intracellular signaling molecules. Some of these targets include Ras, mitogen-activated protein kinase (MAPK), Jak/Stat, phosphoinositide 3-kinase (PI3K), nuclear factor κB (NFκB), and protein kinase C (PKC), highlighting the diversity of downstream effects one might anticipate following activation of members of this pathway. Enhanced expression of the EGFR has been noted in multiple human malignancies including colon, breast, lung, bladder, prostate, brain, ovarian, and head and neck cancers.

The link between EGFR activation and eventual nuclear translocation of β-catenin involves a kinase signaling cascade that leads to the dissociation of β-catenin from α-catenin at the adherens junction (Ji et al. 2009). Upon EGFR activation, two phosphorylation events lead to the dissociation of β-catenin from α-catenin. The first event is activation of ERK2, which directly binds to casein kinase (CK2) on its α-subunit and induces phosphorylation at threonine-360 and serine-362. This phosphorylation event enhances CK2α activity, which has the capacity to phosphorylate serine-641 on α-catenin. Once α-catenin is phosphorylated, β-catenin is released into the cytoplasm and can now translocate to the nucleus. In addition to direct kinase signaling, EGFR activation results in downregulation of the endocytosis protein caveolin-1 (Lu et al. 2003). Overexpression of caveolin-1 induces negative feedback by inhibiting EGF-mediated phosphorylation of α-catenin; thus, its downregulation by EGFR activity prevents the negative feedback loop and further enhances EGF signaling. EGF-mediated transactivation of β-catenin likely plays a role in tumor metastasis as it leads to an increase in tumor cell invasion (Lu et al. 2003). Furthermore, α-catenin phosphorylation is observed in a significant subset of WHO grade IV primary glioblastoma multiforme (GBM), suggesting this is a mechanism for β-catenin activation in these tumors. Additionally, comparison of α-catenin phosphorylation levels between this group and low-grade diffuse astrocytoma shows higher levels in GBM thus presenting a positive association between α-catenin phosphorylation and higher tumor grade.

Another factor that is involved in EGF-induced activation of β-catenin is histone deacetylase 6 (HDAC6). Li et al. dissected the involvement of HDAC6 in β-catenin stabilization and target gene expression in colorectal cancer cell lines (Li et al. 2008a). Treatment with EGF stimulated HDAC6 to relocate to the plasma membrane, where it deacetylates β-catenin at Lys-49. This deacetylation prevents phosphorylation of β-catenin at serine-45, which is the priming step for eventual ubiquitination and degradation of the protein. Prevention of serine-45 phosphorylation leads to nuclear translocation of β-catenin and increased expression of the target gene c-myc in colon cancer cells.

There also seems to be an interaction between another member of the EGFR family, ErbB2, and β-catenin. This interaction was first identified by coimmunoprecipitation studies where β-catenin and the E-cadherin complex were pulled down with ErbB2 (Ochiai et al. 1994). This association was further shown to be direct through ErbB2's cytoplasmic domain core region, and it is this interaction which allows ErbB2 to phosphorylate tyrosine-654 in the 11th armadillo repeat of β-catenin (Kanai et al. 1995; Shomori et al. 2009). Interestingly, tyrosine-654 phosphorylated β-catenin was observed in colon cancer cells at the invasive cancer front, suggesting a role for this crosstalk in the invasive potential of these cells and in tumor progression. In support of this, treatment of melanoma cells expressing proteasome-resistant β-catenin with geldanamycin, an ErbB2 destabilizer, induced tyrosine dephosphorylation of β-catenin as well as redistribution of β-catenin from the nucleus to the membrane where it associated with E-cadherin (Bonvini et al. 2001). This study also reported a substantial decrease in cellular motility after geldanamycin treatment implicating a dependence of these melanoma cells on the interaction between ErbB2 and β-catenin for metastasis. Similar findings were observed in breast cancer cells as geldanamycin treatment induced redistribution of β-catenin from the nucleus to the membrane, as well as decreasing proliferation and motility of SKBr3 human breast cancer cells (Wang et al. 2007). Studies have reported an association between ErbB2 and β-catenin in several other cancers including gastric, liver, and ovarian, suggesting that targeting this association may have widespread therapeutic potential (Bourguignon et al. 2007; Liu et al. 2009; Ougolkov et al. 2000).

Just as EGF is capable of transactivating β-catenin, it appears that Wnt is capable of inducing transactivation of ERK. Observations from breast cancer tumor cell lines show that exposure to Wnt1 and Wnt5a result in activation of ErbB1 and ERK (Civenni et al. 2003). An autocrine Wnt signaling loop in this cell line promotes breast cancer cell proliferation that is, at least partly, mediated by transactivation of EGFR (Schlange et al. 2007). While the mechanism for this transactivation is yet to be fully elucidated, it occurs in a metalloprotease- and Src-dependent manner. Interestingly, the proproliferative effects of this autocrine loop are dependent on EGFR as the ability of Wnt1 to rescue breast cancer cells from 4-hydroxytamoxifen treatment is blocked by an EGFR tyrosine kinase inhibitor. It has also been observed that EGFR is a target of Wnt signaling in liver (Tan et al. 2005). Overexpression of β-catenin in the liver led to an increase in RNA and protein levels of EGFR. Promoter analysis revealed a binding site for Tcf upstream of EGFR, and a reporter assay confirmed EGFR activation after treatment with Wnt3a. In parallel to these findings, 7 out of 10 hepatoblastomas showed upregulation of β-catenin and EGFR. Furthermore, it was shown that EGFR expression is highest in the pure fetal subtype of hepatoblastomas, a finding associated with high levels of two well-known downstream targets of the Wnt pathway, glutamine synthetase and cyclin D1 (Lopez-Terrada et al. 2009). Therefore, evidence supports a model where Wnt and EGF can collaborate with one another to potentiate their effects in the development of cancer.

4.1.2   HGF

The EGF pathway is not the only tyrosine kinase signaling pathway that is involved in crosstalk with the Wnt pathway. HGF signaling can also effectively transactivate β-catenin. The receptor for HGF is Met, which is capable of tyrosine phosphorylation of multiple effectors including GRB2, SHC, SRC, and PI3K, ultimately playing a role in cell growth, motility, proliferation, and survival. Another well-defined interaction for Met is that it directly binds to β-catenin. Following binding of HGF, Met is involved in phosphorylation of β-catenin at tyrosine residues 654 and 670 with subsequent nuclear translocation of β-catenin (Monga et al. 2002; Shibamoto et al. 1994; Zeng et al. 2006). Prior to HGF stimulation, β-catenin exists in a complex with the HGF receptor, Met, at the membrane which becomes dissociated upon binding of the Met receptors, ligand. It is likely that such growth factor stimulation of β-catenin plays a role in various cancers. Indeed, Met and β-catenin cooperate to promote proliferation and invasiveness of colorectal cancer cells via a positive feedback loop (Rasola et al. 2007). Likewise, expression of the Met gene is increased by Wnt stimulation in dysplastic aberrant crypt foci (Boon et al. 2002). Thus, a positive feedback loop can occur where HGF stimulates nuclear translocation of β-catenin, which can promote increased transcription of the receptor Met. Increased levels of Met then further potentiate this circuit providing more receptor for HGF to induce its own downstream targets, as well as further promoting the proproliferative effects of activated β-catenin. Given that tyrosine phosphorylation of residue 654 is a common feature shared between dissociation of β-catenin from Met and dissociation of β-catenin from E-cadherin, it is believed that the two may not be mutually exclusive. It is possible that a trimeric complex forms between β-catenin, E-cadherin, and Met bringing together the two cellular functions of adhesion and growth factor signaling with β-catenin as the central player. Future work will need to address whether or not such an interaction exists and what, if any, implications it may have in the setting of cancer.

Colorectal cancer is not the only tumor for which an association between HGF signaling and β-catenin has been observed. In invasive breast carcinoma, a significant correlation exists between expression, of c-met and abnormal β-catenin expression, implicating crosstalk between the two in breast cancer (Nakopoulou et al. 2000). The presence of abnormal β-catenin suggests poor prognosis in many tumors; however, abnormal expression of β-catenin and c-met in breast cancer tumors from this study was a predictor of a favorable outcome. A connection has also been made in liver cancer where cooperation between activated Met and constitutively active forms of β-catenin induced development of HCC in mice

(Tward et al. 2007). While many of the proproliferative effects of β-catenin are mediated by expression of cyclin D1, Met and β-catenin cooperation in liver tumor development seems to be independent of cyclin D1 expression (Patil et al. 2009). Such cooperation between signaling pathways may also be important in human tumors as an association between phosphorylated Met and mutated β-catenin was observed in a subset of human HCC (Tward et al. 2007). Currently, the best available chemotherapy for liver cancer is sorafenib, a multiple tyrosine kinase inhibitor (Llovet et al. 2008). Given the capacity for both EGF and HGF tyrosine kinase pathways to transactivate β-catenin, it is plausible that sorafenib may have an indirect effect on β-catenin by downregulating the pathways that transactivate it.

4.1.3 TGFβ

A very well-documented crosstalk exists between the Wnt pathway and the TGFβ cytokine family pathway. This family includes TGFβ and the bone morphogenetic proteins (BMPs), which share a signaling cascade that involves two types of receptors (type I and II) as well as a common set of signal transducers known as Smads. Upon ligand binding to the type II receptor, the type I receptor is recruited to form a heterodimer complex. The complex phosphorylates the C-terminus of receptor-regulated Smads (Smad 1, 2, 3, 5, and 8), which are then able to complex with the common Smad partner, Smad4. This complex then translocates to the nucleus, binds to DNA, and regulates target gene expression. Smads regulate multiple genes involved in a multitude of cellular events including proliferation, motility, differentiation, apoptosis, and the immune response. This pathway has also been linked to various human malignancies and may be a feasible target for therapy (reviewed in Dumont and Arteaga 2003).

Crosstalk between the Wnt and TGFβ pathways is quite complex with several interactions occurring at the molecular level between the two pathways. First of all, ligand production for these two pathways is under regulation by the other. For instance, BMP4 expression in human colon cancer cells is dependent on the expression of oncogenic β-catenin (Kim et al. 2002). In addition, colon cancer cells with mutated Apc overexpress and secrete BMP4, suggesting that stabilization of β-catenin upregulates BMP4 expression. However, β-catenin also activates transcription of BAMBI, a BMP inhibitor, in colorectal cancer, indicating that the Wnt pathway interferes with TGF-β-mediated growth arrest (Sekiya et al. 2004). Work in chick embryos shows that Wnt8 regulates production of Nodal, while conversely BMP2/4 is capable of regulating production of Wnt8 (Hoppler and Moon 1998; Rodriguez-Esteban et al. 2001). In the initial stages of tumor formation, inhibition of BMP signaling increases the expression of Wnt ligands in a model of skin cancer (Sharov et al. 2009). This regulation of ligands for the other's pathway allows each pathway to amplify the activity of the other. However, this response seems to be context dependent as active Wnt signaling represses BMP4 during xenopus embryonic development (Baker et al. 1999).

The second level of crosstalk between Wnt and TGFβ occurs in the nucleus where Smad and β-catenin/TCF form a complex that binds to DNA and regulates shared target gene expression. This interaction was identified in Xenopus with the two converging in the promoter region of the Spemann's organizer gene Xtwn, a finding also later shown in mammalian cells (Labbe et al. 2000; Nishita et al. 2000). Joint regulation of genes by these two pathways has also been noted in different cancer cells. In embryonic carcinoma cells, Wnt3a and BMP4 synergistically induce expression of several genes, Id2, Msx1, and Msx2 (Willert et al. 2002). Cotransfection of Smad3/4 and β-catenin induces gastrin expression in gastric cancer cells (Lei et al. 2004). In mouse models of intestinal and mammary tumorigenesis resulting from Wnt pathway activation, it was shown that a set of genes synergistically regulated by Wnt and TGFβ were increased, and treatment with dominant negative TGFβ type II receptor (DNIIR) delayed the onset of mammary tumor development (Labbe et al. 2007). Interestingly, another study showed the opposite in that DNIIR enhanced tumor growth in the mammary gland, suggesting that TGFβ may act as a tumor suppressor (Roarty et al. 2009). This study pointed to Wnt5a, which is capable of downregulating canonical Wnt signaling, as a downstream target of TGFβ signaling and the mechanism for this tumor suppression. One possible explanation for the different findings here may involve temporal differences in signaling pathways throughout tumor progression. Synergism between the two pathways may be important for the initial formation of tumors, whereas unimpeded canonical Wnt signaling independent of TGFβ may support enhanced tumor growth.

Interaction between the Wnt and TGFβ pathways has been noted in various other types of cancer. In the prostate, stromal cells play a tumor suppressive role that seems to be mediated by TGFβ-induced downregulation of Wnt3a expression. TGFβRII knockout specifically in the stromal cells leads to increased expression of Wnt3a and development of prostatic adenocarcinoma (Bhowmick et al. 2004; Li et al. 2008b). These studies implicate a paracrine effect where stromal cells secrete Wnt3a to promote growth and proliferation of neighboring epithelial cells. Targeting of Wnt3a with a neutralizing antibody inhibited tumor progression in this model. TGFβ signaling also modulates β-catenin activity in tumor fibroblast cell lines (Amini Nik et al. 2007). These two pathways are also linked in pancreatic cancer via cooperation between Smad4 and β-catenin. Blockade of Smad4 in Panc-1 cells induces degradation of β-catenin and attenuates its transcriptional activity with Tcf (Romero et al. 2008). This response translated to a decrease in tumorigenic potential of Panc-1 cells. The converse seemed to be true in an in vivo study, which showed that heterozygous inactivating mutations of Smad4 and Apc led to an increase in the incidence of carcinogen-induced pancreatic tumors (Cullingworth et al. 2002). The differences between these studies can be explained by the fact that Panc-1 cells harbor normal APC; thus, the loss of Smad4 is protumorigenic in the absence of APC and tumor suppressive in the presence of normal APC.

An association in colon cancer also exists in that a similar effect was observed for intestinal tumorigenesis as mice with mutation of both Smad4 and Apc developed colorectal tumors that were larger in size and more invasive than what is observed with Apc mutation alone (Takaku et al. 1998). Likewise, inactivation of TGFβRII promotes malignant transformation and invasion of intestinal tumors initiated by mutation of APC (Munoz et al. 2006). In a more regionally specific manner, Smad3 deficiency promotes tumorigenesis in APC^{min} mice almost exclusively in the distal colon providing a model very similar to the pathology observed in familial adenomatous polyposis (FAP) syndrome (Sodir et al. 2006). Further, colorectal cancer cell lines are resistant to BMP-4-induced differentiation and growth suppression (Nishanian et al. 2004). An association has also been observed in liver tumors as mice overexpressing c-myc and TGFβ harbor mutation and/or nuclear translocation of β-catenin in 33% of liver tumors (Calvisi et al. 2001).

A third level of interaction between the pathways occurs in the cytoplasm where Smad7 and either β-catenin or Axin can physically interact with each other. Smad7 can directly bind to β-catenin and induce its degradation by the recruitment of Smurf2 (Han et al. 2006). Conversely, in prostate cancer cells, Smad7 was found to physically associate with β-catenin and lead to an accumulation of β-catenin, which is important for TGF-β-induced, β-catenin-regulated apoptotic responses in these cells (Edlund et al. 2005). Smad7 can also directly bind to Axin, which induces disassembly of the degradation complex and subsequent stabilization of β-catenin at the adherens junction (Tang et al. 2008). This apparent dual role for Smad7 as well as any association in cancer will need to be addressed in future studies.

4.1.4   IGF

Then insulin/insulin-like growth factor (IGF) signaling pathway plays a key role in energy metabolism and growth, but has also been implicated in cancer development. The ligands for this pathway, insulin and IGF-1 or 2, bind their respective receptor at the membrane and induce activation of intracellular insulin receptor substrates (IRS). IRSs then activate several intracellular signaling pathways including the PI3K/Akt and the Ras/MAPK pathways to mediate downstream effects on the cell. In relation to the Wnt pathway, it was identified that insulin receptor substrate 1 (IRS-1) is a downstream target of β-catenin/Tcf and that increased IRS-1 is observed in colorectal carcinomas and ovarian endometriod adenocarcinomas, which harbor nuclear localization of β-catenin (Bommer et al. 2010). Additionally, it was reported that inactivation of IRS-1 in Apc^{min} mice decreases the number of intestinal adenomatous polyps that form, suggesting that this downstream effector plays a key role in intestinal tumorigenesis in association with activated β-catenin (Ramocki et al. 2008). Interestingly, IRS-1 was associated with regulating Sox9 expression in this study, a known downstream target of Wnt signaling (Ramocki et al. 2008). The interaction of IRS-1 with the Wnt pathway may also exist in the development of hepatocellular carcinoma in the setting of chronic hepatitis B virus infection. Overexpression of IRS-1 simultaneously with the HBx antigen in mice induces a significant increase in dysplasia compared to overexpression of either individually (Longato et al. 2009). Tumors from mice overexpressing both also show a clear increase in cytoplasmic and nuclear localization of β-catenin. A subset of phyllodes tumors and breast fibroadenomas show overexpression of IGF in association with nuclear accumulation of β-catenin, although no causal relationship was noted in this study (Sawyer et al. 2003). Conversely, IGF-1 treatment did not enhance β-catenin/Tcf-mediated transcription in esophageal cancer cells (Kiely et al. 2007). IGF1 treatment of several different cancer cell lines induces β-catenin/Tcf-mediated transcription. In the human hepatoma cell line, HepG2, Desbois-Mouthon et al. showed that IGF1 or insulin treatment increased β-catenin/Tcf-mediated transcription and cytoplasmic stabilization of β-catenin (Desbois-Mouthon et al. 2001). IGF-1 also induced stabilization of β-catenin in prostate cancer and early melanoma cells (Satyamoorthy et al. 2001; Verras and Sun 2005). While multiple associations between these two pathways have been noted in several types of cancer, no definitive mechanism for the link has been elucidated. Future studies will be important to identify the mechanism for this crosstalk and whether or not it can be targeted effectively for therapy.

4.1.5 VEGF

Just as EGFR was identified as a downstream target of Wnt, VEGF was found to be a downstream target in colon cancer cells and benign colonic adenomas (Zhang et al. 2001). A more recent study examined the effect of VEGFR-targeted therapy on the Wnt pathway. Naik et al. found that targeting VEGFR led to a decrease in Wnt pathway activity (Naik et al. 2009). Furthermore, such therapy was effective in inducing cell death in colon cancer cells, which harbor mutations in the Wnt pathway that lead to β-catenin stabilization while not affecting cells that have a normal Wnt pathway. While this work is preliminary, a link between these two pathways in cancer likely exists potentially creating a positive connection between cellular proliferation and angiogenesis.

4.1.6 FGF

FGFs have diverse roles in regulating cell proliferation, migration, and differentiation during embryonic development (Ornitz and Itoh 2001). Genomic analyses have demonstrated that many components of the FGF signaling pathway are controlled by β-catenin (Chamorro et al. 2005; Shimokawa et al. 2003), and loss-of-function mutations in FGF9 are found in a subset of colorectal carcinomas (Abdel-Rahman et al. 2008). FGF19 increases β-catenin transcriptional activity in colon cancer cells and in transgenic mice (Pai et al. 2008; Nicholes et al. 2002). Coactivation of the Wnt and FGF pathways in colorectal carcinogenesis leads to a more malignant phenotype (Katoh and Katoh 2006a). FGFs also cooperate with Wnt-1 in MMTV-induced mammary tumorigenesis (Clausse et al. 1993; MacArthur et al. 1995; Shackleford et al. 1993; Lee et al. 1995). Finally, the interaction of the Wnt and FGF signaling pathways may control directional migration of clusters of cancer cells through chemokine receptor expression (Aman and Piotrowski 2008).

4.2 Developmental Pathways

4.2.1 Notch Pathway

The Notch signaling pathway is highly conserved among metazoans and is essential for development, patterning, and tissue homeostasis (Fortini 2009; Artavanis-Tsakonas et al. 1999). In addition, the Notch pathway has also been implicated in the balance between cell proliferation and apoptosis (Artavanis-Tsakonas et al. 1999; Miele 2006), and its deregulation can lead to uncontrolled self-renewal in human carcinomas (Miele 2006; Wang et al. 2008, 2009). Unlike many other receptor signaling pathways, Notch signals are transduced through direct cell-to-cell contact and require activation at the cell surface by ligands of the DSL (Delta and Serrate/Jagged) family. This interaction causes cleavage of the Notch receptor through intramembrane proteolysis. The resulting product, termed the Notch intracellular domain (NICD), then translocates to the nucleus and activates downstream target genes (Kopan and Ilagan 2009; Gordon et al. 2008). Because it controls many diverse functions, it is perhaps not surprising that Notch must work in conjunction with other signaling pathways to assure proper integration of developmental signals. Indeed, crosstalk between the Notch and Wnt pathways has been noted in processes as diverse as somitogenesis, intestinal epithelial cell fate, and hematopoietic stem cell maintenance (Galceran et al. 2004; Nakamura et al. 2007; Duncan et al. 2005). The Notch pathway represses Wnt signaling during development and homeostasis by associating with and regulating the transcription of β-catenin (Hayward et al. 2005). Likewise, stimulation of the Wnt pathway can antagonize Notch signaling through Disheveled (Axelrod et al. 1996). Understanding the balance between these two networks, both of which regulate tumorigenesis, requires elucidating the link between Wnt and Notch signaling and deregulation in cancer.

As in embryogenesis, many reports have detailed an opposing role for the Wnt and Notch pathways in tumorigenesis, where expression of Notch causes suppression of Wnt. Notch can function as a tumor suppressor by inhibiting β-catenin-mediated signaling in the skin, and its deletion or inhibition results in basal cell carcinoma (BCC) associated with enhanced β-catenin expression (Nicolas et al. 2003; Proweller et al. 2006). An activator of the Delta-Notch pathway induces inhibitors of the Wnt pathway in neuroblastoma cells (Revet et al. 2010). Further, Notch activation in a human tongue cancer cell line led to cell cycle arrest and apoptosis through suppression of the Wnt pathway (Duan et al. 2006).

In other models of cancer, especially those occurring in the gastrointestinal tract, evidence suggests a positive feedback mechanism, where the two pathways cooperate in accelerating tumor initiation and progression. The Wnt and Notch pathways work synergistically in the development of intestinal adenomas, as activation of Notch in Apc mutant mice hyperactive for Wnt signaling accelerates adenoma development (Fre et al. 2009). The activation of the Notch pathway in response to Wnt signaling is also seen in colorectal tumors (van Es et al. 2005). Likewise, Maml1, a coactivator of the Notch pathway, can also modulate Wnt activity independently of Notch signaling in colon carcinoma (Alves-Guerra et al. 2007). In hepatoblastomas, mutation in the CTNNB1 gene is commonly found in the presence of increased expression of the Notch ligand Dlk1. Further, the ratio of Notch to Wnt expression has been suggested to indicate prognosis, where a low Notch expression/high Wnt activation is characteristic of a more aggressive phenotype (Lopez-Terrada et al. 2009).

Wnt and Notch appear to operate synergistically in other cancer types as well. In prostate cancer, for example, it is hypothesized that Wnt activates Notch signaling through regulation of the transcription factors HOXC6 and SOX4 (Moreno 2010). Increased Wnt expression in breast epithelial cells triggers an oncogenic conversion through Notch activation, which is required for transformation to a tumorigenic state (Ayyanan et al. 2006; Collu and Brennan 2007). Cooperation between the two pathways is also suggested in the self-renewal of hematopoietic stem cells as well as the induction of T-cell leukemia, where simultaneous deregulation of Wnt and Notch signaling is thought to increase proliferation while maintaining cells in an undifferentiated state (Duncan et al. 2005; Weerkamp et al. 2006). Hyperactivated Hedgehog-dependent Wnt signaling in the presence of deregulated Notch leads to chronic myeloid leukemia, although a direct link between the two pathways is not specified (Sengupta et al. 2007).

Jagged1, a Notch receptor ligand, has been reported to be transcriptionally activated by β-catenin (Estrach et al. 2006; Katoh and Katoh 2006b), and may represent the physical link between Wnt and Notch signaling in cancer. However, reports of a direct correspondence between the two pathways are contradictory. Although one group demonstrated that increased Jagged1 expression correlated with increased Notch activation in the Apc mouse model, they were unable to show a direct correlation between nuclear β-catenin levels and Jagged1 expression in colon tumors (Guilmeau et al. 2010). However, another group found that Notch is downstream of Wnt in colorectal cancer and is mediated by direct activation of Jagged1 through β-catenin. Further, they concluded that Notch is essential for tumorigenesis in the intestine, and that Wnt and Notch work synergistically to promote proliferation in tumors (Rodilla et al. 2009). A third group showed that inhibition of Wnt signaling also decreased Notch signaling through decreased transcription of Jagged1 in colorectal cancer cells, and that restoration of Jagged1-activated Tcf-4 transcription, suggesting the presence of a feedback loop between Notch and Wnt signaling (Pannequin et al. 2009).

4.2.2   Hedgehog Pathway

Like the Notch pathway, the Hedgehog pathway is essential for embryonic development and the maintenance of stem cell populations, as it is a key mediator in tissue
growth, patterning, and morphogenesis (Ingham and McMahon 2001). The three
mammalian Hedgehog genes, Sonic, Indian, and Desert hedgehog (*Shh*, *Ihh*, and
Dhh), encode for secreted proteins that undergo cleavage and lipid modification to
become an active signaling molecule (Zardawi et al. 2009). Binding of a Hedgehog
(Hh) ligand to its receptor, Patched, derepresses the transmembrane protein
Smoothened (Smo), which then causes a signal cascade resulting in the stabilization
of Gli proteins (Taipale and Beachy 2001; Hooper and Scott 2005). These proteins
mediate Hedgehog activity by activating transcription of target genes (Ingham and
McMahon 2001). Increased Hedgehog signaling has also been implicated in numerous
cancers, including the skin, cerebellum, pancreas, and intestinal tract (McMahon
et al. 2003; Pasca di Magliano and Hebrok 2003). Given the similarities in signals
and responses between the Wnt and Hedgehog pathways (Lum and Beachy 2004;
Zhou and Hung 2005), it is not surprising that activation of both pathways can lead
to increased incidence and lethality of specific cancers (Beachy et al. 2004). In fact,
Hedgehog or Wnt pathway activation could be important in up to one third of
cancers (Rubin and de Sauvage 2006).

   The first evidence that the Wnt and Hedgehog pathways are linked in cancer was
discovered in BCCs, which showed elevated levels of Wnt pathway components in
response to Hedgehog signaling abnormalities and Gli1 expression (Bonifas et al.
2001; Yang et al. 2008; Yamazaki et al. 2001; Li et al. 2007). Similar results were
found in endometrial cancers, where elevated Gli1 expression led to accumulation
of nuclear β-catenin (Liao et al. 2009). An analysis of binding elements in the promoters of *WNT2A* and *WNT5A* suggests that Hedgehog signaling both directly and
indirectly upregulates Wnt expression (Katoh and Katoh 2009a, b). However, other
groups found a heterogeneous activation of β-catenin in BCC in response to constitutively active Hedgehog signaling, which suggests that although Wnt signaling
may contribute to the pathogenesis of a subset of BCC, a causal link between Hh
pathway deregulation and Wnt overexpression remains to be confirmed (Salto-
Tellez et al. 2006; Saldanha et al. 2004; El-Bahrawy et al. 2003).

   A significant crosstalk between the Hedgehog and Wnt pathways has also been
reported in gastrointestinal cancers, with several reports indicating that Wnt
signaling can enhance Hedgehog activity. A product of Wnt signaling, CRD-BP,
stabilizes Gli1 mRNA, leading to increased Hedgehog signaling and survival of
colorectal cancer cells (Noubissi et al. 2009). Inhibition of Smo rescues the lethality
of Apc mice, suggesting that Hedgehog is activated in parallel with or downstream
of Wnt signaling (Varnat et al. 2010). Further, β-catenin enhances the transcriptional activity of Gli1 in gastric and colon carcinoma cell lines (Maeda et al. 2006).
The inverse has been reported as well where Hedgehog signaling was shown to
positively regulate the Wnt pathway (Kim and Choi 2009). Reduced expression of
Smo in Apc mice suppressed β-catenin-dependent transcription in intestinal

adenoma cells independently of the canonical Hedgehog pathway, which suggests that activation of Smo contributes to tumorigenesis through regulating Wnt signaling (Arimura et al. 2009). In addition, activation of the Hedgehog pathway through Smo or Gli2 increases Wnt activity in pancreatic adenocarcinoma (Pasca di Magliano et al. 2007).

Other groups, however, have shown that in colorectal cancer, Wnt and Hedgehog act antagonistically (van den Brink and Hardwick 2006). Blocking Wnt activation in colon cancer cells restored Hedgehog signaling (van den Brink et al. 2004), while transfection with Gli1 antagonizes constitutive activation of Wnt-stimulated proliferation (Akiyoshi et al. 2006). sFRP-1, an antagonist of Wnt signaling and a target of the Hedgehog pathway, has been implicated in the mechanism of this interaction (He et al. 2006). Further, Wnt and Hedgehog signaling has been inversely correlated in gastric cancer specimens, and overexpression of Gli1 suppressed Wnt signaling in a gastric cancer cell line (Yanai et al. 2008). There is some indication that the disparate regulation of these two pathways is stage-specific, with stronger Hedgehog expression correlating with Wnt suppression in well-differentiated gastric cancer tissues (Kim et al. 2010).

Correlation of Wnt and Hedgehog expression is also implicated in other forms of cancer. Expression of both Wnt and Notch components appears to be downstream of Hedgehog signaling in medulloblastoma; alternatively, Wnt may be activated by loss of Sufu, a downstream negative regulator of the Hedgehog pathway that also exports β-catenin from the nucleus (Taylor et al. 2004). However, the relevance of these interactions between pathways as it relates to medulloblastoma tumor initiation and progression is presently unclear (Dakubo et al. 2006). Activation of the canonical Wnt pathway in a mouse model of breast cancer correlates with induction of the Hedgehog pathway and may be a critical component in tumor formation (Teissedre et al. 2009). Finally, smoke-induced lung tumors are also driven by simultaneous activation of these two pathways (Lemjabbar-Alaoui et al. 2006) (Fig. 4.2).

4.3 Wnt and Other Networks

4.3.1 Prostaglandin/Cox-2 Pathway

Cyclooxygenase-2 (Cox-2) is an enzyme that converts arachidonic acid to prostaglandin, a lipid compound that controls a wide variety of biological functions, such as inflammation, hormone regulation, and wound healing (Dubois et al. 1998). Upregulation of Cox-2 also contributes to carcinogenesis and invasiveness through increased production of prostaglandins (Dempke et al. 2001). It has been suggested that Cox-2 may be a direct target of β-catenin transcriptional activation (Goss and Groden 2000). In a human hepatoma cell line, Cox-2 activity was demonstrated to be decreased by APC and upregulated by nuclear β-catenin accumulation

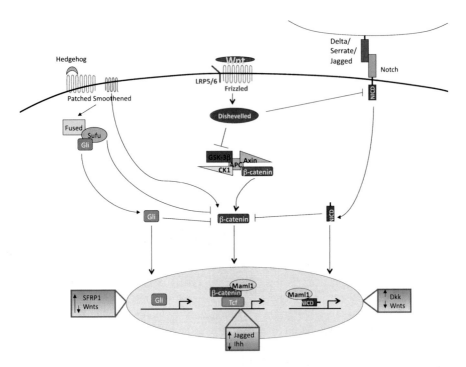

Fig. 4.2 The Hedgehog, Notch, and Wnt pathways are key regulators of cell fate, differentiation, and proliferation, and signaling crosstalk occurs frequently in both development and cancer. Hedgehog signaling occurs when a Hedgehog (Hh) ligand binds to its receptor, Patched, causing derepression of the transmembrane protein Smoothened (Smo). Smo transduces the signal by activating a cascade resulting in the release of Gli from its inactivating complex. Gli then translocates to the nucleus where it activates target gene expression. Crosstalk with the Wnt pathway occurs at the posttranslational as well as the transcriptional levels. Smo is known to increase Wnt signaling through β-catenin, while Gli and Sufu, a negative regulator of the Hedgehog pathway, both inhibit β-catenin translocation to the nucleus. In the nucleus, Gli-mediated transcription can act to either restrict or enhance the expression of Wnt targets, depending on cellular context. Constitutive activation of Wnt signaling causes loss of expression of Ihh, a Hedgehog ligand. Binding of Notch to its membrane-bound ligand Delta/Serrate/Jagged causes intramembrane cleavage of Notch and release of the NICD, which translocates to the nucleus and activates target gene expression. NICD can directly inhibit β-catenin nuclear translocation. Additionally, Notch both downregulates Wnt expression and upregulates Dkk, a negative inhibitor of the Wnt pathway. Wnt upregulates expression of the Notch ligand Jagged, enhancing Notch signaling. Maml1, a coactivator of the Notch pathway, can also modulate β-catenin transcription

(Araki et al. 2003). However, efforts to repeat this result in other cell types have failed to show regulation of Cox-2 by β-catenin (Eisinger et al. 2007). Another group found that mediators of the Wnt pathway activate the Cox-2 promoter, which contributes to transformation in colorectal cancer (Howe et al. 2001; Carlson et al. 2003). Thus, Wnt may activate Cox-2 through an indirect mechanism, although it has also been suggested that β-catenin can directly bind to and stabilize Cox-2 mRNA (Kawasaki et al. 2007). Additionally, prostaglandin E2 has also been shown to stimulate β-catenin in colon cancer cells, establishing a positive feedback loop between the Wnt and Cox-2 pathways (Castellone et al. 2005; Shao et al. 2005;

Buchanan and DuBois 2006). Another current hypothesis is that mutations in APC result in upregulation of Cox-2 through impaired retinoic acid biosynthesis and elevated levels of C/EBP-β, which increases prostaglandin accumulation driving activation of Wnt target genes. In any case, it appears that crosstalk between the Wnt and Cox-2/prostaglandin pathways accelerates the progression of cancer, although the precise mechanisms remain to be elucidated.

The crosstalk between the two pathways has been extensively studied in gastrointestinal cancers. In a mouse model, simultaneous activation of the Wnt and prostaglandin E2 pathways resulted in gastric adenocarcinomas, which recapitulated that seen in human gastric cancer (Itadani et al. 2009; Oshima et al. 2006; Takasu et al. 2008). Likewise, suppression of signaling by proline oxidase expression led to a simultaneous decrease in prostaglandin production and β-catenin transcription (Liu et al. 2008). However, in patients with urothelial carcinoma, there was an inverse relationship between Wnt activation and Cox-2 expression, which might be the result of tissue-specific differences in expression patterns (Kastritis et al. 2009). Wnt and Cox-2 also synergize to further coactivate other cell signaling pathways. For example, alterations in the Wnt pathway can trigger the Cox-2 pathway to constitutively activate PDGFRA/B, a hallmark of aggressive fibromatosis (Signoroni et al. 2007). Further, induction of the prostaglandin E2 pathway and subsequent Wnt activation in the presence of suppressed BMP expression may accelerate the promotion of tumor formation in the gastric mucosa (Oshima et al. 2009).

Blocking the activation of the Cox-2/Wnt pathway is an attractive and efficacious target of many current cancer therapies. Omega-3 polyunsaturated fatty acids inhibit cell growth through simultaneously blocking β-catenin and Cox-2 pathways in both hepatocellular carcinoma and cholangiocarcinoma (Lim et al. 2008, 2009). Polyphenols derived from black tea decrease levels of both Cox-2 and β-catenin downstream targets (Patel et al. 2008). In addition, multiple studies have demonstrated that Cox-2 inhibitors, a class of nonsteroidal anti-inflammatory drugs (NSAIDs) that have chemopreventive activity, also suppress β-catenin signaling, resulting in decreased proliferation and apoptosis of various cellular malignancies (Suh et al. 2009; Sakoguchi-Okada et al. 2007; Behari et al. 2007; Boon et al. 2004; Humar et al. 2008; Tuynman et al. 2008; Lu et al. 2009). However, it has been shown that certain NSAIDS can negatively regulate Wnt activity without affecting Cox-2. R-Etodolac, an enantiomer of a known NSAID, lacks the ability to inhibit Cox-2 but still robustly decreases β-catenin activity along with survival and proliferation in hepatoma cells (Behari et al. 2007). Future studies will likely clarify any benefit to targeting β-catenin independently of Cox-2 with this class of drugs.

4.3.2   PI3K/AKT Pathway

The PI3K pathway is a class of signal transducers that regulate cell proliferation, survival, metabolism, and membrane trafficking (Leevers et al. 1999). Because Akt can phosphorylate and inactivate GSK-3β (Cross et al. 1995), a critical negative regulator of the Wnt pathway, its crosstalk with Wnt in cancer is well documented. However, a recent study has challenged this notion showing that Axin compartmentalizes GSK3 prohibiting crosstalk between the PI3K and Wnt pathways (Ng et al. 2009). Future studies will be essential to rectify the differences between these two studies and definitively explore whether such crosstalk exists. In relation to cancer, PTEN, a tumor suppressor, regulates translocation of β-catenin to the nucleus, and β-catenin is constitutively active in tumor cells with PTEN null mutations (Persad et al. 2001). PTEN expression also reduces β-catenin-mediated augmentation of androgen receptor transactivation in prostate cancer (Sharma et al. 2002). Inhibition of the PI3K pathway in a model of medulloblastoma abrogated Wnt signaling by activation of GSK-3β activity (Baryawno et al. 2010). Akt, a kinase activated by the PI3K pathway which is frequently mutated in cancers, can directly phosphorylate β-catenin, resulting in nuclear translocation, increased transcription, and promotion of tumor cell invasion (Fang et al. 2007). In turn, β-catenin can regulate Akt activation in colorectal and prostate cancer (Dihlmann et al. 2005; Ohigashi et al. 2005). In the context of activated Wnt signaling, PTEN suppresses progression to mammary carcinoma as well as adenocarcinoma through modulation of Akt levels (Marsh et al. 2008; Li et al. 2001; Zhao et al. 2005). There is also a synergistic effect of dysregulated PI3K and Wnt signaling in the development and progression of granulosa cell tumor and testicular cancer (Boyer et al. 2009; Lague et al. 2008). Thus, it appears that PI3K and Wnt can crossregulate via PTEN, GSK3-β, and/or Akt in many different cancer types (Mulholland et al. 2006).

The Wnt and PI3K pathways can also be comodulated by other cellular pathways in the context of tumorigenesis. Reexpression of Glypican-3, a proteoglycan implicated in cell survival, inhibits Wnt and PI3K signaling in a model of mammary adenocarcinoma (Buchanan et al. 2010). Administration of adiponectin also mediated a decrease in PI3K and Wnt signaling in breast cancer through blocking phosphorylation of Akt and GSK-3β (Wang et al. 2006). Galectin-3, β-galactoside-binding protein that has been correlated with metastasis in colon cancer, exacerbates tumor progression by positively regulating Akt and GSK-3β (Song et al. 2009). Insulin-like growth factor 1 can activate the β-catenin pathway through mediation of the PI3K/AKT pathway in both melanoma and hepatoma cells (Desbois-Mouthon et al. 2001; Satyamoorthy et al. 2001). Finally, IL-1β also inactivates GSK-3β by activation of AKT, thus stimulating the Wnt pathway in colon cancer cells (Kaler et al. 2009) (Fig. 4.3).

4.3.3   mTOR

The mammalian target of rapamycin (mTOR) pathway is a serine/threonine kinase cascade that belongs to the PI3K family. mTOR signaling is regulated by various upstream signals including nutrient and energy status, growth factors, and cellular stress. mTOR is a component of two complexes (mTORC1 and mTORC2) that act as serine/threonine kinases for downstream targets. Both complexes contain mTOR

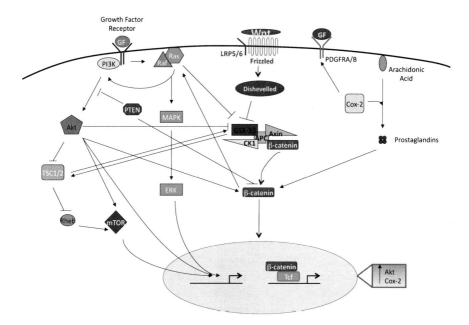

Fig. 4.3 The PI3K/Akt and Ras/MAPK pathways crosstalk with Wnt signaling in several ways. Activation of PI3K through growth factor binding to its cognate receptor triggers activation of Akt, a critical mediator of the pathway that is involved in regulation of the cell cycle, cell survival, and metabolism. Akt can both directly and indirectly activate β-catenin either by triggering its nuclear translocation or by inactivating GSK-3β. In turn, Akt expression is regulated by Wnt/β-catenin signaling. Akt also inhibits TSC1/2, a negative regulator of mTOR, a cellular switch that integrates and transduces nutrient and growth factor signals. GSK-3β phosphorylation of TSC1/2 also contributes to the negative regulation of mTOR, and TSC1/2 in turn negatively regulates β-catenin signaling activity through GSK-3β. Wnt signaling activates the mTOR pathway by inhibiting GSK-3β. PTEN, which inhibits the activation of Akt, also negatively regulates β-catenin nuclear translocation. The Ras/MAPK pathway, which is activated in response to receptor tyrosine kinase signaling, can cross-activate the PI3K pathway, in addition to many other cell processes and pathways. Ras can indirectly activate β-catenin through GSK-3β inhibition. In turn, Wnt/β-catenin signaling can regulate Ras stability by decreasing ubiquitination and degradation. The Cox-2/prostaglandin pathway has recently emerged as a key pathway in the development of many cancers and also demonstrates crosstalk with the Wnt pathway. Cox-2 converts arachidonic acid to prostaglandins, which can increase the nuclear accumulation of β-catenin through several mechanisms. In addition, Cox-2 is a direct target of β-catenin transcription, and Cox-2 expression through the Wnt pathway activates PDGFRA/B

and mLST8, while mTORC1 includes raptor as the third component and mTORC2 includes rictor. mTORC1 can be induced by Rheb to phosphorylate S6 kinase and 4E-BP1, which enhance translation of a subset of mRNAs. Conversely, mTORC2 is involved in Akt phosphorylation and regulation of the actin cytoskeleton.

A link between mTOR and β-catenin was explored after it was identified that renal tumors from Eker rats, which contain a mutation in TSC2, had increased levels of β-catenin and cyclin D1(Kenerson et al. 2002; Mak et al. 2003). The crosstalk involves an interaction between the TSC1/2 complex and GSK3β, which promotes degradation of β-catenin. Mutation of the TSC1/2 complex in patients leads to the disease tuberous sclerosis, which is associated with a variety of tumors including subependymal giant cell astrocytomas (SEGAs). Increased levels of β-catenin were indeed observed in a set of SEGAs (Jozwiak et al. 2007). This increase was associated with cytoplasm/nuclear translocation of β-catenin and upregulation of the target gene c-myc. It has also been reported that TSC-related angiomyolipomas and lymphangioleiomyomatosis exhibit increases in levels of β-catenin as well as two downstream effectors, cyclin D1 and connexin 43 (Mak et al. 2005). A link between the two pathways has also been explored in colon cancer. It was shown that the mTOR pathway is activated in intestinal polyps from Apc(Delta716) heterozygous mutant mice, a model for human FAP (Fujishita et al. 2008). Interestingly, suppression of mTORC1 activity inhibited proliferation of intestinal tumor adenoma cells and decreased tumor angiogenesis. This effect significantly reduced the number of polyps as well as tumor size suggesting the mTOR inhibitors may be an effective therapy for treating intestinal tumors that are positive for Wnt pathway activation.

Crosstalk in the other direction has also been noted as Wnt stimulation induced activation of mTOR and did so independent of β-catenin via GSK3β inhibition (Inoki et al. 2006). GSK3β normally inhibits mTOR via phosphorylation of TSC2. Upon stimulation with Wnt, GSK3β is inhibited thus freeing the mTOR pathway from this negative regulation. Hyperinsulinemia synergistically activates both the mTOR pathway and the Wnt/β-catenin pathway in colorectal tumor formation (Sun and Jin 2008). Chemotherapeutic inhibition of the mTOR pathway also inhibits β-catenin signaling in osteosarcoma (Gazitt et al. 2009). Finally, treatment with rapamycin inhibits growth of MMTV-driven Wnt-1 mammary tumors through inhibition of mTOR (Svirshchevskaya et al. 2008). It will be important to further explore this crosstalk in other types of cancer and examine whether or not treatment with rapamycin has the same effect in these tumors.

4.3.4   Ras Pathway

The Ras family encodes small GTPases, which function as signal transducers inside the cell. The Ras pathway regulates cell growth, proliferation, and differentiation, and as such, is frequently mutated in cancers (Goodsell 1999; Hancock 2003). The Ras and Wnt pathways appear to function concurrently in tumorigenesis, with some evidence of direct regulation. Synchronous activation of K-ras and β-catenin significantly reduced survival in a compound mouse model of prostate cancer, reflecting accelerated tumorigenesis (Pearson et al. 2009). Activating mutations in Kras2 or Hras1 also strongly synergize with Wnt-1 in mammary tumorigenesis (Jang et al. 2006). Similarly, synergistic cooperation between the K-ras and Wnt pathways was observed in models of intestinal, colon, liver, and renal carcinomas (Luo et al. 2009; Sansom et al. 2006; Janssen et al. 2006; D'Abaco et al. 1996; Harada et al. 2004). Wnt and K-ras also synergize in colon cancer to regulate VEGF and gastrin (Zhang et al. 2001; Koh et al. 2000; Chakladar et al. 2005). Direct crosstalk between the pathways has been demonstrated in colon cancer, where oncogenic K-ras activates Wnt signaling through GSK-3β inhibition (Li et al. 2005). Conversely, Wnt/β-catenin signaling can also regulate Ras stability (Kim et al. 2009). These two studies provide a potential mechanistic basis for the synergism between the Wnt/β-catenin and Ras pathways that results in tumorigenesis (Kim et al. 2009).

4.3.5   Miscellaneous Signaling Pathways

Finally, several other cellular pathways exhibit crosstalk with Wnt in cancer. The Wnt and cell adhesion pathways cooperate in many aspects of development as well as in cancer progression (Schambony et al. 2004). In myeloma cells, for example, Wnt contributes to cell adhesion-mediated drug resistance (Kobune et al. 2007). Conversely, in acute myeloid leukemia, these pathways act in opposition, as both adhesion to fibronectin and administration of Wnt antagonists induced chemotherapeutic resistance (De Toni et al. 2006). Inhibition of integrin-linked kinase (ILK), a component of anchorage-independent growth, suppresses nuclear translocation of β-catenin (Oloumi et al. 2006; Tan et al. 2001), while overexpression of Wnt increases ILK activity (D'Amico et al. 2000).

The fibrinolysis, inflammatory, and nitric oxide pathways also exhibit cross-regulation with Wnt signaling in cancer. The plasminogen activator system, which is involved in the breakdown of blood clots, can activate β-catenin in ECV304 carcinoma cells (Maupas-Schwalm et al. 2005). β-catenin signaling inversely correlates with cytokine-induced iNOS, Fas, and other NF-κB-dependent genes in inflammation-associated carcinogenesis (Du et al. 2009). Increased expression of TNF-α in a model of gastrointestinal adenoma induced β-catenin transcription, suggesting that TNF-α can directly regulate the Wnt pathway (Tselepis et al. 2002; Oguma et al. 2008). Finally, β-catenin signaling can inhibit death receptor-mediated apoptosis in squamous cell carcinoma, leukemia, and colorectal cancer (De Toni et al. 2008; Yang et al. 2006; Doubravska et al. 2008; Senthivinayagam et al. 2009).

4.4   Conclusion

Multiple networks have the capacity to interact with Wnt pathway in cancer providing positive and/or negative regulation for expression of downstream targets. The same is true for the effects of Wnt signaling on many of these pathways. Such crosstalk between networks clearly plays an important role in many cancers being involved in transformation, promoting tumor cell proliferation, and inducing motility in metastatic disease. A continued effort in elucidating which crosstalks are the most important will be key for the development of new and effective therapies. Results from these studies will provide the groundwork for a combination therapy approach targeting multiple pathways which will likely be more effective than targeting one pathway alone.

References

Abdel-Rahman WM, Kalinina J, Shoman S, Eissa S, Ollikainen M, Elomaa O, Eliseenkova AV et al (2008) Somatic FGF9 mutations in colorectal and endometrial carcinomas associated with membranous beta-catenin. Hum Mutat 29:390–397

Akiyoshi T, Nakamura M, Koga K, Nakashima H, Yao T, Tsuneyoshi M, Tanaka M et al (2006) Gli1, downregulated in colorectal cancers, inhibits proliferation of colon cancer cells involving Wnt signalling activation. Gut 55:991–999

Alves-Guerra MC, Ronchini C, Capobianco AJ (2007) Mastermind-like 1 Is a specific coactivator of beta-catenin transcription activation and is essential for colon carcinoma cell survival. Cancer Res 67:8690–8698

Aman A, Piotrowski T (2008) Wnt/beta-catenin and Fgf signaling control collective cell migration by restricting chemokine receptor expression. Dev Cell 15:749–761

Amini Nik S, Ebrahim RP, Van Dam K, Cassiman JJ, Tejpar S (2007) TGF-beta modulates beta-catenin stability and signaling in mesenchymal proliferations. Exp Cell Res 313:2887–2895

Araki Y, Okamura S, Hussain SP, Nagashima M, He P, Shiseki M, Miura K et al (2003) Regulation of cyclooxygenase-2 expression by the Wnt and ras pathways. Cancer Res 63:728–734

Arimura S, Matsunaga A, Kitamura T, Aoki K, Aoki M, Taketo MM (2009) Reduced level of smoothened suppresses intestinal tumorigenesis by down-regulation of Wnt signaling. Gastroenterology 137:629–638

Artavanis-Tsakonas S, Rand MD, Lake RJ (1999) Notch signaling: cell fate control and signal integration in development. Science 284:770–776

Axelrod JD, Matsuno K, Artavanis-Tsakonas S, Perrimon N (1996) Interaction between Wingless and Notch signaling pathways mediated by dishevelled. Science 271:1826–1832

Ayyanan A, Civenni G, Ciarloni L, Morel C, Mueller N, Lefort K, Mandinova A et al (2006) Increased Wnt signaling triggers oncogenic conversion of human breast epithelial cells by a Notch-dependent mechanism. Proc Natl Acad Sci U S A 103:3799–3804

Baker JC, Beddington RS, Harland RM (1999) Wnt signaling in Xenopus embryos inhibits bmp4 expression and activates neural development. Genes Dev 13:3149–3159

Baryawno N, Sveinbjornsson B, Eksborg S, Chen CS, Kogner P, Johnsen JI (2010) Small-molecule inhibitors of phosphatidylinositol 3-kinase/Akt signaling inhibit Wnt/beta-catenin pathway cross-talk and suppress medulloblastoma growth. Cancer Res 70:266–276

Beachy PA, Karhadkar SS, Berman DM (2004) Tissue repair and stem cell renewal in carcinogenesis. Nature 432:324–331

Behari J, Zeng G, Otruba W, Thompson MD, Muller P, Micsenyi A, Sekhon SS et al (2007) R-Etodolac decreases beta-catenin levels along with survival and proliferation of hepatoma cells. J Hepatol 46:849–857

Bhowmick NA, Chytil A, Plieth D, Gorska AE, Dumont N, Shappell S, Washington MK et al (2004) TGF-beta signaling in fibroblasts modulates the oncogenic potential of adjacent epithelia. Science 303:848–851

Bommer GT, Feng Y, Iura A, Giordano TJ, Kuick R, Kadikoy H, Sikorski D et al (2010) IRS1 regulation by Wnt/beta-catenin signaling and varied contribution of IRS1 to the neoplastic phenotype. J Biol Chem 285:1928–1938

Bonifas JM, Pennypacker S, Chuang PT, McMahon AP, Williams M, Rosenthal A, De Sauvage FJ et al (2001) Activation of expression of hedgehog target genes in basal cell carcinomas. J Invest Dermatol 116:739–742

Bonvini P, An WG, Rosolen A, Nguyen P, Trepel J, Garcia de Herreros A, Dunach M et al (2001) Geldanamycin abrogates ErbB2 association with proteasome-resistant beta-catenin in melanoma cells, increases beta-catenin-E-cadherin association, and decreases beta-catenin-sensitive transcription. Cancer Res 61:1671–1677

Boon EM, van der Neut R, van de Wetering M, Clevers H, Pals ST (2002) Wnt signaling regulates expression of the receptor tyrosine kinase met in colorectal cancer. Cancer Res 62: 5126–5128

Boon EM, Keller JJ, Wormhoudt TA, Giardiello FM, Offerhaus GJ, van der Neut R, Pals ST (2004) Sulindac targets nuclear beta-catenin accumulation and Wnt signalling in adenomas of patients with familial adenomatous polyposis and in human colorectal cancer cell lines. Br J Cancer 90:224–229

Bourguignon LY, Peyrollier K, Gilad E, Brightman A (2007) Hyaluronan-CD44 interaction with neural Wiskott-Aldrich syndrome protein (N-WASP) promotes actin polymerization and ErbB2 activation leading to beta-catenin nuclear translocation, transcriptional up-regulation, and cell migration in ovarian tumor cells. J Biol Chem 282:1265–1280

Boyer A, Paquet M, Lague MN, Hermo L, Boerboom D (2009) Dysregulation of WNT/CTNNB1 and PI3K/AKT signaling in testicular stromal cells causes granulosa cell tumor of the testis. Carcinogenesis 30:869–878

Buchanan FG, DuBois RN (2006) Connecting COX-2 and Wnt in cancer. Cancer Cell 9:6–8

Buchanan C, Stigliano I, Garay-Malpartida HM, Rodrigues Gomes L, Puricelli L, Sogayar MC, Bal de Kier Joffe E et al (2010) Glypican-3 reexpression regulates apoptosis in murine adenocarcinoma mammary cells modulating PI3K/Akt and p38MAPK signaling pathways. Breast Cancer Res Treat 119:559–574

Calvisi DF, Factor VM, Loi R, Thorgeirsson SS (2001) Activation of beta-catenin during hepatocarcinogenesis in transgenic mouse models: relationship to phenotype and tumor grade. Cancer Res 61:2085–2091

Carlson ML, Wilson ET, Prescott SM (2003) Regulation of COX-2 transcription in a colon cancer cell line by Pontin52/TIP49a. Mol Cancer 2:42

Castellone MD, Teramoto H, Williams BO, Druey KM, Gutkind JS (2005) Prostaglandin E2 promotes colon cancer cell growth through a Gs-axin-beta-catenin signaling axis. Science 310:1504–1510

Chakladar A, Dubeykovskiy A, Wojtukiewicz LJ, Pratap J, Lei S, Wang TC (2005) Synergistic activation of the murine gastrin promoter by oncogenic Ras and beta-catenin involves SMAD recruitment. Biochem Biophys Res Commun 336:190–196

Chamorro MN, Schwartz DR, Vonica A, Brivanlou AH, Cho KR, Varmus HE (2005) FGF-20 and DKK1 are transcriptional targets of beta-catenin and FGF-20 is implicated in cancer and development. Embo J 24:73–84

Civenni G, Holbro T, Hynes NE (2003) Wnt1 and Wnt5a induce cyclin D1 expression through ErbB1 transactivation in HC11 mammary epithelial cells. EMBO Rep 4:166–171

Clausse N, Baines D, Moore R, Brookes S, Dickson C, Peters G (1993) Activation of both Wnt-1 and Fgf-3 by insertion of mouse mammary tumor virus downstream in the reverse orientation: a reappraisal of the enhancer insertion model. Virology 194:157–165

Collu GM, Brennan K (2007) Cooperation between Wnt and Notch signalling in human breast cancer. Breast Cancer Res 9:105

Cross DA, Alessi DR, Cohen P, Andjelkovich M, Hemmings BA (1995) Inhibition of glycogen synthase kinase-3 by insulin mediated by protein kinase B. Nature 378:785–789

Cullingworth J, Hooper ML, Harrison DJ, Mason JO, Sirard C, Patek CE, Clarke AR (2002) Carcinogen-induced pancreatic lesions in the mouse: effect of Smad4 and Apc genotypes. Oncogene 21:4696–4701

D'Abaco GM, Whitehead RH, Burgess AW (1996) Synergy between Apc min and an activated ras mutation is sufficient to induce colon carcinomas. Mol Cell Biol 16:884–891

D'Amico M, Hulit J, Amanatullah DF, Zafonte BT, Albanese C, Bouzahzah B, Fu M et al (2000) The integrin-linked kinase regulates the cyclin D1 gene through glycogen synthase kinase 3beta and cAMP-responsive element-binding protein-dependent pathways. J Biol Chem 275:32649–32657

Dakubo GD, Mazerolle CJ, Wallace VA (2006) Expression of Notch and Wnt pathway components and activation of Notch signaling in medulloblastomas from heterozygous patched mice. J Neurooncol 79:221–227

De Toni F, Racaud-Sultan C, Chicanne G, Mas VM, Cariven C, Mesange F, Salles JP et al (2006) A crosstalk between the Wnt and the adhesion-dependent signaling pathways governs the chemosensitivity of acute myeloid leukemia. Oncogene 25:3113–3122

De Toni EN, Thieme SE, Herbst A, Behrens A, Stieber P, Jung A, Blum H et al (2008) OPG is regulated by beta-catenin and mediates resistance to TRAIL-induced apoptosis in colon cancer. Clin Cancer Res 14:4713–4718

Dempke W, Rie C, Grothey A, Schmoll HJ (2001) Cyclooxygenase-2: a novel target for cancer chemotherapy? J Cancer Res Clin Oncol 127:411–417

Desbois-Mouthon C, Cadoret A, Blivet-Van Eggelpoel MJ, Bertrand F, Cherqui G, Perret C, Capeau J (2001) Insulin and IGF-1 stimulate the beta-catenin pathway through two signalling cascades involving GSK-3beta inhibition and Ras activation. Oncogene 20:252–259

Dihlmann S, Kloor M, Fallsehr C, von Knebel Doeberitz M (2005) Regulation of AKT1 expression by beta-catenin/Tcf/Lef signaling in colorectal cancer cells. Carcinogenesis 26:1503–1512

Doubravska L, Simova S, Cermak L, Valenta T, Korinek V, Andera L (2008) Wnt-expressing rat embryonic fibroblasts suppress Apo2L/TRAIL-induced apoptosis of human leukemia cells. Apoptosis 13:573–587

Du Q, Zhang X, Cardinal J, Cao Z, Guo Z, Shao L, Geller DA (2009) Wnt/beta-catenin signaling regulates cytokine-induced human inducible nitric oxide synthase expression by inhibiting nuclear factor-kappaB activation in cancer cells. Cancer Res 69:3764–3771

Duan L, Yao J, Wu X, Fan M (2006) Growth suppression induced by Notch1 activation involves Wnt-beta-catenin down-regulation in human tongue carcinoma cells. Biol Cell 98:479–490

Dubois RN, Abramson SB, Crofford L, Gupta RA, Simon LS, Van De Putte LB, Lipsky PE (1998) Cyclooxygenase in biology and disease. Faseb J 12:1063–1073

Dumont N, Arteaga CL (2003) Targeting the TGF beta signaling network in human neoplasia. Cancer Cell 3:531–536

Duncan AW, Rattis FM, DiMascio LN, Congdon KL, Pazianos G, Zhao C, Yoon K et al (2005) Integration of Notch and Wnt signaling in hematopoietic stem cell maintenance. Nat Immunol 6:314–322

Edlund S, Lee SY, Grimsby S, Zhang S, Aspenstrom P, Heldin CH, Landstrom M (2005) Interaction between Smad7 and beta-catenin: importance for transforming growth factor beta-induced apoptosis. Mol Cell Biol 25:1475–1488

Eisinger AL, Prescott SM, Jones DA, Stafforini DM (2007) The role of cyclooxygenase-2 and prostaglandins in colon cancer. Prostaglandins Other Lipid Mediat 82:147–154

El-Bahrawy M, El-Masry N, Alison M, Poulsom R, Fallowfield M (2003) Expression of beta-catenin in basal cell carcinoma. Br J Dermatol 148:964–970

Estrach S, Ambler CA, Lo Celso C, Hozumi K, Watt FM (2006) Jagged 1 is a beta-catenin target gene required for ectopic hair follicle formation in adult epidermis. Development 133:4427–4438

Fang D, Hawke D, Zheng Y, Xia Y, Meisenhelder J, Nika H, Mills GB et al (2007) Phosphorylation of beta-catenin by AKT promotes beta-catenin transcriptional activity. J Biol Chem 282:11221–11229

Fortini ME (2009) Notch signaling: the core pathway and its posttranslational regulation. Dev Cell 16:633–647

Fre S, Pallavi SK, Huyghe M, Lae M, Janssen KP, Robine S, Artavanis-Tsakonas S et al (2009) Notch and Wnt signals cooperatively control cell proliferation and tumorigenesis in the intestine. Proc Natl Acad Sci U S A 106:6309–6314

Fujishita T, Aoki K, Lane HA, Aoki M, Taketo MM (2008) Inhibition of the mTORC1 pathway suppresses intestinal polyp formation and reduces mortality in ApcDelta716 mice. Proc Natl Acad Sci U S A 105:13544–13549

Galceran J, Sustmann C, Hsu SC, Folberth S, Grosschedl R (2004) LEF1-mediated regulation of Delta-like1 links Wnt and Notch signaling in somitogenesis. Genes Dev 18:2718–2723

Gazitt Y, Kolaparthi V, Moncada K, Thomas C, Freeman J (2009) Targeted therapy of human osteosarcoma with 17AAG or rapamycin: characterization of induced apoptosis and inhibition of mTOR and Akt/MAPK/Wnt pathways. Int J Oncol 34:551–561

Goodsell DS (1999) The molecular perspective: the ras oncogene. Stem Cells 17:235–236

Gordon WR, Arnett KL, Blacklow SC (2008) The molecular logic of Notch signaling – a structural and biochemical perspective. J Cell Sci 121:3109–3119

Goss KH, Groden J (2000) Biology of the adenomatous polyposis coli tumor suppressor. J Clin Oncol 18:1967–1979

Guilmeau S, Flandez M, Mariadason JM, Augenlicht LH (2010) Heterogeneity of Jagged1 expression in human and mouse intestinal tumors: implications for targeting Notch signaling. Oncogene 29:992–1002

Han G, Li AG, Liang YY, Owens P, He W, Lu S, Yoshimatsu Y et al (2006) Smad7-induced beta-catenin degradation alters epidermal appendage development. Dev Cell 11:301–312

Hancock JF (2003) Ras proteins: different signals from different locations. Nat Rev Mol Cell Biol 4:373–384

Harada N, Oshima H, Katoh M, Tamai Y, Oshima M, Taketo MM (2004) Hepatocarcinogenesis in mice with beta-catenin and Ha-ras gene mutations. Cancer Res 64:48–54

Hayward P, Brennan K, Sanders P, Balayo T, DasGupta R, Perrimon N, Martinez Arias A (2005) Notch modulates Wnt signalling by associating with Armadillo/beta-catenin and regulating its transcriptional activity. Development 132:1819–1830

He J, Sheng T, Stelter AA, Li C, Zhang X, Sinha M, Luxon BA et al (2006) Suppressing Wnt signaling by the hedgehog pathway through sFRP-1. J Biol Chem 281:35598–35602

Hooper JE, Scott MP (2005) Communicating with Hedgehogs. Nat Rev Mol Cell Biol 6:306–317

Hoppler S, Moon RT (1998) BMP-2/-4 and Wnt-8 cooperatively pattern the Xenopus mesoderm. Mech Dev 71:119–129

Howe LR, Crawford HC, Subbaramaiah K, Hassell JA, Dannenberg AJ, Brown AM (2001) PEA3 is up-regulated in response to Wnt1 and activates the expression of cyclooxygenase-2. J Biol Chem 276:20108–20115

Humar B, McNoe L, Dunbier A, Heathcott R, Braithwaite AW, Reeve AE (2008) Heterogeneous gene expression changes in colorectal cancer cells share the WNT pathway in response to growth suppression by APHS-mediated COX-2 inhibition. Biologics 2:329–337

Ingham PW, McMahon AP (2001) Hedgehog signaling in animal development: paradigms and principles. Genes Dev 15:3059–3087

Inoki K, Ouyang H, Zhu T, Lindvall C, Wang Y, Zhang X, Yang Q et al (2006) TSC2 integrates Wnt and energy signals via a coordinated phosphorylation by AMPK and GSK3 to regulate cell growth. Cell 126:955–968

Itadani H, Oshima H, Oshima M, Kotani H (2009) Mouse gastric tumor models with prostaglandin E2 pathway activation show similar gene expression profiles to intestinal-type human gastric cancer. BMC Genomics 10:615

Jang JW, Boxer RB, Chodosh LA (2006) Isoform-specific ras activation and oncogene dependence during MYC- and Wnt-induced mammary tumorigenesis. Mol Cell Biol 26:8109–8121

Janssen KP, Alberici P, Fsihi H, Gaspar C, Breukel C, Franken P, Rosty C et al (2006) APC and oncogenic KRAS are synergistic in enhancing Wnt signaling in intestinal tumor formation and progression. Gastroenterology 131:1096–1109

Ji H, Wang J, Nika H, Hawke D, Keezer S, Ge Q, Fang B et al (2009) EGF-induced ERK activation promotes CK2-mediated disassociation of alpha-catenin from beta-catenin and transactivation of beta-catenin. Mol Cell 36:547–559

Jozwiak J, Kotulska K, Grajkowska W, Jozwiak S, Zalewski W, Oldak M, Lojek M et al (2007) Upregulation of the WNT pathway in tuberous sclerosis-associated subependymal giant cell astrocytomas. Brain Dev 29:273–280

Kaler P, Godasi BN, Augenlicht L, Klampfer L (2009) The NF-kappaB/AKT-dependent Induction of Wnt signaling in colon cancer cells by macrophages and IL-1beta. Cancer Microenviron 2:69–80

Kanai Y, Ochiai A, Shibata T, Oyama T, Ushijima S, Akimoto S, Hirohashi S (1995) c-erbB-2 gene product directly associates with beta-catenin and plakoglobin. Biochem Biophys Res Commun 208:1067–1072

Kastritis E, Murray S, Kyriakou F, Horti M, Tamvakis N, Kavantzas N, Patsouris ES et al (2009) Somatic mutations of adenomatous polyposis coli gene and nuclear b-catenin accumulation have prognostic significance in invasive urothelial carcinomas: evidence for Wnt pathway implication. Int J Cancer 124:103–108

Katoh M, Katoh M (2006a) Cross-talk of WNT and FGF signaling pathways at GSK3beta to regulate beta-catenin and SNAIL signaling cascades. Cancer Biol Ther 5:1059–1064

Katoh M, Katoh M (2006b) Notch ligand, JAG1, is evolutionarily conserved target of canonical WNT signaling pathway in progenitor cells. Int J Mol Med 17:681–685

Katoh M, Katoh M (2009a) Transcriptional regulation of WNT2B based on the balance of Hedgehog, Notch, BMP and WNT signals. Int J Oncol 34:1411–1415

Katoh M, Katoh M (2009b) Transcriptional mechanisms of WNT5A based on NF-kappaB, Hedgehog, TGFbeta, and Notch signaling cascades. Int J Mol Med 23:763–769

Kawasaki T, Nosho K, Ohnishi M, Suemoto Y, Kirkner GJ, Dehari R, Meyerhardt JA et al (2007) Correlation of beta-catenin localization with cyclooxygenase-2 expression and CpG island methylator phenotype (CIMP) in colorectal cancer. Neoplasia 9:569–577

Kenerson HL, Aicher LD, True LD, Yeung RS (2002) Activated mammalian target of rapamycin pathway in the pathogenesis of tuberous sclerosis complex renal tumors. Cancer Res 62:5645–5650

Kiely B, O'Donovan RT, McKenna SL, O'Sullivan GC (2007) Beta-catenin transcriptional activity is inhibited downstream of nuclear localisation and is not influenced by IGF signalling in oesophageal cancer cells. Int J Cancer 121:1903–1909

Kim BM, Choi MY (2009) New insights into the role of Hedgehog signaling in gastrointestinal development and cancer. Gastroenterology 137:422–424

Kim JS, Crooks H, Dracheva T, Nishanian TG, Singh B, Jen J, Waldman T (2002) Oncogenic beta-catenin is required for bone morphogenetic protein 4 expression in human cancer cells. Cancer Res 62:2744–2748

Kim SE, Yoon JY, Jeong WJ, Jeon SH, Park Y, Yoon JB, Park YN et al (2009) H-Ras is degraded by Wnt/beta-catenin signaling via beta-TrCP-mediated polyubiquitylation. J Cell Sci 122:842–848

Kim JH, Shin HS, Lee SH, Lee I, Lee YS, Park JC, Kim YJ et al (2010) Contrasting activity of Hedgehog and Wnt pathways according to gastric cancer cell differentiation: relevance of crosstalk mechanisms. Cancer Sci 101:328–335

Kobune M, Chiba H, Kato J, Kato K, Nakamura K, Kawano Y, Takada K et al (2007) Wnt3/RhoA/ROCK signaling pathway is involved in adhesion-mediated drug resistance of multiple myeloma in an autocrine mechanism. Mol Cancer Ther 6:1774–1784

Koh TJ, Bulitta CJ, Fleming JV, Dockray GJ, Varro A, Wang TC (2000) Gastrin is a target of the beta-catenin/TCF-4 growth-signaling pathway in a model of intestinal polyposis. J Clin Invest 106:533–539

Kopan R, Ilagan MX (2009) The canonical Notch signaling pathway: unfolding the activation mechanism. Cell 137:216–233

Labbe E, Letamendia A, Attisano L (2000) Association of Smads with lymphoid enhancer binding factor 1/T cell-specific factor mediates cooperative signaling by the transforming growth factor-beta and wnt pathways. Proc Natl Acad Sci U S A 97:8358–8363

Labbe E, Lock L, Letamendia A, Gorska AE, Gryfe R, Gallinger S, Moses HL et al (2007) Transcriptional cooperation between the transforming growth factor-beta and Wnt pathways in mammary and intestinal tumorigenesis. Cancer Res 67:75–84

Lague MN, Paquet M, Fan HY, Kaartinen MJ, Chu S, Jamin SP, Behringer RR et al (2008) Synergistic effects of Pten loss and WNT/CTNNB1 signaling pathway activation in ovarian granulosa cell tumor development and progression. Carcinogenesis 29:2062–2072

Lee FS, Lane TF, Kuo A, Shackleford GM, Leder P (1995) Insertional mutagenesis identifies a member of the Wnt gene family as a candidate oncogene in the mammary epithelium of int-2/Fgf-3 transgenic mice. Proc Natl Acad Sci U S A 92:2268–2272

Leevers SJ, Vanhaesebroeck B, Waterfield MD (1999) Signalling through phosphoinositide 3-kinases: the lipids take centre stage. Curr Opin Cell Biol 11:219–225

Lei S, Dubeykovskiy A, Chakladar A, Wojtukiewicz L, Wang TC (2004) The murine gastrin promoter is synergistically activated by transforming growth factor-beta/Smad and Wnt signaling pathways. J Biol Chem 279:42492–42502

Lemjabbar-Alaoui H, Dasari V, Sidhu SS, Mengistab A, Finkbeiner W, Gallup M, Basbaum C (2006) Wnt and Hedgehog are critical mediators of cigarette smoke-induced lung cancer. PLoS One 1:e93

Li Y, Podsypanina K, Liu X, Crane A, Tan LK, Parsons R, Varmus HE (2001) Deficiency of Pten accelerates mammary oncogenesis in MMTV-Wnt-1 transgenic mice. BMC Mol Biol 2:2

Li J, Mizukami Y, Zhang X, Jo WS, Chung DC (2005) Oncogenic K-ras stimulates Wnt signaling in colon cancer through inhibition of GSK-3beta. Gastroenterology 128:1907–1918

Li X, Deng W, Lobo-Ruppert SM, Ruppert JM (2007) Gli1 acts through Snail and E-cadherin to promote nuclear signaling by beta-catenin. Oncogene 26:4489–4498

Li Y, Zhang X, Polakiewicz RD, Yao TP, Comb MJ (2008a) HDAC6 is required for epidermal growth factor-induced beta-catenin nuclear localization. J Biol Chem 283:12686–12690

Li X, Placencio V, Iturregui JM, Uwamariya C, Sharif-Afshar AR, Koyama T, Hayward SW et al (2008b) Prostate tumor progression is mediated by a paracrine TGF-beta/Wnt3a signaling axis. Oncogene 27:7118–7130

Liao X, Siu MK, Au CW, Chan QK, Chan HY, Wong ES, Ip PP et al (2009) Aberrant activation of hedgehog signaling pathway contributes to endometrial carcinogenesis through beta-catenin. Mod Pathol 22:839–847

Lim K, Han C, Xu L, Isse K, Demetris AJ, Wu T (2008) Cyclooxygenase-2-derived prostaglandin E2 activates beta-catenin in human cholangiocarcinoma cells: evidence for inhibition of these signaling pathways by omega 3 polyunsaturated fatty acids. Cancer Res 68:553–560

Lim K, Han C, Dai Y, Shen M, Wu T (2009) Omega-3 polyunsaturated fatty acids inhibit hepatocellular carcinoma cell growth through blocking beta-catenin and cyclooxygenase-2. Mol Cancer Ther 8:3046–3055

Liu Y, Borchert GL, Surazynski A, Phang JM (2008) Proline oxidase, a p53-induced gene, targets COX-2/PGE2 signaling to induce apoptosis and inhibit tumor growth in colorectal cancers. Oncogene 27:6729–6737

Liu J, Ahiekpor A, Li L, Li X, Arbuthnot P, Kew M, Feitelson MA (2009) Increased expression of ErbB-2 in liver is associated with hepatitis B x antigen and shorter survival in patients with liver cancer. Int J Cancer 125:1894–1901

Llovet JM, Ricci S, Mazzaferro V, Hilgard P, Gane E, Blanc JF, de Oliveira AC et al (2008) Sorafenib in advanced hepatocellular carcinoma. N Engl J Med 359:378–390

Longato L, de la Monte S, Kuzushita N, Horimoto M, Rogers AB, Slagle BL, Wands JR (2009) Overexpression of insulin receptor substrate-1 and hepatitis Bx genes causes premalignant alterations in the liver. Hepatology 49:1935–1943

Lopez-Terrada D, Gunaratne PH, Adesina AM, Pulliam J, Hoang DM, Nguyen Y, Mistretta TA et al (2009) Histologic subtypes of hepatoblastoma are characterized by differential canonical Wnt and Notch pathway activation in DLK+ precursors. Hum Pathol 40:783–794

Lu Z, Ghosh S, Wang Z, Hunter T (2003) Downregulation of caveolin-1 function by EGF leads to the loss of E-cadherin, increased transcriptional activity of beta-catenin, and enhanced tumor cell invasion. Cancer Cell 4:499–515

Lu W, Tinsley HN, Keeton A, Qu Z, Piazza GA, Li Y (2009) Suppression of Wnt/beta-catenin signaling inhibits prostate cancer cell proliferation. Eur J Pharmacol 602:8–14

Lum L, Beachy PA (2004) The Hedgehog response network: sensors, switches, and routers. Science 304:1755–1759

Luo F, Brooks DG, Ye H, Hamoudi R, Poulogiannis G, Patek CE, Winton DJ et al (2009) Mutated K-ras(Asp12) promotes tumourigenesis in Apc(Min) mice more in the large than the small intestines, with synergistic effects between K-ras and Wnt pathways. Int J Exp Pathol 90:558–574

MacArthur CA, Shankar DB, Shackleford GM (1995) Fgf-8, activated by proviral insertion, cooperates with the Wnt-1 transgene in murine mammary tumorigenesis. J Virol 69:2501–2507

Maeda O, Kondo M, Fujita T, Usami N, Fukui T, Shimokata K, Ando T et al (2006) Enhancement of GLI1-transcriptional activity by beta-catenin in human cancer cells. Oncol Rep 16:91–96

Mak BC, Takemaru K, Kenerson HL, Moon RT, Yeung RS (2003) The tuberin-hamartin complex negatively regulates beta-catenin signaling activity. J Biol Chem 278:5947–5951

Mak BC, Kenerson HL, Aicher LD, Barnes EA, Yeung RS (2005) Aberrant beta-catenin signaling in tuberous sclerosis. Am J Pathol 167:107–116

Marsh V, Winton DJ, Williams GT, Dubois N, Trumpp A, Sansom OJ, Clarke AR (2008) Epithelial Pten is dispensable for intestinal homeostasis but suppresses adenoma development and progression after Apc mutation. Nat Genet 40:1436–1444

Maupas-Schwalm F, Robinet C, Auge N, Thiers JC, Garcia V, Cambus JP, Salvayre R et al (2005) Activation of the {beta}-catenin/T-cell-specific transcription factor/lymphoid enhancer factor-1 pathway by plasminogen activators in ECV304 carcinoma cells. Cancer Res 65: 526–532

McMahon AP, Ingham PW, Tabin CJ (2003) Developmental roles and clinical significance of hedgehog signaling. Curr Top Dev Biol 53:1–114

Miele L (2006) Notch signaling. Clin Cancer Res 12:1074–1079

Monga SP, Mars WM, Pediaditakis P, Bell A, Mule K, Bowen WC, Wang X et al (2002) Hepatocyte growth factor induces Wnt-independent nuclear translocation of beta-catenin after Met-beta-catenin dissociation in hepatocytes. Cancer Res 62:2064–2071

Moreno CS (2010) The sex-determining region Y-Box 4 and homeobox C6 transcriptional networks in prostate cancer progression. Crosstalk with the Wnt, Notch, and PI3K pathways. Am J Pathol 176:518–527

Mulholland DJ, Dedhar S, Wu H, Nelson CC (2006) PTEN and GSK3beta: key regulators of progression to androgen-independent prostate cancer. Oncogene 25:329–337

Munoz NM, Upton M, Rojas A, Washington MK, Lin L, Chytil A, Sozmen EG et al (2006) Transforming growth factor beta receptor type II inactivation induces the malignant transformation of intestinal neoplasms initiated by Apc mutation. Cancer Res 66:9837–9844

Naik S, Dothager RS, Marasa J, Lewis CL, Piwnica-Worms D (2009) Vascular endothelial growth factor receptor-1 is synthetic lethal to aberrant {beta}-catenin activation in colon cancer. Clin Cancer Res 15:7529–7537

Nakamura T, Tsuchiya K, Watanabe M (2007) Crosstalk between Wnt and Notch signaling in intestinal epithelial cell fate decision. J Gastroenterol 42:705–710

Nakopoulou L, Gakiopoulou H, Keramopoulos A, Giannopoulou I, Athanassiadou P, Mavrommatis J, Davaris PS (2000) c-met tyrosine kinase receptor expression is associated with abnormal beta-catenin expression and favourable prognostic factors in invasive breast carcinoma. Histopathology 36:313–325

Ng SS, Mahmoudi T, Danenberg E, Bejaoui I, de Lau W, Korswagen HC, Schutte M et al (2009) Phosphatidylinositol 3-kinase signaling does not activate the wnt cascade. J Biol Chem 284:35308–35313

Nicholes K, Guillet S, Tomlinson E, Hillan K, Wright B, Frantz GD, Pham TA et al (2002) A mouse model of hepatocellular carcinoma: ectopic expression of fibroblast growth factor 19 in skeletal muscle of transgenic mice. Am J Pathol 160:2295–2307

Nicolas M, Wolfer A, Raj K, Kummer JA, Mill P, van Noort M, Hui CC et al (2003) Notch1 functions as a tumor suppressor in mouse skin. Nat Genet 33:416–421

Nishanian TG, Kim JS, Foxworth A, Waldman T (2004) Suppression of tumorigenesis and activation of Wnt signaling by bone morphogenetic protein 4 in human cancer cells. Cancer Biol Ther 3:667–675

Nishita M, Hashimoto MK, Ogata S, Laurent MN, Ueno N, Shibuya H, Cho KW (2000) Interaction between Wnt and TGF-beta signalling pathways during formation of Spemann's organizer. Nature 403:781–785

Noubissi FK, Goswami S, Sanek NA, Kawakami K, Minamoto T, Moser A, Grinblat Y et al (2009) Wnt signaling stimulates transcriptional outcome of the Hedgehog pathway by stabilizing GLI1 mRNA. Cancer Res 69:8572–8578

Ochiai A, Akimoto S, Kanai Y, Shibata T, Oyama T, Hirohashi S (1994) c-erbB-2 gene product associates with catenins in human cancer cells. Biochem Biophys Res Commun 205:73–78

Oguma K, Oshima H, Aoki M, Uchio R, Naka K, Nakamura S, Hirao A et al (2008) Activated macrophages promote Wnt signalling through tumour necrosis factor-alpha in gastric tumour cells. Embo J 27:1671–1681

Ohigashi T, Mizuno R, Nakashima J, Marumo K, Murai M (2005) Inhibition of Wnt signaling downregulates Akt activity and induces chemosensitivity in PTEN-mutated prostate cancer cells. Prostate 62:61–68

Oloumi A, Syam S, Dedhar S (2006) Modulation of Wnt3a-mediated nuclear beta-catenin accumulation and activation by integrin-linked kinase in mammalian cells. Oncogene 25:7747–7757

Ornitz DM, Itoh N (2001) Fibroblast growth factors. Genome Biol 2:Reviews3005

Oshima H, Matsunaga A, Fujimura T, Tsukamoto T, Taketo MM, Oshima M (2006) Carcinogenesis in mouse stomach by simultaneous activation of the Wnt signaling and prostaglandin E2 pathway. Gastroenterology 131:1086–1095

Oshima H, Oguma K, Du YC, Oshima M (2009) Prostaglandin E2, Wnt, and BMP in gastric tumor mouse models. Cancer Sci 100:1779–1785

Ougolkov A, Mai M, Takahashi Y, Omote K, Bilim V, Shimizu A, Minamoto T (2000) Altered expression of beta-catenin and c-erbB-2 in early gastric cancer. J Exp Clin Cancer Res 19:349–355

Pai R, Dunlap D, Qing J, Mohtashemi I, Hotzel K, French DM (2008) Inhibition of fibroblast growth factor 19 reduces tumor growth by modulating beta-catenin signaling. Cancer Res 68:5086–5095

Pannequin J, Bonnans C, Delaunay N, Ryan J, Bourgaux JF, Joubert D, Hollande F (2009) The wnt target jagged-1 mediates the activation of notch signaling by progastrin in human colorectal cancer cells. Cancer Res 69:6065–6073

Pasca di Magliano M, Hebrok M (2003) Hedgehog signalling in cancer formation and maintenance. Nat Rev Cancer 3:903–911

Pasca di Magliano M, Biankin AV, Heiser PW, Cano DA, Gutierrez PJ, Deramaudt T, Segara D et al (2007) Common activation of canonical Wnt signaling in pancreatic adenocarcinoma. PLoS One 2:e1155

Patel R, Ingle A, Maru GB (2008) Polymeric black tea polyphenols inhibit 1, 2-dimethylhydrazine induced colorectal carcinogenesis by inhibiting cell proliferation via Wnt/beta-catenin pathway. Toxicol Appl Pharmacol 227:136–146

Patil MA, Lee SA, Macias E, Lam ET, Xu C, Jones KD, Ho C et al (2009) Role of cyclin D1 as a mediator of c-Met- and beta-catenin-induced hepatocarcinogenesis. Cancer Res 69:253–261

Pearson HB, Phesse TJ, Clarke AR (2009) K-ras and Wnt signaling synergize to accelerate prostate tumorigenesis in the mouse. Cancer Res 69:94–101

Persad S, Troussard AA, McPhee TR, Mulholland DJ, Dedhar S (2001) Tumor suppressor PTEN inhibits nuclear accumulation of beta-catenin and T cell/lymphoid enhancer factor 1-mediated transcriptional activation. J Cell Biol 153:1161–1174

Proweller A, Tu L, Lepore JJ, Cheng L, Lu MM, Seykora J, Millar SE et al (2006) Impaired notch signaling promotes de novo squamous cell carcinoma formation. Cancer Res 66:7438–7444

Ramocki NM, Wilkins HR, Magness ST, Simmons JG, Scull BP, Lee GH, McNaughton KK et al (2008) Insulin receptor substrate-1 deficiency promotes apoptosis in the putative intestinal crypt stem cell region, limits Apcmin/+ tumors, and regulates Sox9. Endocrinology 149:261–267

Rasola A, Fassetta M, De Bacco F, D'Alessandro L, Gramaglia D, Di Renzo MF, Comoglio PM (2007) A positive feedback loop between hepatocyte growth factor receptor and beta-catenin sustains colorectal cancer cell invasive growth. Oncogene 26:1078–1087

Revet I, Huizenga G, Koster J, Volckmann R, van Sluis P, Versteeg R, Geerts D (2010) MSX1 induces the Wnt pathway antagonist genes DKK1, DKK2, DKK3, and SFRP1 in neuroblastoma cells, but does not block Wnt3 and Wnt5A signalling to DVL3. Cancer Lett 289:195–207

Roarty K, Baxley SE, Crowley MR, Frost AR, Serra R (2009) Loss of TGF-beta or Wnt5a results in an increase in Wnt/beta-catenin activity and redirects mammary tumour phenotype. Breast Cancer Res 11:R19

Rodilla V, Villanueva A, Obrador-Hevia A, Robert-Moreno A, Fernandez-Majada V, Grilli A, Lopez-Bigas N et al (2009) Jagged1 is the pathological link between Wnt and Notch pathways in colorectal cancer. Proc Natl Acad Sci U S A 106:6315–6320

Rodriguez-Esteban C, Capdevila J, Kawakami Y, Izpisua Belmonte JC (2001) Wnt signaling and PKA control Nodal expression and left-right determination in the chick embryo. Development 128:3189–3195

Romero D, Iglesias M, Vary CP, Quintanilla M (2008) Functional blockade of Smad4 leads to a decrease in beta-catenin levels and signaling activity in human pancreatic carcinoma cells. Carcinogenesis 29:1070–1076

Rubin LL, de Sauvage FJ (2006) Targeting the Hedgehog pathway in cancer. Nat Rev Drug Discov 5:1026–1033

Sakoguchi-Okada N, Takahashi-Yanaga F, Fukada K, Shiraishi F, Taba Y, Miwa Y, Morimoto S et al (2007) Celecoxib inhibits the expression of survivin via the suppression of promoter activity in human colon cancer cells. Biochem Pharmacol 73:1318–1329

Saldanha G, Ghura V, Potter L, Fletcher A (2004) Nuclear beta-catenin in basal cell carcinoma correlates with increased proliferation. Br J Dermatol 151:157–164

Salto-Tellez M, Peh BK, Ito K, Tan SH, Chong PY, Han HC, Tada K et al (2006) RUNX3 protein is overexpressed in human basal cell carcinomas. Oncogene 25:7646–7649

Sansom OJ, Meniel V, Wilkins JA, Cole AM, Oien KA, Marsh V, Jamieson TJ et al (2006) Loss of Apc allows phenotypic manifestation of the transforming properties of an endogenous K-ras oncogene in vivo. Proc Natl Acad Sci U S A 103:14122–14127

Satyamoorthy K, Li G, Vaidya B, Patel D, Herlyn M (2001) Insulin-like growth factor-1 induces survival and growth of biologically early melanoma cells through both the mitogen-activated protein kinase and beta-catenin pathways. Cancer Res 61:7318–7324

Sawyer EJ, Hanby AM, Poulsom R, Jeffery R, Gillett CE, Ellis IO, Ellis P et al (2003) Beta-catenin abnormalities and associated insulin-like growth factor overexpression are important in phyllodes tumours and fibroadenomas of the breast. J Pathol 200:627–632

Schambony A, Kunz M, Gradl D (2004) Cross-regulation of Wnt signaling and cell adhesion. Differentiation 72:307–318

Schlange T, Matsuda Y, Lienhard S, Huber A, Hynes NE (2007) Autocrine WNT signaling contributes to breast cancer cell proliferation via the canonical WNT pathway and EGFR transactivation. Breast Cancer Res 9:R63

Sekiya T, Adachi S, Kohu K, Yamada T, Higuchi O, Furukawa Y, Nakamura Y et al (2004) Identification of BMP and activin membrane-bound inhibitor (BAMBI), an inhibitor of transforming growth factor-beta signaling, as a target of the beta-catenin pathway in colorectal tumor cells. J Biol Chem 279:6840–6846

Sengupta A, Banerjee D, Chandra S, Banerji SK, Ghosh R, Roy R, Banerjee S (2007) Deregulation and cross talk among Sonic hedgehog, Wnt, Hox and Notch signaling in chronic myeloid leukemia progression. Leukemia 21:949–955

Senthivinayagam S, Mishra P, Paramasivam SK, Yallapragada S, Chatterjee M, Wong L, Rana A et al (2009) Caspase-mediated cleavage of beta-catenin precedes drug-induced apoptosis in resistant cancer cells. J Biol Chem 284:13577–13588

Shackleford GM, MacArthur CA, Kwan HC, Varmus HE (1993) Mouse mammary tumor virus infection accelerates mammary carcinogenesis in Wnt-1 transgenic mice by insertional activation of int-2/Fgf-3 and hst/Fgf-4. Proc Natl Acad Sci U S A 90:740–744

Shao J, Jung C, Liu C, Sheng H (2005) Prostaglandin E2 Stimulates the beta-catenin/T cell factor-dependent transcription in colon cancer. J Biol Chem 280:26565–26572

Sharma M, Chuang WW, Sun Z (2002) Phosphatidylinositol 3-kinase/Akt stimulates androgen pathway through GSK3beta inhibition and nuclear beta-catenin accumulation. J Biol Chem 277:30935–30941

Sharov AA, Mardaryev AN, Sharova TY, Grachtchouk M, Atoyan R, Byers HR, Seykora JT et al (2009) Bone morphogenetic protein antagonist noggin promotes skin tumorigenesis via stimulation of the Wnt and Shh signaling pathways. Am J Pathol 175:1303–1314

Shibamoto S, Hayakawa M, Takeuchi K, Hori T, Oku N, Miyazawa K, Kitamura N et al (1994) Tyrosine phosphorylation of beta-catenin and plakoglobin enhanced by hepatocyte growth factor and epidermal growth factor in human carcinoma cells. Cell Adhes Commun 1:295–305

Shimokawa T, Furukawa Y, Sakai M, Li M, Miwa N, Lin YM, Nakamura Y (2003) Involvement of the FGF18 gene in colorectal carcinogenesis, as a novel downstream target of the beta-catenin/T-cell factor complex. Cancer Res 63:6116–6120

Shomori K, Ochiai A, Akimoto S, Ino Y, Shudo K, Ito H, Hirohashi S (2009) Tyrosine-phosphorylation of the 12th armadillo-repeat of beta-catenin is associated with cadherin dysfunction in human cancer. Int J Oncol 35:517–524

Signoroni S, Frattini M, Negri T, Pastore E, Tamborini E, Casieri P, Orsenigo M et al (2007) Cyclooxygenase-2 and platelet-derived growth factor receptors as potential targets in treating aggressive fibromatosis. Clin Cancer Res 13:5034–5040

Sodir NM, Chen X, Park R, Nickel AE, Conti PS, Moats R, Bading JR et al (2006) Smad3 deficiency promotes tumorigenesis in the distal colon of ApcMin/+ mice. Cancer Res 66:8430–8438

Song S, Mazurek N, Liu C, Sun Y, Ding QQ, Liu K, Hung MC et al (2009) Galectin-3 mediates nuclear beta-catenin accumulation and Wnt signaling in human colon cancer cells by regulation of glycogen synthase kinase-3beta activity. Cancer Res 69:1343–1349

Suh Y, Afaq F, Johnson JJ, Mukhtar H (2009) A plant flavonoid fisetin induces apoptosis in colon cancer cells by inhibition of COX2 and Wnt/EGFR/NF-kappaB-signaling pathways. Carcinogenesis 30:300–307

Sun J, Jin T (2008) Both Wnt and mTOR signaling pathways are involved in insulin-stimulated proto-oncogene expression in intestinal cells. Cell Signal 20:219–229

Svirshchevskaya EV, Mariotti J, Wright MH, Viskova NY, Telford W, Fowler DH, Varticovski L (2008) Rapamycin delays growth of Wnt-1 tumors in spite of suppression of host immunity. BMC Cancer 8:176

Taipale J, Beachy PA (2001) The Hedgehog and Wnt signalling pathways in cancer. Nature 411:349–354

Takaku K, Oshima M, Miyoshi H, Matsui M, Seldin MF, Taketo MM (1998) Intestinal tumorigenesis in compound mutant mice of both Dpc4 (Smad4) and Apc genes. Cell 92:645–656

Takasu S, Tsukamoto T, Cao XY, Toyoda T, Hirata A, Ban H, Yamamoto M et al (2008) Roles of cyclooxygenase-2 and microsomal prostaglandin E synthase-1 expression and beta-catenin activation in gastric carcinogenesis in N-methyl-N-nitrosourea-treated K19-C2mE transgenic mice. Cancer Sci 99:2356–2364

Tan C, Costello P, Sanghera J, Dominguez D, Baulida J, de Herreros AG, Dedhar S (2001) Inhibition of integrin linked kinase (ILK) suppresses beta-catenin-Lef/Tcf-dependent transcription and expression of the E-cadherin repressor, snail, in APC-/- human colon carcinoma cells. Oncogene 20:133–140

Tan X, Apte U, Micsenyi A, Kotsagrelos E, Luo JH, Ranganathan S, Monga DK et al (2005) Epidermal growth factor receptor: a novel target of the Wnt/beta-catenin pathway in liver. Gastroenterology 129:285–302

Tang Y, Liu Z, Zhao L, Clemens TL, Cao X (2008) Smad7 stabilizes beta-catenin binding to E-cadherin complex and promotes cell-cell adhesion. J Biol Chem 283:23956–23963

Taylor MD, Zhang X, Liu L, Hui CC, Mainprize TG, Scherer SW, Wainwright B et al (2004) Failure of a medulloblastoma-derived mutant of SUFU to suppress WNT signaling. Oncogene 23:4577–4583

Teissedre B, Pinderhughes A, Incassati A, Hatsell SJ, Hiremath M, Cowin P (2009) MMTV-Wnt1 and -DeltaN89beta-catenin induce canonical signaling in distinct progenitors and differentially activate Hedgehog signaling within mammary tumors. PLoS One 4:e4537

Tselepis C, Perry I, Dawson C, Hardy R, Darnton SJ, McConkey C, Stuart RC et al (2002) Tumour necrosis factor-alpha in Barrett's oesophagus: a potential novel mechanism of action. Oncogene 21:6071–6081

Tuynman JB, Vermeulen L, Boon EM, Kemper K, Zwinderman AH, Peppelenbosch MP, Richel DJ (2008) Cyclooxygenase-2 inhibition inhibits c-Met kinase activity and Wnt activity in colon cancer. Cancer Res 68:1213–1220

Tward AD, Jones KD, Yant S, Cheung ST, Fan ST, Chen X, Kay MA et al (2007) Distinct pathways of genomic progression to benign and malignant tumors of the liver. Proc Natl Acad Sci U S A 104:14771–14776

van den Brink GR, Hardwick JC (2006) Hedgehog Wnteraction in colorectal cancer. Gut 55:912–914

van den Brink GR, Bleuming SA, Hardwick JC, Schepman BL, Offerhaus GJ, Keller JJ, Nielsen C et al (2004) Indian Hedgehog is an antagonist of Wnt signaling in colonic epithelial cell differentiation. Nat Genet 36:277–282

van Es JH, van Gijn ME, Riccio O, van den Born M, Vooijs M, Begthel H, Cozijnsen M et al (2005) Notch/gamma-secretase inhibition turns proliferative cells in intestinal crypts and adenomas into goblet cells. Nature 435:959–963

Varnat F, Zacchetti G, Ruiz IAA (2010) Hedgehog pathway activity is required for the lethality and intestinal phenotypes of mice with hyperactive Wnt signaling. Mech Dev 127:73–81

Verras M, Sun Z (2005) Beta-catenin is involved in insulin-like growth factor 1-mediated transactivation of the androgen receptor. Mol Endocrinol 19:391–398

Wang Y, Lam JB, Lam KS, Liu J, Lam MC, Hoo RL, Wu D et al (2006) Adiponectin modulates the glycogen synthase kinase-3beta/beta-catenin signaling pathway and attenuates mammary tumorigenesis of MDA-MB-231 cells in nude mice. Cancer Res 66:11462–11470

Wang K, Ma Q, Ren Y, He J, Zhang Y, Chen W (2007) Geldanamycin destabilizes HER2 tyrosine kinase and suppresses Wnt/beta-catenin signaling in HER2 overexpressing human breast cancer cells. Oncol Rep 17:89–96

Wang Z, Li Y, Banerjee S, Sarkar FH (2008) Exploitation of the Notch signaling pathway as a novel target for cancer therapy. Anticancer Res 28:3621–3630

Wang Z, Li Y, Banerjee S, Sarkar FH (2009) Emerging role of Notch in stem cells and cancer. Cancer Lett 279:8–12

Weerkamp F, van Dongen JJ, Staal FJ (2006) Notch and Wnt signaling in T-lymphocyte development and acute lymphoblastic leukemia. Leukemia 20:1197–1205

Willert J, Epping M, Pollack JR, Brown PO, Nusse R (2002) A transcriptional response to Wnt protein in human embryonic carcinoma cells. BMC Dev Biol 2:8

Yamazaki F, Aragane Y, Kawada A, Tezuka T (2001) Immunohistochemical detection for nuclear beta-catenin in sporadic basal cell carcinoma. Br J Dermatol 145:771–777

Yanai K, Nakamura M, Akiyoshi T, Nagai S, Wada J, Koga K, Noshiro H et al (2008) Crosstalk of hedgehog and Wnt pathways in gastric cancer. Cancer Lett 263:145–156

Yang F, Zeng Q, Yu G, Li S, Wang CY (2006) Wnt/beta-catenin signaling inhibits death receptor-mediated apoptosis and promotes invasive growth of HNSCC. Cell Signal 18:679–687

Yang SH, Andl T, Grachtchouk V, Wang A, Liu J, Syu LJ, Ferris J et al (2008) Pathological responses to oncogenic Hedgehog signaling in skin are dependent on canonical Wnt/beta3-catenin signaling. Nat Genet 40:1130–1135

Zardawi SJ, O'Toole SA, Sutherland RL, Musgrove EA (2009) Dysregulation of Hedgehog, Wnt and Notch signalling pathways in breast cancer. Histol Histopathol 24:385–398

Zeng G, Apte U, Micsenyi A, Bell A, Monga SP (2006) Tyrosine residues 654 and 670 in beta-catenin are crucial in regulation of Met-beta-catenin interactions. Exp Cell Res 312:3620–3630

Zhang X, Gaspard JP, Chung DC (2001) Regulation of vascular endothelial growth factor by the Wnt and K-ras pathways in colonic neoplasia. Cancer Res 61:6050–6054

Zhao H, Cui Y, Dupont J, Sun H, Hennighausen L, Yakar S (2005) Overexpression of the tumor suppressor gene phosphatase and tensin homologue partially inhibits wnt-1-induced mammary tumorigenesis. Cancer Res 65:6864–6873

Zhou BP, Hung MC (2005) Wnt, hedgehog and snail: sister pathways that control by GSK-3beta and beta-Trcp in the regulation of metastasis. Cell Cycle 4:772–776

Chapter 5
Dysregulation of the Wnt Pathway in Solid Tumors

Jenifer R. Prosperi, Hue H. Luu, and Kathleen H. Goss

Abstract Activation of the WNT signaling pathway has long been implicated in driving cancer pathogenesis from compelling evidence derived from complementary in vitro and animal studies. Moreover, there are extensive data supporting the nuclear localization of β-catenin, a surrogate marker frequently used as a read-out of WNT pathway activation, in addition to the overexpression of pathway activators and loss of pathway inhibitors in human cancers. Despite being most often linked with colorectal cancer, WNT pathway activation has now been associated with virtually every type of solid cancer that occurs in humans, although the frequency can vary dramatically among tumor subtypes and specific pathway components. These findings have significant implications regarding the mechanisms by which pathway activation might drive tumor development in specific tumor subtypes as well as the potential utility and impact of targeting this pathway therapeutically. In this chapter, we will summarize, both by tumor type and pathway components, the expansive evidence suggesting that the pathway is dysregulated in nearly half of all the most common types of human malignancies.

Abbreviations

APC	Adenomatous polyposis coli
BCC	Basal cell carcinoma
CNS	Central nervous system
CtBP	c-Terminal binding protein
DKK	Dickkopf
DVL	Disheveled
EBV	Epstein-Barr virus
ESCC	Esophageal squamous cell carcinoma
FAP	Familial adenomatous polyposis

K.H. Goss (✉)
Department of Surgery, University of Chicago, Chicago, IL 60637, USA
e-mail: kgoss@uchicago.edu

K.H. Goss and M. Kahn (eds.), *Targeting the Wnt Pathway in Cancer*,
DOI 10.1007/978-1-4419-8023-6_5, © Springer Science+Business Media, LLC 2011

FVPC	Follicular variant of papillary carcinoma
FZD	Frizzled
GSK3β	Glycogen synthase kinase 3 beta
HCC	Hepatocellular carcinomas
HNSCC	Head and neck squamous cell carcinoma
LEF-1	Leukemia enhancer-binding factor 1
L-FLAC	Low-grade adenocarcinoma of the fetal type
LOH	Loss of heterozygosity
LRP	Lipoprotein receptor-related protein
LTR	Long terminal repeat
MCR	Mutation cluster region
MMTV	Mouse mammary tumor virus
MSI	Microsatellite instability
NKD	Naked cuticle homolog
NSCLC	Non-small cell lung cancer
OEA	Ovarian endometrial adenocarcinoma
PanIN	Pancreatic intraepithelial neoplasia
PNET	Primitive neuroectodermal tumor
PSA	Prostate-specific antigen
PTC	Parathyroid carcinoma
SFRP	Secreted frizzled-related protein
TCF	T-cell factor
WDFA	Well-differentiated fetal adenocarcinoma
Wg	Wingless
WIF-1	WNT inhibitory factor 1
WT 1	Wilms' tumor 1

5.1 Introduction

The canonical WNT pathway is a signaling network that is conserved from flies to humans, and its activity is associated with numerous biological processes, including embryonic and tissue development, maintenance of the stem cell nice, the epithelial-to-mesenchymal transition, and tumorigenesis. The first hint that WNT signaling might be involved in the pathogenesis of cancer came in 1982 when Int-1 was identified as being an integration site of the mouse mammary tumor virus (MMTV), and subsequently found to be homologous to wingless (Wg) signaling peptide in *Drosophila* (Nusse and Varmus 1982). It was renamed as the first member of the WNT family of secreted proteins, WNT-1 (Nusse et al. 1991; Rijsewijk et al. 1987). The expression of both WNT-1 and WNT-3 is strongly induced by proviral insertion in mouse mammary tumors (Nusse and Varmus 1982; Roelink et al. 1990). Demonstrating that WNT-1 overexpression was causally involved in mammary tumorigenesis, Int-1/WNT-1 transgene expression driven by the MMTV long terminal repeat (LTR) was sufficient for metastatic mammary tumor development in mice (Li et al. 2000; Tsukamoto et al. 1988). Since then, numerous lines of evidence from rodent models and in vitro studies support the hypothesis that ectopic WNT pathway activation drives tumor pathogenesis in the mammary gland (reviewed recently in Prosperi and Goss 2010). While the precise role of WNT/β-catenin activity in human breast cancer is not completely understood, several components of the pathway are dysregulated, including the WNT ligands, receptors, antagonists, and downstream effectors.

Nearly 10 years after ectopic WNT expression was first linked to breast cancer, the *adenomatous polyposis coli* (*APC*) tumor suppressor gene, localized to human chromosome 5q, was identified as the gene mutated in the inherited colorectal cancer syndrome familial adenomatous polyposis (FAP) through linkage analysis of large affected families (Bodmer et al. 1987; Leppert et al. 1987) and conventional positional cloning strategies (Groden et al. 1991; Joslyn et al. 1991; Kinzler et al. 1991; Nishisho et al. 1991). FAP is a rare, autosomal dominant syndrome charac-terized by the development of hundreds to thousands of colorectal adenomas at a young age, some of which will progress to metastatic colorectal adenocarcinomas if not removed. Common extracolonic tumors associated with FAP include tumors of the duodenum, stomach, pancreas, thyroid, liver, and central nervous system (CNS), as well as osteomas and desmoid tumors. Like other tumor suppressors, *APC* mutation follows the classical "two-hit" model in that patients with FAP inherit one germline mutation and develop tumors from those cells in which a sec-ond hit, or loss of the wildtype allele of *APC*, is somatically acquired, and mutation location often dictates the FAP phenotype (reviewed in Goss and Groden 2000). Importantly, identifying *APC* as the gene responsible for FAP has also revealed a common mechanism for the development of sporadic colorectal cancer. *APC* mutations are the earliest known oncogenic events in colorectal cancer progression, as they have been identified in some aberrant crypt foci and frequently in both adenomas and adenocarcinomas (reviewed in Goss and Groden 2000).

A few years after APC was identified as the "gatekeeper" of colorectal cancer, its role as a potent negative regulator of canonical WNT signaling was unveiled and associated with cancer. Cancers may selectively enhance WNT signaling by upreg-ulating the activators or inactivating the inhibitors to potentiate cancer pathogenesis in the colon and other tissues to provide them with a growth advantage and ability to migrate and maintain stem cell properties. In this chapter, we will provide an overview of the evidence for aberrant WNT/β-catenin pathway activation in com-mon human solid tumors (Table 5.1). For clarity, we will categorize specific path-way alterations by whether they generally result in pathway activation through gain of function or through loss of function, despite the fact that it may be unclear what the actual outcome is (e.g., some WNTs can inhibit canonical signaling by activat-ing noncanonical pathways). Pathway dysregulation in individual tumor subtypes will be discussed separately when possible. By convention, we will designate the signaling components with capital letters since this chapter refers mostly to the human gene or protein, unless otherwise noted. Relevant to the data presented here, but beyond the scope of this review and covered in other chapters of the book, there is abundant evidence supporting the requirement for WNT/β-catenin signaling

Table 5.1 Summary of alterations of Wnt/β-catenin pathway components in solid tumors

Pathway component	Tumor type	Common alterations
Wnts		
WNT-1	Breast, lung, gastric, prostate, pancreatic, liver, skin, gynecological, pituitary	Increased expression
WNT-2	Colorectal, breast, lung, gastric, prostate, skin, CNS	Increased expression
	Skin, gynecological[a]	Decreased expression[a]
WNT-3	Liver	Increased expression
	Gynecological[a]	Decreased expression[a]
WNT-4	Liver, pituitary	Increased expression
	Gynecological[a]	Decreased expression[a]
WNT-5A	Colorectal, breast, lung, gastric, head/neck, prostate, liver, skin, CNS, musculoskeletal, gynecological, thyroid, pituitary	Increased expression
	Liver, skin, gynecological[a]	Decreased expression[a]
WNT-6	Prostate	Increased expression
WNT-7A	Lung, head/neck	Decreased expression
WNT-7B	Breast, bladder, skin	Increased expression
WNT-9B	Gynecological	Increased expression
WNT-10A	Gastric	Increased expression
WNT-10B	Breast, skin, CNS, musculoskeletal, gynecological, pituitary	Increased expression
WNT-13	CNS, musculoskeletal, pituitary	Increased expression
WNT-14	Head/neck	Increased expression
Secreted Wnt antagonists		
SFRP1	Colorectal, breast, lung, head/neck, prostate, pancreatic, liver, kidney, bladder, CNS, gynecological, esophageal	Decreased expression Promoter methylation
SFRP2	Colorectal, breast, head/neck, pancreatic, liver, kidney, bladder, CNS, gynecological, esophageal, pituitary	Decreased expression Promoter methylation
SFRP3/FRZB	Gastric, kidney, CNS	Decreased expression
SFRP4	Colorectal, breast, lung, head/neck, pancreatic, kidney, bladder, CNS, gynecological, esophageal, pituitary	Decreased expression Promoter methylation
SFRP5	Colorectal, breast, lung, head/neck, pancreatic, liver, kidney, bladder, CNS, gynecological, esophageal	Decreased expression Promoter methylation
WIF-1	Colorectal, breast, lung, head/neck, prostate, pancreatic, liver, kidney, bladder, CNS, esophageal, pituitary	Decreased expression Promoter methylation
DKK-1	Colorectal, breast, gastric, skin, CNS, gynecological, esophageal	Decreased expression
	Lung, pancreatic, kidney[a]	Promoter methylation Increased expression[a]
DKK-2	Colorectal, gastric, kidney, skin	Decreased expression Promoter methylation
DKK-3	Colorectal, lung, gastric, prostate, liver, kidney, bladder, skin, CNS, gynecological	Decreased expression Promoter methylation

Table 5.1 (continued)

Pathway component	Tumor type	Common alterations
Wnt receptors/coreceptors		
FZD1	Colorectal, gynecological	Increased expression
FZD2	Colorectal, gastric, head/neck, pancreatic, CNS	Increased expression
FZD4	Colorectal	Increased expression
FZD5	Head/neck, kidney	Increased expression
FZD6	Colorectal, liver	Increased expression
FZD7	Gastric, liver	Increased expression
FZD8	Gastric, kidney	Increased expression
FZD9/3	Gastric, head/neck, liver	Increased expression
LRP5	Breast, musculoskeletal, parathyroid	Increased expression
		Alternative isoforms
LRP6	Breast	Increased expression
Pathway regulators		
DVL-1	Lung, head/neck, prostate, gynecological	Increased expression
DVL-3	Lung, CNS	Increased expression
Prickle-1	Liver	Decreased expression
CK2	Breast	Increased expression
FRAT1	CNS, gynecological,	Increased expression
β-TrCP	Esophageal	Decreased expression
Destruction complex components		
β-catenin	Colon, breast, lung, gastric, head/neck, prostate, pancreatic, liver, kidney, bladder, skin, CNS, musculoskeletal, gynecological, esophageal, adrenal, thyroid	Stabilizing mutation N/C accumulation
GSK3β	Gynecological	Increased expression
	Parathyroid[a]	Decreased expression[a]
APC	Colorectal, breast, lung, gastric, head/neck, prostate, pancreatic, liver, bladder, skin, CNS, musculoskeletal, gynecological, esophageal, adrenal, thyroid, parathyroid	Inactivating mutation Decreased expression Promoter methylation
AXIN1	Gastric, prostate, liver, CNS, gynecological, esophageal, thyroid	Inactivating mutation Decreased expression
AXIN2	Colorectal, lung, gastric, liver, skin, gynecological	Inactivating mutation Promoter methylation
TCF/LEF transcription factors		
LEF-1	Colorectal, pancreatic, liver, CNS	Increased expression
		Alternative isoforms
TCF-3	Skin	Increased expression
TCF-4	Colorectal, lung, gastric, prostate, liver, CNS, gynecological	Increased expression Mutation

Please see text for references and details

[a] Unusual or unexpected alterations in the corresponding tumor types

for tumor development using both cell culture and animal models. It is clear from the extensive pathway alterations found in most tumor types that the promise of therapeutic efficacy for WNT/β-catenin pathway inhibitors extends beyond colon cancer and may provide opportunities for drug development for cancers that have few options currently.

5.2 Colorectal Cancer

5.2.1 Upregulation of Pathway Activators

While the expression of most WNT ligands is not changed in colorectal cancers compared to normal colonic mucosa, WNT-2 and, to a lesser extent, WNT-5A are significantly upregulated in malignant tissue (Holcombe et al. 2002; Vider et al. 1996). Several frizzled (FZD) WNT receptors, including FZD1, FZD2, FZD4, and FZD6, are overexpressed in colorectal cancers, and in the case of FZD1 and FZD2, are upregulated at the invasive front of poorly differentiated, advanced colon cancers only (Gregorieff and Clevers 2005; Holcombe et al. 2002). Particularly in tumors that do not carry an *APC* mutation, β-catenin (the *CTNNB1* gene) is mutated in some sporadic colorectal cancers, most often in exon 3 that encodes the residues phosphorylated by glycogen synthase kinase 3 beta (GSK3β) (Liu et al. 2002). *CTNNB1* mutations have been observed in approximately 20% of colorectal tumors with high microsatellite instability (MSI), but only in 2% of MSI-low or -stable tumors (Fukushima et al. 2001). The β-catenin transcription factor partner leukemia enhancer-binding factor 1 (LEF-1) is overexpressed in a majority of sporadic colorectal cancers (Hovanes et al. 2001; Porfiri et al. 1997), and the related T-cell factor 4 (TCF-4) transcription factor (encoded by the *TCF7L2* gene) is mutated in as many as 39–44% of MSI-high but not in MSI-low or stable tumors (Duval et al. 1999; Fukushima et al. 2001). This activating frameshift mutation in *TCF7L2* is thought to facilitate resistance to transcriptional repression by c-terminal binding protein (CtBP) (Cuilliere-Dartigues et al. 2006).

5.2.2 Loss of Pathway Inhibitors

The secreted WNT antagonists that compete with FZD receptors for WNT binding including WNT inhibitory factor 1 (WIF-1), secreted frizzled-related protein 1 (SFRP1), SFRP2, SFRP4, and SFRP5 are silenced by CpG hypermethylation and downregulated in 40–82% of colorectal carcinomas compared to normal mucosa (Aguilera et al. 2006; Caldwell et al. 2004; Qi et al. 2007; Taniguchi et al. 2005). Like APC loss, some of these events occur early in colorectal cancer progression. SFRP1 hypermethylation is also detectable in most adenomas (Caldwell et al. 2006), and SFRP2 methylation is increased in stool samples from patients with hyperplastic polyps and adenomas (Oberwalder et al. 2008). The secreted dickkopf (DKK)-1, -2, and -3 proteins that inhibit WNT signaling through coreceptor binding are frequently silenced by CpG island hypermethylation in colorectal cancers (Aguilera et al. 2006; Sato et al. 2007; Yu et al. 2009), and DKK-1 expression is reduced specifically in advanced stage tumors (Aguilera et al. 2006). Interestingly, a recent study also reported that DKK-2 and-4 were upregulated in human colorectal cancers compared to adjacent normal tissues (Matsui et al. 2009). Loss of *APC* is by far the most common genetic alteration in sporadic colorectal cancer. The frequency of *APC* inactivation has been reported to be between 25–88% of sporadic colorectal adenomas and 31–83% of adenocarcinomas, depending on the specific study, type of alteration, and patient cohort (De Filippo et al. 2002; Diergaarde et al. 2003; Fukushima et al. 2001; Huang et al. 1996; Konishi et al. 1996; Luchtenborg et al. 2005; Miyaki et al. 1994; Miyoshi et al. 2002; Powell et al. 1992; Rowan et al. 2000; Tsai et al. 2002; Yashima et al. 1994; Yu and Wang 1998). The frequency of *APC* loss in sporadic adenomas is 59–78% (Lamlum et al. 2000; Miyaki et al. 1994; Powell et al. 1992; Takayama et al. 2001). More than 1,400 germline and somatic mutations in *APC* have been associated with FAP and sporadic colorectal cancer (reviewed in Goss and Groden 2000), and approximately 60% of reported somatic mutations occur in the mutation cluster region (MCR) in the middle of the coding region (Miyoshi et al. 1992). Interestingly, the "two hits" in *APC* in colorectal cancers are interdependent such that mutations within the MCR in sporadic and FAP tumors are typically associated with allelic loss as the "second hit," while mutations outside the region tend to have truncating mutations on the other allele (Lamlum et al. 1999; Rowan et al. 2000). *APC* inactivation can also be accomplished through epigenetic silencing of the promoter through hypermethylation. The *APC* gene promoter is hypermethylated in 18–45% of primary sporadic colorectal adenomas and carcinomas, although there is some debate whether this is dependent on the presence, number, or position of *APC* mutations and loss of heterozygosity (LOH) in sporadic or FAP colorectal cancers (Arnold et al. 2004; Esteller et al. 2000; Hiltunen et al. 1997; Lind et al. 2004; Segditsas et al. 2008). Some *APC* alleles, such as APCI1307K that is commonly found in the Ashkenazi Jewish population at an increased risk of colon cancer, are also associated with increased breast cancer risk within the same population (Redston et al. 1995). Like APC, the *AXIN2* tumor suppressor is inactivated by mutation in some colon cancers (Lammi et al. 2004; Liu et al. 2000) and is silenced by promoter methylation in others, for example in approximately 50% of MSI-positive tumors (Koinuma et al. 2006).

5.3 Breast Cancer

5.3.1 Upregulation of Pathway Activators

WNT-2, -4, -5A, -7B, and -10B are overexpressed in malignant breast tissue compared to normal breast (Bui et al. 1997a; Huguet et al. 1994; Iozzo et al. 1995; Lejeune et al. 1995; Watanabe et al. 2004), and the WNT coreceptor low-density lipoprotein receptor-related protein 6 (LRP6) is upregulated in some breast cancers (Lindvall et al. 2009). Further, an aberrantly spliced LRP5 isoform resistant to DKK-1 inhibition is expressed in human breast cancers, but not normal tissue (Bjorklund et al. 2009). Nuclear and cytosolic accumulation of β-catenin has been observed in as many as 60% of human breast cancers and is associated with poor prognosis (Khramtsov et al. 2010; Lin et al. 2000; Lopez-Knowles et al. 2010). Recently, our laboratory demonstrated that β-catenin cytoplasmic and nuclear accumulation is most frequently observed in triple-negative basal-like invasive breast cancers compared to other subtypes (Khramtsov et al. 2010), consistent with a recently identified WNT gene signature derived from a lung metastasis model that was strongly associated with basal-like breast cancers (DiMeo et al. 2009). Mutations in the amino-terminal domain of β-catenin have been also observed in triple-negative metaplastic carcinomas, some of which also had point mutations in *APC* (Hayes et al. 2008). Stabilizing mutations in *CTNNB1* are observed in almost 50% of cases of breast fibromatosis (Abraham et al. 2002b) and in 25% of metaplastic carcinomas (Hayes et al. 2008), but have not been detected in other types of invasive breast cancers (Kizildag et al. 2008; Ozaki et al. 2005; Sarrio et al. 2003; Ueda et al. 2001). Two other proteins that potentiate WNT/β-catenin signaling by affecting β-catenin stabilization, protein kinase CK2 and Pin1, are also overexpressed in human breast cancers and associated with β-catenin accumulation (Landesman-Bollag et al. 2001; Ryo et al. 2001). Phospho-β-catenin has been localized to both the cytosol and nuclei of breast cancer cells in situ, and these distinct pools were differentially associated with patient prognosis (Nakopoulou et al. 2006).

5.3.2 Loss of Pathway Inhibitors

WIF-1, *SFRP1*, *SFRP2*, *SFRP5*, and *DKK-1* are transcriptionally silenced through promoter methylation in 40–83% of human breast cancers (Ai et al. 2006; Suzuki et al. 2008; Veeck et al. 2008). Specifically, *SFRP1* and *SFRP5* hypermethylation are observed in 61–73% of primary breast cancers and associated with reduced overall survival (Veeck et al. 2006, 2008). SFRP1 is lost in more than 80% of invasive human breast tumors (Ugolini et al. 2001) and its inactivation in early-stage tumors is associated with poor prognosis (Klopocki et al. 2004). DKK-1 expression is lost from more than 70% of breast cancers (Forget et al. 2007). Despite the observations that *AXIN* sequence variants can be detected in breast cancer samples (Webster et al. 2000) and that chromosome 17q23-24, the locus encoding AXIN2, shows LOH in breast cancer (Mai et al. 1999), *AXIN1* and *AXIN2* do not appear to be commonly inactivated in this tumor type. Both epigenetic and genetic alterations in *APC* have also been identified in human breast cancer. In some breast cancer tissues with nuclear or cytosolic accumulation of β-catenin, *APC* mutations have been identified or decreased expression was observed (Abraham et al. 2002b; Jonsson et al. 2000; Ozaki et al. 2005).

Unlike colorectal cancer, most *APC* mutations that occur in sporadic human breast cancer have been identified outside of the MCR (Abraham et al. 2002b; Furuuchi et al. 2000; Ho et al. 1999; Kashiwaba et al. 1994; Wada et al. 1997). *APC* promoter methylation generally occurs more frequently than mutation and is observed in as many as 70% of human breast cancers (Dulaimi et al. 2004; Jin et al. 2001; Prasad et al. 2008; Sarrio et al. 2003; Van der Auwera et al. 2008; Virmani et al. 2001) and in some in situ cancers (Dulaimi et al. 2004). Although some studies have failed to find a correlation between *APC* status and clinical parameters (Jin et al. 2001; Kashiwaba et al. 1994), others have demonstrated that epigenetic silencing is associated with advanced tumor stage and size (Virmani et al. 2001), poor prognosis as well as disease-free and overall survival (Prasad et al. 2008). Interestingly, APC expression is frequently silenced in 50% of invasive lobular carcinomas, but β-catenin is not transcriptionally active in this subset of tumors (Sarrio et al. 2003). Promoter methylation is also observed in more than 70% of inflammatory breast cancer cases, a rare but especially aggressive form of breast cancer (Van der Auwera et al. 2008), thus suggesting that APC may be preferentially inactivated in distinct breast cancer subtypes.

5.4   Lung Cancer

5.4.1   Upregulation of Pathway Activators

In lung tumors, WNT-1 expression is associated with poor prognosis and high β-catenin levels (Huang et al. 2008). Non-small cell lung cancers (NSCLCs) frequently overexpress WNT-1 and WNT-2, in 40 and 88% of tumors, respectively (Nakashima et al. 2008; You et al. 2004), and patients with WNT-1 positive tumors demonstrate reduced survival (Nakashima et al. 2008). WNT-5A is overexpressed in lung cancer (Iozzo et al. 1995) and preferentially expressed in squamous cell carcinomas rather than adenocarcinomas and correlates with proliferative index (Huang et al. 2005). WNT-7A expression is decreased in 100% of NSCLCs compared to normal lung (Winn et al. 2005). Disheveled (DVL) and DVL-3 are also upregulated in more than half of NSCLCs (Uematsu et al. 2003a; Wei et al. 2008) and associated with poor tumor differentiation (Wei et al. 2008). Although only 4% of primary lung tumors carry mutations in exon 3 of β-catenin (Sunaga et al. 2001), loss of membrane β-catenin and/or cytoplasmic accumulation in lung cancer is associated with high tumor stage, large tumor size, and decreased survival (Kren et al. 2003). In contrast, other studies have found that high cytoplasmic and nuclear expression of β-catenin was a favorable prognostic factor in lung cancer, specifically in nonsquamous cell carcinomas (Hommura et al. 2002). In a specific subtype of lung cancer, low-grade adenocarcinoma of the fetal type (L-FLAC)/well-differentiated fetal adenocarcinoma (WDFA), 100% of cases studied demonstrated nuclear/cytoplasmic expression of β-catenin and some carried exon 3 mutations in *CTNNB1* (Nakatani et al. 2002). TCF-4 is highly expressed in 80% of lung cancers and is associated with advanced stage (Xu et al. 2007).

5.4.2   Loss of Pathway Inhibitors

Several WNT antagonists are hypermethylated in primary lung adenocarcinoma (Licchesi et al. 2008), including *SFRP1* which is methylated in 55% of *NSCLCs* (Fukui et al. 2005). WIF-1 protein expression is downregulated (Wissmann et al. 2003), and it is subjected to promoter methylation in 83% of lung cancers (Mazieres et al. 2004), particularly in NSCLC patients with malignant pleural effusions (Yang et al. 2009). DKK-1 is expressed in approximately 48% of lung tumors (Forget et al. 2007) and, although DKK-1 is downregulated in many tumor types, there is a significant increase in serum DKK-1 concentration that correlates with lung cancer progression and decreased survival (Sheng et al. 2009). DKK-3 mRNA expression is decreased in 63% of NSCLCs, specifically in adenocarcinomas and squamous cell carcinomas (Nozaki et al. 2001), and *DKK-3* methylation is predictive of poor outcome (Suzuki et al. 2007). Mutations within the MCR of *APC* are observed in only 4% of lung cancers (Ohgaki et al. 2004); yet, *APC* promoter methylation, detectable in patient serum or plasma, has been identified in more than 95% of primary lung cancers, including NSCLC, and associated with reduced survival (Brabender et al. 2001; Usadel et al. 2002). Silencing of *APC* by methylation is more common in lung primary adenocarcinomas than metastases, in contrast to *SFRP1* and *WIF-1* that are more frequently methylated in metastases (Tang et al. 2006). AXIN expression is negatively correlated with TCF-4 expression and is more frequently preserved in well-differentiated tumors (Xu et al. 2007), and an *AXIN2* single nucleotide polymorphism (Pro50Ser) is associated with lung cancer risk in a Japanese population (Kanzaki et al. 2006).

5.4.3   Mesothelioma

Using WNT-specific microarray analysis of malignant pleural mesothelioma tissues, multiple pathway components were found to be up- and downregulated, including frequent overexpression of WNT-2 (Mazieres et al. 2005). Nuclear and/ or cytoplasmic localization of β-catenin is observed in 78–100% early- and late-stage malignant mesotheliomas (Abutaily et al. 2003; Dai et al. 2005; Uematsu et al. 2003b), although no stabilizing mutations in *CTNNB1* have been detected (Abutaily et al. 2003; Uematsu et al. 2003b). DVL-3 is also upregulated in malignant mesotheliomas (Uematsu et al. 2003b). *SFRP1*, *SFRP4*, *SFRP5*, and *WIF-1* are methylated in greater than 80% of malignant pleural mesothelioma (Batra et al. 2006; Lee et al. 2004). Approximately one quarter of malignant mesotheliomas show loss of staining with a carboxy-terminal APC antibody compared to hyperplastic cases, but no change when using an animo-terminal antibody, thus supporting the presence of mutant APC rather than loss of expression (Abutaily et al. 2003).

5.5   Gastric Cancer

5.5.1   *Upregulation of Pathway Activators*

By expression profiling, the WNT/β-catenin pathway was activated in 46% of primary gastric cancers, and high activation was associated with worse overall survival (Ooi et al. 2009). Several WNT ligands are overexpressed frequently in gastric cancers, including WNT-1 (Zhang and Xue 2008), WNT-2 (Huang et al. 2006; Katoh 2001; Vider et al. 1996), WNT-5A (Kurayoshi et al. 2006; Saitoh et al. 2002a), WNT-8B (Saitoh et al. 2002b), and WNT-10A (Kirikoshi et al. 2001a, d). WNT-1 upregulation is significantly associated with several clinical parameters including 5-year survival, and WNT-5A expression correlates with advanced stage and poor prognosis (Kurayoshi et al. 2006). FZD7 is overexpressed in a wide range (17–75%) of gastric carcinomas (Kirikoshi et al. 2001c; To et al. 2001). FZD2 and -8 are upregulated in approximately 40% gastric cancers, while FZD9 is overexpressed in 20% of cases (Kirikoshi et al. 2001b). Nuclear accumulation of β-catenin has been observed in 17–87% of gastric adenocarcinomas (Chen et al. 2005; Clements et al. 2002; Grabsch et al. 2001; Kim et al. 2003, 2010; Nabais et al. 2003; To et al. 2001; Woo et al. 2001). Nuclear β-catenin localization in gastric cancers is associated with WNT-2 overexpression (Cheng et al. 2005; Han et al. 2007), and its overexpression is correlated with tumor size, stage, invasion, lymph node metastasis, and 5-year survival (Zhang and Xue 2008). Gastric cancers of the intestinal phenotype are particularly enriched in *CTNNB1* mutations and β-catenin nuclear accumulation (Ogasawara et al. 2006). TCF-4 overexpression, concomitant with nuclear β-catenin, is frequently observed in both primary gastric cancers and metastases (Chen et al. 2005).

5.5.2   *Loss of Pathway Inhibitors*

WIF-1, *SFRP1*, *SFRP2*, *SFRP3* (also known as *FRZB*), and *SFRP5* are hypermethylated and/or downregulated in 44–96% primary gastric cancer specimens (Byun et al. 2005; Dahl et al. 2007; Nojima et al. 2007; Taniguchi et al. 2005; To et al. 2001; Zhao et al. 2007, 2009). DKK antagonists are underexpressed in up to

84% of gastric cancers due to promoter hypermethylation (Sato et al. 2007; Yu et al. 2009) and associated with poor survival (Yu et al. 2009). *APC* mutations have been reported in up to 60% gastric cancer cases, particularly of the intestinal-type (Ebert et al. 2002; Horii et al. 1992; Lee et al. 2002). Loss of APC expression in tumors is associated with p21 status and more frequent in Epstein-Barr virus (EBV)-positive cancers (Kim et al. 2010). Mutations in at least one WNT pathway gene, including *AXIN1, AXIN2,* and *CTNNB1,* have been observed in 7% of gastric cancer cases (Pan et al. 2008).

5.6   Head and Neck Cancer

5.6.1   Upregulation of Pathway Activators

In head and neck squamous cell carcinoma (HNSCC), multiple components of the WNT/β-catenin signaling pathway, including FZD2, FZD3/9, DVL-1, and β-catenin, are highly expressed at the mRNA level (Leethanakul et al. 2000). Of all the WNTs, WNT-5A and WNT-14 are among the most highly expressed in malignant HNSCCs, while WNT-10B expression is observed exclusively in undifferentiated areas of the tumors (Baker et al. 2005; Diaz Prado et al. 2009). Interestingly, altered expressions of WNT-7A and FZD5 predict survival of HNSCC patients (Diaz Prado et al. 2009). Although no mutations in *CTNNB1* have been identified, alterations in β-catenin expression have been observed in HNSCC and are correlated with advance tumor stage (Goto et al. 2010; Lo Muzio et al. 2005). β-Catenin reduction or absence, particularly at the invasive front of tumors, is correlated with poor prognosis (Mahomed et al. 2007; Ueda et al. 2006). In fact, β-catenin accumulation in the cytosol and nuclei is observed in a majority of adenoid cystic carcinoma and polymorphous low-grade adenocarcinoma, subtypes of salivary gland cancer (Ferrazzo et al. 2009).

5.6.2   Loss of Pathway Inhibitors

SFRP1, SFRP2, SFRP4, and *SFRP5* promoter hypermethylation occurs in approximately one third (29–35%) of HNSCC cases and is correlated with several risk factors (e.g., smoking, drinking, and HPV infection), but is not associated with survival (Marsit et al. 2006). *SFRP1, SFRP2,* and *SFRP5* are also methylated in 16–36% of primary oral squamous cell carcinomas (Sogabe et al. 2008), and WIF-1 is downregulated in cell lines established from primary salivary gland tumors (Queimado et al. 2008). Reduced APC mRNA expression has been observed in 39% of HNSCC cases (Chang et al. 2000), perhaps due to LOH or epigenetic silencing of the *APC* gene (Chang et al. 2000; Worsham et al. 2006).

5.7   Prostate Cancer

5.7.1   *Upregulation of Pathway Activators*

WNT-1, -5A, and -6 are highly expressed in primary prostate cancers compared to normal prostate (Chen et al. 2004; Hall et al. 2005; Iozzo et al. 1995), and WNT-2 is increased in metastases relative to primary prostate tumors (Hall et al. 2005). Abnormal expression of WNT-5A and β-catenin has been observed in up to 28 and 71% of prostate tumor specimens, respectively, but there is simultaneous expression in only 5% of these cases (Chesire et al. 2000; de la Taille et al. 2003; Yamamoto et al. 2010). Some studies have shown that β-catenin accumulation is associated with high Gleason scores and prostate-specific antigen (PSA) levels (Chen et al. 2004; de la Taille et al. 2003; Whitaker et al. 2008), while others have failed to find an association between stage or biochemical relapse with β-catenin but did so with WNT-1 or WNT-5A expression (Chen et al. 2004; Yamamoto et al. 2010). One mechanism attributable to WNT-5A upregulation is promoter hypomethylation, which is observed in 65% of primary prostate cancers (Wang et al. 2007). *CTNNB1* mutations are observed in only 4–9% of advanced prostate cancer cases (Chesire et al. 2000; Gerstein et al. 2002; Voeller et al. 1998; Yardy et al. 2009). DVL-1 is significantly overexpressed in prostate cancers and increased with grade (Mizutani et al. 2005). Interestingly, men homozygous for a *TCF-4* SNP have an elevated relative risk of aggressive prostate cancer (Agalliu et al. 2008).

5.7.2   *Loss of Pathway Inhibitors*

The *SFRP1* and *DKK-3* genes are hypermethylated in as many as 83 and 68% of primary prostate cancers, respectively (Coutinho-Camillo et al. 2006; Lodygin et al. 2005), resulting in decreased expression in tumor cells (Coutinho-Camillo et al. 2006; Kawano et al. 2006; Zenzmaier et al. 2008). Both SFRP1 and DKK-3, however, are upregulated in the stroma of prostate tumors (Joesting et al. 2005; Zenzmaier et al. 2008). DKK-1 expression is decreased in prostate cancers compared to normal prostate tissue and is downregulated during progression to metastasis (Hall et al. 2005, 2008). WIF-1 is downregulated at the mRNA and protein levels in 23% and 64% of prostate cancers, respectively (Wissmann et al. 2003), and SFRP4 expression predicts good prognosis in prostate cancers (Horvath et al. 2004, 2007). *APC* appears to be commonly inactivated in prostate cancer. Somatic loss occurs in 2–43% cancers (Brewster et al. 1994; Gerstein et al. 2002; Phillips et al. 1994; Yardy et al. 2009), while promoter hypermethylation is observed in as many as 90% of prostate cancers (Bastian et al. 2005; Jeronimo et al. 2004; Yegnasubramanian et al. 2004) and is an independent predictor of unfavorable outcome (Henrique et al. 2007).

Mutations in *AXIN1* have also been detected in 14% of advanced prostate cancers (Yardy et al. 2009).

5.8 Pancreatic Cancer

5.8.1 Upregulation of Pathway Activators

Through microarray gene expression profiling approaches, several WNT pathway genes have been associated with advanced pancreatic cancer (Campagna et al. 2008), often with expression localized to the stroma rather than tumor cells (Pilarsky et al. 2008). At the protein level, WNT-1 and FZD2 are overexpressed in advanced pancreatic adenocarcinomas (Zeng et al. 2006). More than half of pancreatic cancers have reduced membrane-associated β-catenin, and 65% of advanced pancreatic adenocarcinomas have increased β-catenin (Zeng et al. 2006). Nuclear or cytosolic β-catenin accumulation has been described in 4–51% of pancreatic carcinomas (Al-Aynati et al. 2004; Lowy et al. 2003; Wang et al. 2009a), but mutations are fairly uncommon (Zeng et al. 2006). β-catenin stabilization might be a relatively early event in tumor progression since high-grade pancreatic intraepithelial neoplasia (PanIN) lesions show increased nuclear localization (Al-Aynati et al. 2004). Nuclear β-catenin and *CTNNB1* mutations are observed in more than 90% of solid pseudopapillary tumors of the pancreas in contrast to ductal adenocarcinomas (Abraham et al. 2002a; Min Kim et al. 2006; Nishimori et al. 2006; Tiemann et al. 2007). β-catenin mutation and accumulation have also been observed in intraductal papillary mucinous neoplasms, in solid and cystic tumor of the pancreas, and pancreatoblastomas (Abraham et al. 2001; Chetty et al. 2006; Miao et al. 2003). Increased LEF-1 expression, and that of transcript variants, in pancreatic cancer correlates with advanced tumor stage (Jesse et al. 2010).

5.8.2 Loss of Pathway Inhibitors

Promoter hypermethylation and concomitant downregulation of expression of SFRP1, SFRP2, SFRP4, and SFRP5 are observed in 48–77% of pancreatic cancer samples (Bu et al. 2008). WIF-1 is downregulated in 75% of pancreatic cancer samples (Taniguchi et al. 2005), while DKK-1 mRNA is actually overexpressed in ductal adenocarcinomas (Takahashi et al. 2010). *APC* mutations have been described in pancreatic carcinomas (Yashima et al. 1994), including 18% of acinar cell carcinomas (Abraham et al. 2002c). In solid pseudopapillary tumors, LOH of the *APC* locus 5q22.1 (Min Kim et al. 2006) and AXIN2 overexpression have been observed (Cavard et al. 2009). Like β-catenin dysregulation, APC loss has been associated with intraductal papillary mucinous neoplasms and pancreatoblastomas (Abraham et al. 2001; Chetty et al. 2006).

5.9 Hepatocellular Carcinoma and Hepatoblastoma

5.9.1 Upregulation of Pathway Activators

Upregulation of WNT-3 and -4, and FZD3, FZD6, and FZD7 is observed in 95% of hepatocellular carcinomas (HCC) as compared to normal liver (Bengochea et al. 2008). FZD7, in particular, is overexpressed in 90% of HCC and is associated with chronic hepatitis B virus infection (Merle et al. 2004) and β-catenin nuclear accumulation (Merle et al. 2005). There are conflicting data about WNT-5A such that both upregulation and loss of expression have been reported in 80–90% of HCC (Bengochea et al. 2008; Liu et al. 2008). *CTNNB1* mutations have been detected in 3–44% HCC (Boyault et al. 2007; Cui et al. 2003; de La Coste et al. 1998; Edamoto et al. 2003; Ishizaki et al. 2004; Kim et al. 2008; Nhieu et al. 1999; Park et al. 2005; Prange et al. 2003; Wong et al. 2001; Zucman-Rossi et al. 2007). HCCs frequently demonstrate nuclear localization of β-catenin (in 17–43% of cases) that is correlated with grade, poor differentiation, hepatitis B surface antigen and increased proliferative index (Kim et al. 2008; Nhieu et al. 1999; Schmitt-Graeff et al. 2005; Suzuki et al. 2002; Tien et al. 2005; Wang et al. 2009b; Wong et al. 2001). High WNT-1 expression in hepatitis-associated HCC is correlated with nuclear β-catenin and increased recurrence after tumor resection (Lee et al. 2009b). TCF-4 and LEF-1 are often overexpressed or even mutated in those HCCs that show β-catenin accumulation (Cui et al. 2003; Jiang et al. 2002; Schmitt-Graeff et al. 2005). Activation of the pathway may be even more common in hepatoblastomas, such that as many as 75% carry *CTNNB1* mutations (Blaker et al. 1999; Jeng et al. 2000; Koch et al. 1999; Park et al. 2001b; Takayasu et al. 2001; Taniguchi et al. 2002; Udatsu et al. 2001; Wei et al. 2000).

5.9.2 Loss of Pathway Inhibitors

Promoter methylation of *SFRP1*, *SFRP2*, and *SFRP5* occurs in 30–76% of primary HCCs (Bengochea et al. 2008; Huang et al. 2007; Shih et al. 2006, 2007; Takagi et al. 2008). Other WNT pathway antagonists, including DKK-3, WIF-1, and Prickle-1, are methylated and/or downregulated in HCC compared to adjacent and control normal tissues (Chan et al. 2006; Ding et al. 2009). Despite the fact that HCC is reported in some FAP patients (Cetta et al. 1997; Gruner et al. 1998; Hughes and Michels 1992; Kurahashi et al. 1995; Su et al. 2001), *APC* is not frequently mutated in sporadic HCC as it is in hepatoblastoma (Kurahashi et al. 1995; Oda et al. 1996; Park et al. 2001b). In contrast, mutations of *AXIN1* or *AXIN2* have been described in 6–25% of HCCs (Kim et al. 2008; Park et al. 2005; Satoh et al. 2000; Taniguchi et al. 2002; Zucman-Rossi et al. 2007), including more than half of those tumors with nuclear β-catenin (Ishizaki et al. 2004). Mutations in *AXIN1*, but not *AXIN2*, have been identified in hepatoblastomas (Miao et al. 2003; Taniguchi et al. 2002).

5.10   Kidney Cancer

5.10.1   Upregulation of Pathway Activators

In pediatric and adult Wilms' tumor, also known as nephroblastoma, nuclear accumulation of β-catenin is frequently observed, ranging from 25 to 67% (Koesters et al. 2003; Su et al. 2008). *CTNNB1* mutations, even some outside of exon 3 (Li et al. 2004), are observed in many tumors that have nuclear β-catenin and almost always in Wilms' tumors that carry a Wilms' tumor (*WT1*) mutation (Koesters et al. 1999, 2003; Kusafuka et al. 2002; Maiti et al. 2000; Su et al. 2008), but also in some without a *WT1* mutation (Fukuzawa et al. 2008). Both β-catenin accumulation and mutation appear to occur in about a quarter of clear cell renal carcinomas, but rarely in papillary or chromophobe renal cancers (Kim et al. 2000). Expression of both FZD5 and FZD8 is increased in a majority of renal cell carcinomas (Janssens et al. 2004).

5.10.2   Loss of Pathway Inhibitors

SFRP1 is downregulated in the vast majority (i.e., 89–97%) of renal cell carcinomas (Awakura et al. 2008; Dahl et al. 2007), especially clear cell carcinomas, likely through both promoter methylation and LOH (Awakura et al. 2008; Dahl et al. 2007; Saini et al. 2009). In fact, *SFRP1* methylation is a significant independent predictor of outcome (Urakami et al. 2006a). Moreover, SFRP2, SFRP3, SFRP4, SFRP5, WIF-1, DKK-2, and DKK-3 are all significantly downregulated and/or methylated in renal cancers compared to normal renal tissue (Hirata et al. 2009, 2010; Kawakami et al. 2009, 2011; Urakami et al. 2006a). Unexpectedly, DKK-1 is overexpressed in a majority of Wilms' tumors examined (Wirths et al. 2003). LOH of 5q21, the *APC* locus, is infrequent in these tumors (Hoban et al. 1997; Mannens et al. 1990).

5.11   Bladder Cancer

5.11.1   Upregulation of Pathway Activators

WNT-7B is most highly expressed in superficial bladder tumors suggesting that it is involved in early tumor development (Bui et al. 1998). Nuclear accumulation of β-catenin is a predictor of poor survival in bladder cancer (Kastritis et al. 2009). Despite the fact that *CTNNB1* mutations occur infrequently in bladder tumors, they correlate with elevated levels of the target genes *c-myc* and *cyclin D1* (Shiina et al. 2002).

5.11.2 Loss of Pathway Inhibitors

In bladder cancer, deletions of chromosome 8p, the *SFRP1* locus, are correlated with invasive disease, consistent with loss of SFRP1 mRNA and protein in 40% and 70% of tumors, respectively (Stoehr et al. 2004). Promoter methylation of *SFRP1* is also observed in bladder cancer (Stoehr et al. 2004), as is methylation of *SFRP2*, *SFRP4*, and *SFRP5*, *WIF-1*, and *DKK-3* (Marsit et al. 2005, 2006; Urakami et al. 2006b). Importantly, SFRP downregulation in as many as 62% of bladder cancers is associated with advanced tumor stage and poor survival (Marsit et al. 2005, 2006). WIF-1 protein loss is observed in a quarter of bladder tumors and is also correlated with advanced stage (Wissmann et al. 2003). Moreover, *SFRP2* and *DKK-3* methylation levels are predictors of bladder cancer, and methylation can be detected even in the urine of bladder cancer patients (Urakami et al. 2006b). Somatic *APC* missense mutations or frameshift deletions were recently found in approximately 16% of invasive urothelial carcinomas and predicted worse patient outcome (Kastritis et al. 2009).

5.12 Skin Cancer

5.12.1 Upregulation of Pathway Activators

WNT-5A is overexpressed in malignant melanoma, increases with melanoma progression, and best defines a specific subclass of melanoma (Bittner et al. 2000; Carr et al. 2003; Iozzo et al. 1995). Most importantly, WNT-5A expression correlates with reduced metastasis-free and overall survival (Carr et al. 2003; Da Forno et al. 2008). Coexpressed FZD and WNT-5A show a shift from nuclear to cytosolic localization in malignant tumors, and WNT-5A is associated with nuclear β-catenin in cutaneous malignant melanoma (Bachmann et al. 2005). While WNT-2, -5A, -7B, and -10B are overexpressed in some benign nevi as well, there are melanomas that show decreased expression in WNT-2 and WNT-5A (Pham et al. 2003). While *CTNNB1* mutation is infrequent in melanomas (Castiglia et al. 2008), nuclear and cytosolic accumulation of β-catenin is observed in nearly 60% of malignant melanomas (Demunter et al. 2002; Kielhorn et al. 2003; Maelandsmo et al. 2003; Omholt et al. 2001; Pecina-Slaus et al. 2007; Reifenberger et al. 2002; Rimm et al. 1999; Worm et al. 2004). Although some reports indicate nuclear β-catenin does not correlate with melanoma stage or mutation status (Demunter et al. 2002), others indicate that it actually correlates with improved patient survival (Chien et al. 2009). Additional data suggest that nuclear and/or cytosolic β-catenin decreases with melanoma progression (Bachmann et al. 2005; Kageshita et al. 2001; Maelandsmo et al. 2003). In basal cell carcinomas (BCCs), WNT-1 and -5A are frequently overexpressed and β-catenin localization shifts from the membrane to the cytosol (Lo Muzio et al. 2002; Saldanha et al. 2004). Nuclear β-catenin has been observed in as many as 25% of BCC (Doglioni et al. 2003; Saldanha et al. 2004), although β-catenin accumulation has not been observed in all BCC cohorts (Boonchai et al. 2000). Nuclear β-catenin is also observed in Bowen disease, spiroadenomas, and occasionally in squamous cell carcinoma, and high levels of TCF-3 are observed in BCC and spiroadenomas (Doglioni et al. 2003). One third of human sebaceous tumors have mutations in *LEF-1* that impair LEF-1 protein binding to β-catenin (Takeda et al. 2006). WNT pathway activation is particularly common in hair follicle-related tumors, including benign and malignant pilomatrix neoplasms. Mutations and nuclear localization of β-catenin are observed in more than 60% and 90% of pilomatricomas, respectively (Chan et al. 1999; Durand and Moles 1999; Hassanein and Glanz 2004; Lazar et al. 2005; Moreno-Bueno et al. 2001a; Park et al. 2001a; Xia et al. 2006).

5.12.2   Loss of Pathway Inhibitors

DKK-1, -2, and -3 are significantly downregulated in most primary melanoma tissue samples (Kuphal et al. 2006). Both somatic biallelic deletion and silencing by hypermethylation of *APC* are observed in melanoma in as many as 17% of tumors (Castiglia et al. 2008; Korabiowska et al. 2004; Worm et al. 2004). A germline mutation in *AXIN2* has been identified in a melanoma patient (Castiglia et al. 2008).

5.13   Tumors of the Central Nervous System (CNS)

5.13.1   Gliomas

In gliomas, WNT-2, WNT-5A, WNT-10B, WNT-13, and FZD2 are overexpressed (Howng et al. 2002; Pu et al. 2009), and WNT-5A, for example, is more highly expressed in advanced stage tumors, such as glioblastoma multiforme, compared to normal brain and low-grade astrocytoma (Yu et al. 2007). Cytosolic and nuclear accumulation of β-catenin was observed in more than half of astrocytomas examined, and low levels of β-catenin were associated with better prognosis (Zhang et al. 2010). There are also increased levels and cytosolic/nuclear accumulation of β-catenin in tuberous sclerosis-associated subependymal giant cell astrocytomas (Jozwiak et al. 2007). FRAT1, a potent activator of WNT signaling, is expressed in most glioma samples and increases with advanced grade and correlates with β-catenin expression (Guo et al. 2010). β-catenin, DVL-3, LEF-1, and TCF-4 expressions are all upregulated in astrocytomas with cytosolic/nuclear β-catenin accumulation (Sareddy et al. 2009). TCF-4 has several isoforms expressed in brain tumors and most are overexpressed, and *TCF-4* mutations are observed in 23% of brain tumors (Howng et al. 2002). At least one WNT antagonist, including SFRP1, SFRP2, SFRP4, SFRP5, DKK-1, or DKK-3 (as well as naked cuticle homolog 1 and 2 [NKD1 and 2]), is hypermethylated and downregulated in approximately one third of diffuse astrocytomas and anaplastic astrocytomas as well as more than 70% primary and secondary glioblastomas (Gotze et al. 2010). Similarly, WIF-1 is decreased through promoter methylation in astrocytomas and is associated with increased grade (Yang et al. 2010). Mutations, large deletions, and LOH in *AXIN1* have been observed in a small proportion of glioblastomas (Baeza et al. 2003; Dahmen et al. 2001; Nikuseva Martic et al. 2010).

5.13.2 Medulloblastomas

In childhood medulloblastoma, nuclear β-catenin prevalent in 25% of tumors actually predicts good outcome (Ellison et al. 2005), and *CTNNB1* mutations are found in up to 20% of these tumors (Eberhart et al. 2000; Huang et al. 2000; Rogers et al. 2009; Yokota et al. 2002; Zurawel et al. 1998). In fact, WNT signaling and *CTNNB1* mutations characterize a molecular subtype of medulloblastoma (Kool et al. 2008; Thompson et al. 2006). *SFRP1*, *SFRP2*, and *SFRP3* are methylated in 4–24% of primary medulloblastomas (Kongkham et al. 2010), and DKK-1 is silenced by methylation and significantly downregulated in medulloblastoma (Vibhakar et al. 2007). Turcot's syndrome is a subtype of FAP in which patients present with CNS tumors, particularly medulloblastoma. LOH of *APC* is observed in medulloblastoma of Turcot's patients (Hamilton et al. 1995), and *APC* mutations have been identified in sporadic medulloblastomas (Huang et al. 2000; Koch et al. 2001). Like glioblastomas, some reports have identified loss of *AXIN1* in medulloblastomas (Baeza et al. 2003; Dahmen et al. 2001; Nikuseva Martic et al. 2010).

5.13.3 Other CNS Tumors

CNS primitive neuroectodermal tumors (PNETs), pediatric brain tumors histologically similar to medulloblastomas, also show nuclear β-catenin in approximately 36% tumors, but only *CTNNB1* mutations in 4–5% (Koch et al. 2001; Rogers et al. 2009). *CTNNB1* mutations and the expression of WNT pathway components are observed in grade 3 ependymomas, tumors derived from ependymal cells that cover the cerebral ventricles and central canal of the spinal cord (Palm et al. 2009). Meningiomas also frequently have nuclear localization of β-catenin as well as expression of WNT-5A, WNT-10B, and WNT-13 (Howng et al. 2002; Pecina-Slaus et al. 2008). In addition, almost half of all meningiomas demonstrate *APC* LOH and reduced APC protein expression (Pecina-Slaus et al. 2008).

5.14 Musculoskeletal Tumors

5.14.1 Osteosarcoma

Cytoplasmic and nuclear β-catenin accumulation is seen in approximately 70% of the osteosarcoma samples examined, but mutational analysis of *CTNNB1* failed to detect any genetic alterations, suggesting that the potential aberrations may be upstream or in β-catenin degradation (Haydon et al. 2002). Overexpression of LRP5 in 50% of tumors is a marker for disease progression in human osteosarcoma, although sequencing of exon 3 of *LRP5* did not reveal any mutations in selected patient samples (Hoang et al. 2004). Chen et al. examined WNT-10B in osteosarcoma samples and found that increased expression correlated with poor overall survival (Chen et al. 2008). There is evidence to suggest that loss of APC function, especially in combination with MET and TWIST abnormalities, is a significant negative prognostic factor in osteosarcoma (Entz-Werle et al. 2007). Conversely, Cai et al. reported inactivation of the WNT/β-catenin pathway in high-grade osteosarcoma (Cai et al. 2010).

5.14.2 Ewing's Sarcoma

Analysis of nine different Ewing's sarcoma cell lines revealed marked stimulation of the β-catenin/canonical WNT pathway with detection of WNT-10B, WNT-5A, WNT-11, and WNT-13 in nearly all the cells (Uren et al. 2004). Additionally, WNT-3A and DKK-1 stimulate neurite outgrowth in Ewing's sarcoma cells via a FZD3- and c-Jun N terminal kinase (JNK)-dependent mechanism (Endo et al. 2008). Furthermore, the oncogenic fusion gene product commonly seen in Ewing's sarcoma, EWS/FLI1, regulates DKK expression (Navarro et al. 2010).

5.14.3 Soft Tissue Tumors

WNT signaling has also been shown to have an important role in several soft tissue sarcomas such as synovial sarcoma, malignant fibrous histiocytoma, dedifferentiated liposarcoma, and fibrosarcoma (Fukukawa et al. 2009; Guo et al. 2008; Matushansky et al. 2007; Pretto et al. 2006; Sakamoto et al. 2002). Recruitment of β-catenin into the nucleus is observed in synovial sarcoma (Pretto et al. 2006). Furthermore, activation of the noncanonical DVL-Rac1-JNK pathway by FZD10 has also been described in human synovial sarcoma (Fukukawa et al. 2009). In dedifferentiated liposarcoma and malignant fibrous histiocytoma, β-catenin accumulation and *CTNNB1* gene mutations have been reported (Matushansky et al. 2007; Sakamoto et al. 2002). Among the soft tissue tumors involving the musculoskeletal system, the role of APC and β-catenin has been best defined in desmoid tumors (also known as aggressive fibromatosis), a rare soft tissue tumor that has locally invasive features but rarely metastasizes. The findings of desmoid tumors affecting 10–15% of all patients with FAP support a relationship between WNT signaling and this disease (Clark et al. 1999; Couture et al. 2000; Gurbuz et al. 1994; Latchford et al. 2007). Additionally, somatic mutations in *APC* are seen in half of sporadic cases of desmoid tumors (Alman et al. 1997). High levels of β-catenin mRNA and protein in desmoid tumors are commonly observed (Alman et al. 1997; Saito et al. 2002); in fact, β-catenin expression is used as a prognostic indicator for disease-free survival in patients (Gebert et al. 2007). In several cases of sporadic desmoid tumors, somatic mutations in *CTNNB1* have been identified (Lips et al. 2009; Saito et al. 2002).

5.15 Gynecological Cancers

5.15.1 Ovarian Cancer

WNT-1 and WNT-5A expressions are significantly higher in epithelial ovarian cancers than benign tumors and normal ovary, and WNT-5A expression predicts poor outcome (Badiglian Filho et al. 2009). WNT-9B and -10B are specifically upregulated in ovarian endometrial adenocarcinoma (OEA) specimens (Steg et al. 2006), and FZD1 is significantly higher in benign and malignant ovarian tumors than normal ovaries (Badiglian Filho et al. 2009). Nuclear and/or cytoplasmic β-catenin accumulation is common in ovarian adenocarcinomas (Kildal et al. 2005; Rask et al. 2003; Wang et al. 2006), particularly in most cases of endometrioid tumors but not in other subtypes (Kildal et al. 2005; Saegusa and Okayasu 2001; Sarrio et al. 2006; Schlosshauer et al. 2002; Wu et al. 2001), although there are some reports of β-catenin accumulation also in serous adenocarcinomas (Rask et al. 2003; Wang et al. 2006). In a cohort of ovarian carcinomas, β-catenin accumulation is associated with FRAT1 overexpression (Wang et al. 2006). *CTNNB1* mutation, however, is less frequently observed – in 16–38% ovarian cancers and enriched in OEAs (Hendrix et al. 2006; Moreno-Bueno et al. 2001b; Sagae et al. 1999; Sarrio et al. 2006; Wright et al. 1999; Wu et al. 2001, 2007b). The GSK3β kinase, responsible for β-catenin phosphorylation, has also been shown to be overexpressed in ovarian cancer compared to normal ovary (Rask et al. 2003). SFRP1, SFRP2, and SFRP5 are frequently downregulated by hypermethylation in ovarian cancer and associated with recurrence and overall survival (Su et al. 2009, 2010; Takada et al. 2004). SFRP4 specifically has been associated with β-catenin expression in 84% primary serous ovarian tumors (Drake et al. 2009), while WIF-1 is actually upregulated in OEAs (Steg et al. 2006). *APC* biallelic somatic mutations (Wu et al. 2001, 2007a) and LOH have been described in as many as 33% of ovarian cancers (Sarrio et al. 2006), and APC expression is reduced in ovarian cancer (Rask et al. 2003), including serous ovarian carcinomas (Karbova et al. 2002). Mutations in and downregulation of AXIN1 and AXIN2 have also been described (Steg et al. 2006; Wu et al. 2001).

5.15.2   Endometrial Cancer

Unexpectedly, the expression of WNT-2, -3, -4, and -5A is reduced in endometrial carcinomas compared to normal endometrium (Bui et al. 1997b). Nuclear
β-catenin has been described in 16–38% of endometrial carcinomas, particularly endometriod tumors (Fukuchi et al. 1998; Nei et al. 1999; Pijnenborg et al.
2004; Schlosshauer et al. 2002; Scholten et al. 2003), 60% of endometrial
hyperplasias (Nei et al. 1999), and some endometrial sarcomas (Kildal et al.
2009; Kurihara et al. 2010). There is significant coexpression of nuclear
β-catenin and TCF-4 in endometrial carcinomas (Saegusa et al. 2005). Stabilizing
mutations in *CTNNB1* occur in 13–22% of endometrial cancers (Fukuchi et al.
1998; Ikeda et al. 2000; Kobayashi et al. 1999; Konopka et al. 2007; Mirabelli-
Primdahl et al. 1999; Nei et al. 1999; Saegusa et al. 2001; Saegusa and Okayasu
2001), again often in those tumors of the endometriod subtype (Moreno-Bueno
et al. 2001b). SFRP1 and SFRP4 are hypermethylated and downregulated in
endometriod endometrial cancers and associated with MSI (Risinger et al.
2005), and SFRP4 is downregulated in endometrial stromal sarcomas (Hrzenjak
et al. 2004). DKK-1 expression is reduced in endometrial carcinomas compared
to benign tumors (Yi et al. 2009). *APC* LOH and promoter methylation is
observed in 24–47% of endometrial cancers and is associated with the endometriod phenotype and MSI but not nuclear β-catenin (Moreno-Bueno et al.
2001b; Pijnenborg et al. 2004).

5.15.3   Cervical Cancer

Nuclear and cytosolic β-catenin accumulation is observed in 73% of invasive
cervical cancers, while *CTNNB1* mutation is only detectable in approximately 10%
(Shinohara et al. 2001). DVL-1 is overexpressed in two thirds of primary cervical
squamous cell cancers (Okino et al. 2003). *SFRP1*, *SFRP2*, *SFRP4*, and *SFRP5* are
hypermethylated in 53–83% of adenocarcinoma of the cervix tissues (Lin et al.
2009), and *DKK-3* is methylated in 31% of cervical cancer cases (Lee et al. 2009a).
Although infrequent, *AXIN1* mutations have been reported in cervical cancers
(Su et al. 2003).

5.16   Other Tumors

5.16.1   Esophageal Cancer

β-catenin has been shown to be decreased in more than half of esophageal
squamous cell carcinoma (ESCC) tumors and correlated with invasion and

metastasis as well as poor prognosis (Wang et al. 2010). In contrast, overexpression of β-catenin has been described in more than two thirds of ESCC cases (Peng et al. 2009). AXIN and APC are downregulated in approximately 30–50% of ESCC, and reduced AXIN expression is a negative predictor for overall survival (Li et al. 2009; Peng et al. 2009). Interestingly, the E3-ubiquitin ligase β-TrCP is downregulated in approximately 25% of ESCCs (Li et al. 2009), and DKK-1 expression in 42% tumors predicts poor disease-free survival (Makino et al. 2009). In esophageal adenocarcinomas, SFRP1, -2, -4, and -5 and WIF-1 are hypermethylated and downregulated in 73–93% cases (Taniguchi et al. 2005; Zou et al. 2005).

5.16.2   Adrenal Tumors

Adrenal tumors are more common in FAP patients (Smith et al. 2000), suggesting that APC and WNT signaling might be important in this tumor type. β-catenin nuclear/cytoplasmic accumulation has been observed in as many as 45% of adreno-cortical carcinomas and adenomas (Tadjine et al. 2008; Tissier et al. 2005). Additionally, β-catenin accumulation and mutation have also been detected in all primary pigmented nodular adrenocortical disease samples analyzed (Gaujoux et al. 2008).

5.16.3   Thyroid and Parathyroid Tumors

WNT-5A is upregulated in most papillary thyroid cancers and some follicular carcinomas (Kremenevskaja et al. 2005). Nuclear and/or cytosolic β-catenin is observed in more than 75% of all types of well-differentiated thyroid cancers (Weinberger et al. 2007), including thyroid papillary microcarcinoma, parathy-roid carcinoma (PTC), follicular carcinoma, and follicular variant of papillary carcinoma (FVPC) (Lantsov et al. 2005; Rezk et al. 2004). In anaplastic thyroid cancers, *CTNNB1, APC,* and *AXIN* mutations are detectable in 5%, 9%, and 82% tumors, respectively (Kurihara et al. 2004). Cytosolic β-catenin, which correlates with cyclin D1 expression, was observed in 67% papillary thyroid cancers, but only 9% follicular adenomas and 25% follicular cancers (Ishigaki et al. 2002). *CTNNB1* mutations and nuclear β-catenin were found in 21–25% of poorly dif-ferentiated thyroid cancers and 48–66% of undifferentiated carcinomas (Garcia-Rostan et al. 2001). Although parathyroid cancers are very rare, aberrantly spliced LRP5 is expressed in 86–100% of primary parathyroid tumors and is mutually exclusive with *CTNNB1* mutations (Bjorklund et al. 2007). Moreover, the expression of APC and GSK3β is lost in one third and 75% of PTCs, respec-tively (Juhlin et al. 2009).

5.16.4   Pituitary Tumors

WNT-1, -4, -5A, -10B, and -13 and FZD6 are upregulated in pituitary adenomas, but they are not all associated with nuclear β-catenin in these tumors (Howng et al. 2002; Miyakoshi et al. 2008). More than half of pituitary adenomas have nuclear β-catenin (Semba et al. 2001), although there are conflicting reports about the presence of *CTNNB1* mutations (Semba et al. 2001; Sun et al. 2005). There is, however, well-documented downregulation of WIF-1, SFRP2, and SFRP4 mRNA and protein in pituitary tumors and hypermethylation of the *WIF-1* promoter in almost 90% of cases (Elston et al. 2008). Unexpectedly, SFRP1 expression is upregulated in nonfunctional pituitary adenomas and was thought to activate the pathway (Moreno et al. 2005). In pituitary adenomas, nuclear β-catenin accumulation was not associated with *APC*, *AXIN*, or *GSK3β* mutations (Sun et al. 2005).

5.17   Conclusion

In sum, the evidence described in detail here demonstrates that the Wnt pathway is frequently deregulated in the human solid tumors discussed here, ranging from 40–63% among distinct tumor types (Fig. 5.1). In total, we estimate the average occurrence of WNT signaling pathway alterations across cancers to be approximately 48%, placing it as one of the most commonly altered pathways in cancer. Specific tumor subtypes can vary dramatically in the occurrence of WNT pathway alterations, suggesting that pathway activation may be responsible for certain histopathological or prognostic features of those subclasses. Another implication of these data is that specific cancer subtypes might be responsive to therapeutic approaches to abrogate WNT signaling while others may not. Such data are critical in guiding the informative preclinical and early clinical studies necessary to determine the efficacy of these therapies in cell lines, animal models and, ultimately, patients. It is also important to realize that alterations have been described in virtually every component of the WNT pathway in human cancers (Table 5.1), a finding that has compelling implications for the development of therapeutic strategies to target the pathway in vivo and how tumors may adapt to and even bypass WNT pathway inhibition. Lastly, the days of WNT pathway alterations being exclusively associated with colorectal cancer are clearly behind us. The importance of pathway dysregulation in tumor initiation and progression will need to be carefully dissected in the context of tumor types since the possibility remains that the biological consequence of aberrant pathway regulation may differ significantly among tissues.

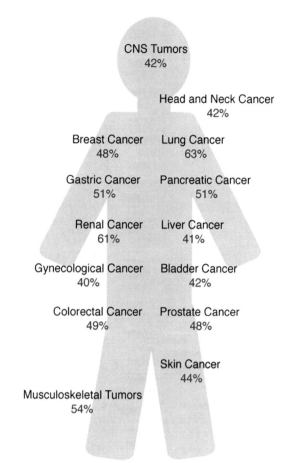

Fig. 5.1 Frequency of WNT pathway alterations in human solid tumors. The mean frequency of pathway dysregulation in each tumor type (irrespective of subtype) was calculated by compiling percentages reported in the literature for all pathway components, regardless of the type of alteration (e.g., increased or decreased expression, mutation, promoter methylation, etc.). If a percentage was not reported in a given study, the study was not included in this analysis. Many, but not all, of these frequencies are described in the text with appropriate references; for simplification, some are reported as a range for a specific alteration

Acknowledgments The authors acknowledge that this was an ambitious task to summarize WNT pathway dysregulation in human cancer and apologize to those investigators whose work was inadvertently omitted from this review of the literature. Work in the senior authors' laboratory has been funded by an American Cancer Society Research Scholar Grant (04-251-01-CCG), an AACR/Komen Career Development Award, and the University of Chicago Breast Cancer SPORE. J.R.P. is funded by an American Cancer Society Postdoctoral Fellowship, and H.H.L. is funded by grants from NIH/NIAMS and the Orthopaedic Research and Education Foundation.

References

Abraham SC, Wu TT, Klimstra DS, Finn LS, Lee JH, Yeo CJ, Cameron JL, Hruban RH (2001) Distinctive molecular genetic alterations in sporadic and familial adenomatous polyposis-associated pancreatoblastomas: frequent alterations in the APC/beta-catenin pathway and chromosome 11p. Am J Pathol 159:1619–1627

Abraham SC, Klimstra DS, Wilentz RE, Yeo CJ, Conlon K, Brennan M, Cameron JL, Wu TT, Hruban RH (2002a) Solid-pseudopapillary tumors of the pancreas are genetically distinct from pancreatic ductal adenocarcinomas and almost always harbor beta-catenin mutations. Am J Pathol 160:1361–1369

Abraham SC, Reynolds C, Lee JH, Montgomery EA, Baisden BL, Krasinskas AM, Wu TT (2002b) Fibromatosis of the breast and mutations involving the APC/beta-catenin pathway. Hum Pathol 33:39–46

Abraham SC, Wu TT, Hruban RH, Lee JH, Yeo CJ, Conlon K, Brennan M, Cameron JL, Klimstra DS (2002c) Genetic and immunohistochemical analysis of pancreatic acinar cell carcinoma: frequent allelic loss on chromosome 11p and alterations in the APC/beta-catenin pathway. Am J Pathol 160:953–962

Abutaily AS, Collins JE, Roche WR (2003) Cadherins, catenins and APC in pleural malignant mesothelioma. J Pathol 201:355–362

Agalliu I, Suuriniemi M, Prokunina-Olsson L, Johanneson B, Collins FS, Stanford JL, Ostrander EA (2008) Evaluation of a variant in the transcription factor 7-like 2 (TCF7L2) gene and prostate cancer risk in a population-based study. Prostate 68:740–747

Aguilera O, Fraga MF, Ballestar E, Paz MF, Herranz M, Espada J, Garcia JM, Munoz A, Esteller M, Gonzalez-Sancho JM (2006) Epigenetic inactivation of the Wnt antagonist DICKKOPF-1 (DKK-1) gene in human colorectal cancer. Oncogene 25:4116–4121

Ai L, Tao Q, Zhong S, Fields CR, Kim WJ, Lee MW, Cui Y, Brown KD, Robertson KD (2006) Inactivation of Wnt inhibitory factor-1 (WIF1) expression by epigenetic silencing is a common event in breast cancer. Carcinogenesis 27:1341–1348

Al-Aynati MM, Radulovich N, Riddell RH, Tsao MS (2004) Epithelial-cadherin and beta-catenin expression changes in pancreatic intraepithelial neoplasia. Clin Cancer Res 10:1235–1240

Alman BA, Li C, Pajerski ME, Diaz-Cano S, Wolfe HJ (1997) Increased beta-catenin protein and somatic APC mutations in sporadic aggressive fibromatoses (desmoid tumors). Am J Pathol 151:329–334

Arnold CN, Goel A, Niedzwiecki D, Dowell JM, Wasserman L, Compton C, Mayer RJ, Bertagnolli MM, Boland CR (2004) APC promoter hypermethylation contributes to the loss of APC expression in colorectal cancers with allelic loss on 5q. Cancer Biol Ther 3:960–964

Awakura Y, Nakamura E, Ito N, Kamoto T, Ogawa O (2008) Methylation-associated silencing of SFRP1 in renal cell carcinoma. Oncol Rep 20:1257–1263

Bachmann IM, Straume O, Puntervoll HE, Kalvenes MB, Akslen LA (2005) Importance of P-cadherin, beta-catenin, and Wnt5a/frizzled for progression of melanocytic tumors and prognosis in cutaneous melanoma. Clin Cancer Res 11:8606–8614

Badiglian Filho L, Oshima CT, De Oliveira LF, De Oliveira CH, De Sousa DR, Gomes TS, Goncalves WJ (2009) Canonical and noncanonical Wnt pathway: a comparison among normal ovary, benign ovarian tumor and ovarian cancer. Oncol Rep 21:313–320

Baeza N, Masuoka J, Kleihues P, Ohgaki H (2003) AXIN1 mutations but not deletions in cerebellar medulloblastomas. Oncogene 22:632–636

Baker H, Patel V, Molinolo AA, Shillitoe EJ, Ensley JF, Yoo GH, Meneses-Garcia A, Myers JN, El-Naggar AK, Gutkind JS, Hancock WS (2005) Proteome-wide analysis of head and neck squamous cell carcinomas using laser-capture microdissection and tandem mass spectrometry. Oral Oncol 41:183–199

Bastian PJ, Ellinger J, Wellmann A, Wernert N, Heukamp LC, Muller SC, von Ruecker A (2005) Diagnostic and prognostic information in prostate cancer with the help of a small set of hypermethylated gene loci. Clin Cancer Res 11:4097–4106

Batra S, Shi Y, Kuchenbecker KM, He B, Reguart N, Mikami I, You L, Xu Z, Lin YC, Clement G, Jablons DM (2006) Wnt inhibitory factor-1, a Wnt antagonist, is silenced by promoter hyperm-ethylation in malignant pleural mesothelioma. Biochem Biophys Res Commun 342:1228–1232

Bengochea A, de Souza MM, Lefrancois L, Le Roux E, Galy O, Chemin I, Kim M, Wands JR, Trepo C, Hainaut P, Scoazec JY, Vitvitski L, Merle P (2008) Common dysregulation of Wnt/Frizzled receptor elements in human hepatocellular carcinoma. Br J Cancer 99:143–150

Bittner M, Meltzer P, Chen Y, Jiang Y, Seftor E, Hendrix M, Radmacher M, Simon R, Yakhini Z, Ben-Dor A, Sampas N, Dougherty E, Wang E, Marincola F, Gooden C, Lueders J, Glatfelter A, Pollock P, Carpten J, Gillanders E, Leja D, Dietrich K, Beaudry C, Berens M, Alberts D, Sondak V (2000) Molecular classification of cutaneous malignant melanoma by gene expres-sion profiling. Nature 406:536–540

Bjorklund P, Akerstrom G, Westin G (2007) An LRP5 receptor with internal deletion in hyperparathy-roid tumors with implications for deregulated WNT/beta-catenin signaling. PLoS Med 4:e328

Bjorklund P, Svedlund J, Olsson AK, Akerstrom G, Westin G (2009) The internally truncated LRP5 receptor presents a therapeutic target in breast cancer. PLoS One 4:e4243

Blaker H, Hofmann WJ, Rieker RJ, Penzel R, Graf M, Otto HF (1999) Beta-catenin accumulation and mutation of the CTNNB1 gene in hepatoblastoma. Genes Chromosomes Cancer 25:399–402

Bodmer WF, Bailey C, Bodmer J, Bussey H, Ellis A, Gorman P, Lucibello F, Murday V, Rider S, Scambler P, Sheer D, Soloman E, Spurr N (1987) Localization of the gene for familial adenoma-tous polyposis on chromosome 5. Nature 328:614–616

Boonchai W, Walsh M, Cummings M, Chenevix-Trench G (2000) Expression of beta-catenin, a key mediator of the WNT signaling pathway, in basal cell carcinoma. Arch Dermatol 136:937–938

Boyault S, Rickman DS, de Reynies A, Balabaud C, Rebouissou S, Jeannot E, Herault A, Saric J, Belghiti J, Franco D, Bioulac-Sage P, Laurent-Puig P, Zucman-Rossi J (2007) Transcriptome clas-sification of HCC is related to gene alterations and to new therapeutic targets. Hepatology 45:42–52

Brabender J, Usadel H, Danenberg KD, Metzger R, Schneider PM, Lord RV, Wickramasinghe K, Lum CE, Park J, Salonga D, Singer J, Sidransky D, Holscher AH, Meltzer SJ, Danenberg PV (2001) Adenomatous polyposis coli gene promoter hypermethylation in non-small cell lung cancer is associated with survival. Oncogene 20:3528–3532

Brewster SF, Browne S, Brown KW (1994) Somatic allelic loss at the DCC, APC, nm23-H1 and p53 tumor suppressor gene loci in human prostatic carcinoma. J Urol 151:1073–1077

Bu XM, Zhao CH, Zhang N, Gao F, Lin S, Dai W (2008) Hypermethylation and aberrant expres-sion of secreted frizzled-related protein genes in pancreatic cancer. World J Gastroenterol 14:3421–3424

Bui TD, Rankin J, Smith K, Huguet EL, Ruben S, Strachan T, Harris AL, Lindsay S (1997a) A novel human Wnt gene, WNT10B, maps to 12q13 and is expressed in human breast carci-nomas. Oncogene 14:1249–1253

Bui TD, Zhang L, Rees MC, Bicknell R, Harris AL (1997b) Expression and hormone regulation of Wnt2, 3, 4, 5a, 7a, 7b and 10b in normal human endometrium and endometrial carcinoma. Br J Cancer 75:1131–1136

Bui TD, O'Brien T, Crew J, Cranston D, Harris AL (1998) High expression of Wnt7b in human superficial bladder cancer vs invasive bladder cancer. Br J Cancer 77:319–324

Byun T, Karimi M, Marsh JL, Milovanovic T, Lin F, Holcombe RF (2005) Expression of secreted Wnt antagonists in gastrointestinal tissues: potential role in stem cell homeostasis. J Clin Pathol 58:515–519

Cai Y, Mohseny AB, Karperien M, Hogendoorn PC, Zhou G, Cleton-Jansen AM (2010) Inactive Wnt/beta-catenin pathway in conventional high-grade osteosarcoma. J Pathol 220:24–33

Caldwell GM, Jones C, Gensberg K, Jan S, Hardy RG, Byrd P, Chughtai S, Wallis Y, Matthews GM, Morton DG (2004) The Wnt antagonist sFRP1 in colorectal tumorigenesis. Cancer Res 64:883–888

Caldwell GM, Jones CE, Taniere P, Warrack R, Soon Y, Matthews GM, Morton DG (2006) The Wnt antagonist sFRP1 is downregulated in premalignant large bowel adenomas. Br J Cancer 94:922–927

Campagna D, Cope L, Lakkur SS, Henderson C, Laheru D, Iacobuzio-Donahue CA (2008) Gene expression profiles associated with advanced pancreatic cancer. Int J Clin Exp Pathol 1:32–43

Carr KM, Bittner M, Trent JM (2003) Gene-expression profiling in human cutaneous melanoma. Oncogene 22:3076–3080

Castiglia D, Bernardini S, Alvino E, Pagani E, De Luca N, Falcinelli S, Pacchiarotti A, Bonmassar E, Zambruno G, D'Atri S (2008) Concomitant activation of Wnt pathway and loss of mismatch repair function in human melanoma. Genes Chromosomes Cancer 47:614–624

Cavard C, Audebourg A, Letourneur F, Audard V, Beuvon F, Cagnard N, Radenen B, Varlet P, Vacher-Lavenu MC, Perret C, Terris B (2009) Gene expression profiling provides insights into the pathways involved in solid pseudopapillary neoplasm of the pancreas. J Pathol 218:201–209

Cetta F, Cetta D, Petracci M, Cama A, Fusco A, Barbarisi A (1997) Childhood hepatocellular tumors in FAP. Gastroenterology 113:1051–1052

Chan EF, Gat U, McNiff JM, Fuchs E (1999) A common human skin tumour is caused by activating mutations in beta-catenin. Nat Genet 21:410–413

Chan DW, Chan CY, Yam JW, Ching YP, Ng IO (2006) Prickle-1 negatively regulates Wnt/beta-catenin pathway by promoting Dishevelled ubiquitination/degradation in liver cancer. Gastroenterology 131:1218–1227

Chang KW, Lin SC, Mangold KA, Jean MS, Yuan TC, Lin SN, Chang CS (2000) Alterations of adenomatous polyposis Coli (APC) gene in oral squamous cell carcinoma. Int J Oral Maxillofac Surg 29:223–226

Chen G, Shukeir N, Potti A, Sircar K, Aprikian A, Goltzman D, Rabbani SA (2004) Up-regulation of Wnt-1 and beta-catenin production in patients with advanced metastatic prostate carcinoma: potential pathogenetic and prognostic implications. Cancer 101:1345–1356

Chen XY, Wang ZC, Li H, Cheng XX, Sun Y, Wang XW, Wu ML, Liu J (2005) Nuclear translocations of beta-catenin and TCF4 in gastric cancers correlate with lymph node metastasis but probably not with CD44 expression. Hum Pathol 36:1294–1301

Chen K, Fallen S, Abaan HO, Hayran M, Gonzalez C, Wodajo F, MacDonald T, Toretsky JA, Uren A (2008) Wnt10b induces chemotaxis of osteosarcoma and correlates with reduced survival. Pediatr Blood Cancer 51:349–355

Cheng XX, Wang ZC, Chen XY, Sun Y, Kong QY, Liu J, Li H (2005) Correlation of Wnt-2 expression and beta-catenin intracellular accumulation in Chinese gastric cancers: relevance with tumour dissemination. Cancer Lett 223:339–347

Chesire DR, Ewing CM, Sauvageot J, Bova GS, Isaacs WB (2000) Detection and analysis of beta-catenin mutations in prostate cancer. Prostate 45:323–334

Chetty R, Serra S, Salahshor S, Alsaad K, Shih W, Blaszyk H, Woodgett JR, Tsao MS (2006) Expression of Wnt-signaling pathway proteins in intraductal papillary mucinous neoplasms of the pancreas: a tissue microarray analysis. Hum Pathol 37:212–217

Chien AJ, Moore EC, Lonsdorf AS, Kulikauskas RM, Rothberg BG, Berger AJ, Major MB, Hwang ST, Rimm DL, Moon RT (2009) Activated Wnt/beta-catenin signaling in melanoma is associated with decreased proliferation in patient tumors and a murine melanoma model. Proc Natl Acad Sci U S A 106:1193–1198

Clark SK, Neale KF, Landgrebe JC, Phillips RK (1999) Desmoid tumours complicating familial adenomatous polyposis. Br J Surg 86:1185–1189

Clements WM, Wang J, Sarnaik A, Kim OJ, MacDonald J, Fenoglio-Preiser C, Groden J, Lowy AM (2002) Beta-catenin mutation is a frequent cause of Wnt pathway activation in gastric cancer. Cancer Res 62:3503–3506

Coutinho-Camillo CM, Miracca EC, dos Santos ML, Salaorni S, Sarkis AS, Nagai MA (2006) Identification of differentially expressed genes in prostatic epithelium in relation to androgen receptor CAG repeat length. Int J Biol Markers 21:96–105

Couture J, Mitri A, Lagace R, Smits R, Berk T, Bouchard HL, Fodde R, Alman B, Bapat B (2000) A germline mutation at the extreme 3' end of the APC gene results in a severe desmoid phenotype and is associated with overexpression of beta-catenin in the desmoid tumor. Clin Genet 57:205–212

Cui J, Zhou X, Liu Y, Tang Z, Romeih M (2003) Wnt signaling in hepatocellular carcinoma: analysis of mutation and expression of beta-catenin, T-cell factor-4 and glycogen synthase kinase 3-beta genes. J Gastroenterol Hepatol 18:280–287

Cuilliere-Dartigues P, El-Bchiri J, Krimi A, Buhard O, Fontanges P, Flejou JF, Hamelin R, Duval A (2006) TCF-4 isoforms absent in TCF-4 mutated MSI-H colorectal cancer cells colocalize with nuclear CtBP and repress TCF-4-mediated transcription. Oncogene 25:4441–4448

Da Forno PD, Pringle JH, Hutchinson P, Osborn J, Huang Q, Potter L, Hancox RA, Fletcher A, Saldanha GS (2008) WNT5A expression increases during melanoma progression and correlates with outcome. Clin Cancer Res 14:5825–5832

Dahl E, Wiesmann F, Woenckhaus M, Stoehr R, Wild PJ, Veeck J, Knuchel R, Klopocki E, Sauter G, Simon R, Wieland WF, Walter B, Denzinger S, Hartmann A, Hammerschmied CG (2007) Frequent loss of SFRP1 expression in multiple human solid tumours: association with aberrant promoter methylation in renal cell carcinoma. Oncogene 26:5680–5691

Dahmen RP, Koch A, Denkhaus D, Tonn JC, Sorensen N, Berthold F, Behrens J, Birchmeier W, Wiestler OD, Pietsch T (2001) Deletions of AXIN1, a component of the WNT/wingless pathway, in sporadic medulloblastomas. Cancer Res 61:7039–7043

Dai Y, Bedrossian CW, Michael CW (2005) The expression pattern of beta-catenin in mesothelial proliferative lesions and its diagnostic utilities. Diagn Cytopathol 33:320–324

De Filippo C, Luceri C, Caderni G, Pacini M, Messerini L, Biggeri A, Mini E, Tonelli F, Cianchi F, Dolara P (2002) Mutations of the APC gene in human sporadic colorectal cancers. Scand J Gastroenterol 37:1048–1053

de La Coste A, Romagnolo B, Billuart P, Renard CA, Buendia MA, Soubrane O, Fabre M, Chelly J, Beldjord C, Kahn A, Perret C (1998) Somatic mutations of the beta-catenin gene are frequent in mouse and human hepatocellular carcinomas. Proc Natl Acad Sci U S A 95:8847–8851

de la Taille A, Rubin MA, Chen MW, Vacherot F, de Medina SG, Burchardt M, Buttyan R, Chopin D (2003) Beta-catenin-related anomalies in apoptosis-resistant and hormone-refractory prostate cancer cells. Clin Cancer Res 9:1801–1807

Demunter A, Libbrecht L, Degreef H, De Wolf-Peeters C, van den Oord JJ (2002) Loss of membranous expression of beta-catenin is associated with tumor progression in cutaneous melanoma and rarely caused by exon 3 mutations. Mod Pathol 15:454–461

Diaz Prado SM, Medina Villaamil V, Aparicio Gallego G, Blanco Calvo M, Lopez Cedrun JL, Sironvalle Soliva S, Valladares Ayerbes M, Garcia Campelo R, Anton Aparicio LM (2009) Expression of Wnt gene family and frizzled receptors in head and neck squamous cell carcinomas. Virchows Arch 455:67–75

Diergaarde B, van Geloof WL, van Muijen GN, Kok FJ, Kampman E (2003) Dietary factors and the occurrence of truncating APC mutations in sporadic colon carcinomas: a Dutch population-based study. Carcinogenesis 24:283–290

DiMeo TA, Anderson K, Phadke P, Fan C, Perou CM, Naber S, Kuperwasser C (2009) A novel lung metastasis signature links Wnt signaling with cancer cell self-renewal and epithelial-mesenchymal transition in basal-like breast cancer. Cancer Res 69:5364–5373

Ding Z, Qian YB, Zhu LX, Xiong QR (2009) Promoter methylation and mRNA expression of DKK-3 and WIF-1 in hepatocellular carcinoma. World J Gastroenterol 15:2595–2601

Doglioni C, Piccinin S, Demontis S, Cangi MG, Pecciarini L, Chiarelli C, Armellin M, Vukosavljevic T, Boiocchi M, Maestro R (2003) Alterations of beta-catenin pathway in non-melanoma skin tumors: loss of alpha-ABC nuclear reactivity correlates with the presence of beta-catenin gene mutation. Am J Pathol 163:2277–2287

Drake J, Shearwood AM, White J, Friis R, Zeps N, Charles A, Dharmarajan A (2009) Expression of secreted frizzled-related protein 4 (SFRP4) in primary serous ovarian tumours. Eur J Gynaecol Oncol 30:133–141

Dulaimi E, Hillinck J, Ibanez de Caceres I, Al-Saleem T, Cairns P (2004) Tumor suppressor gene promoter hypermethylation in serum of breast cancer patients. Clin Cancer Res 10:6189–6193

Durand M, Moles JP (1999) Beta-catenin mutations in a common skin cancer: pilomatricoma. Bull Cancer 86:725–726

Duval A, Gayet J, Zhou XP, Iacopetta B, Thomas G, Hamelin R (1999) Frequent frameshift mutations of the TCF-4 gene in colorectal cancers with microsatellite instability. Cancer Res 59:4213–4215

Eberhart CG, Tihan T, Burger PC (2000) Nuclear localization and mutation of beta-catenin in medulloblastomas. J Neuropathol Exp Neurol 59:333–337

Ebert MP, Fei G, Kahmann S, Muller O, Yu J, Sung JJ, Malfertheiner P (2002) Increased beta-catenin mRNA levels and mutational alterations of the APC and beta-catenin gene are present in intestinal-type gastric cancer. Carcinogenesis 23:87–91

Edamoto Y, Hara A, Biernat W, Terracciano L, Cathomas G, Riehle HM, Matsuda M, Fujii H, Scoazec JY, Ohgaki H (2003) Alterations of RB1, p53 and Wnt pathways in hepatocellular carcinomas associated with hepatitis C, hepatitis B and alcoholic liver cirrhosis. Int J Cancer 106:334–341

Ellison DW, Onilude OE, Lindsey JC, Lusher ME, Weston CL, Taylor RE, Pearson AD, Clifford SC (2005) beta-Catenin status predicts a favorable outcome in childhood medulloblastoma: the United Kingdom Children's Cancer Study Group Brain Tumour Committee. J Clin Oncol 23:7951–7957

Elston MS, Gill AJ, Conaglen JV, Clarkson A, Shaw JM, Law AJ, Cook RJ, Little NS, Clifton-Bligh RJ, Robinson BG, McDonald KL (2008) Wnt pathway inhibitors are strongly down-regulated in pituitary tumors. Endocrinology 149:1235–1242

Endo Y, Beauchamp E, Woods D, Taylor WG, Toretsky JA, Uren A, Rubin JS (2008) Wnt-3a and Dickkopf-1 stimulate neurite outgrowth in Ewing tumor cells via a Frizzled3- and c-Jun N-terminal kinase-dependent mechanism. Mol Cell Biol 28:2368–2379

Entz-Werle N, Lavaux T, Metzger N, Stoetzel C, Lasthaus C, Marec P, Kalifa C, Brugieres L, Pacquement H, Schmitt C, Tabone MD, Gentet JC, Lutz P, Babin A, Oudet P, Gaub MP, Perrin-Schmitt F (2007) Involvement of MET/TWIST/APC combination or the potential role of ossification factors in pediatric high-grade osteosarcoma oncogenesis. Neoplasia 9:678–688

Esteller M, Sparks A, Toyota M, Sanchez-Cespedes M, Capella G, Peinado MA, Gonzalez S, Tarafa G, Sidransky D, Meltzer SJ, Baylin SB, Herman JG (2000) Analysis of adenomatous polyposis coli promoter hypermethylation in human cancer. Cancer Res 60:4366–4371

Ferrazzo KL, Neto MM, dos Santos E, dos Santos PD, de Sousa SO (2009) Differential expression of galectin-3, beta-catenin, and cyclin D1 in adenoid cystic carcinoma and polymorphous low-grade adenocarcinoma of salivary glands. J Oral Pathol Med 38:701–707

Forget MA, Turcotte S, Beauseigle D, Godin-Ethier J, Pelletier S, Martin J, Tanguay S, Lapointe R (2007) The Wnt pathway regulator DKK1 is preferentially expressed in hormone-resistant breast tumours and in some common cancer types. Br J Cancer 96:646–653

Fukuchi T, Sakamoto M, Tsuda H, Maruyama K, Nozawa S, Hirohashi S (1998) Beta-catenin mutation in carcinoma of the uterine endometrium. Cancer Res 58:3526–3528

Fukui T, Kondo M, Ito G, Maeda O, Sato N, Yoshioka H, Yokoi K, Ueda Y, Shimokata K, Sekido Y (2005) Transcriptional silencing of secreted frizzled related protein 1 (SFRP 1) by promoter hypermethylation in non-small-cell lung cancer. Oncogene 24:6323–6327

Fukukawa C, Nagayama S, Tsunoda T, Toguchida J, Nakamura Y, Katagiri T (2009) Activation of the non-canonical Dvl-Rac1-JNK pathway by Frizzled homologue 10 in human synovial sarcoma. Oncogene 28:1110–1120

Fukushima H, Yamamoto H, Itoh F, Horiuchi S, Min Y, Iku S, Imai K (2001) Frequent alterations of the beta-catenin and TCF-4 genes, but not of the APC gene, in colon cancers with high-frequency microsatellite instability. J Exp Clin Cancer Res 20:553–559

Fukuzawa R, Anaka MR, Heathcott RW, McNoe LA, Morison IM, Perlman EJ, Reeve AE (2008) Wilms tumour histology is determined by distinct types of precursor lesions and not epigenetic changes. J Pathol 215:377–387

Furuuchi K, Tada M, Yamada H, Kataoka A, Furuuchi N, Hamada J, Takahashi M, Todo S, Moriuchi T (2000) Somatic mutations of the APC gene in primary breast cancers. Am J Pathol 156:1997–2005

Garcia-Rostan G, Camp RL, Herrero A, Carcangiu ML, Rimm DL, Tallini G (2001) Beta-catenin dysregulation in thyroid neoplasms: down-regulation, aberrant nuclear expression, and CTNNB1 exon 3 mutations are markers for aggressive tumor phenotypes and poor prognosis. Am J Pathol 158:987–996

Gaujoux S, Tissier F, Groussin L, Libe R, Ragazzon B, Launay P, Audebourg A, Dousset B, Bertagna X, Bertherat J (2008) Wnt/beta-catenin and 3', 5'-cyclic adenosine 5'-monophosphate/

protein kinase A signaling pathways alterations and somatic beta-catenin gene mutations in the progression of adrenocortical tumors. J Clin Endocrinol Metab 93:4135–4140

Gebert C, Hardes J, Kersting C, August C, Supper H, Winkelmann W, Buerger H, Gosheger G (2007) Expression of beta-catenin and p53 are prognostic factors in deep aggressive fibromatosis. Histopathology 50:491–497

Gerstein AV, Almeida TA, Zhao G, Chess E, Shih Ie M, Buhler K, Pienta K, Rubin MA, Vessella R, Papadopoulos N (2002) APC/CTNNB1 (beta-catenin) pathway alterations in human prostate cancers. Genes Chromosomes Cancer 34:9–16

Goss KH, Groden J (2000) Biology of the adenomatous polyposis coli tumor suppressor. J Clin Oncol 18:1967–1979

Goto M, Mitra RS, Liu M, Lee J, Henson BS, Carey T, Bradford C, Prince M, Wang CY, Fearon ER, D'Silva NJ (2010) Rap1 stabilizes beta-catenin and enhances beta-catenin-dependent transcription and invasion in squamous cell carcinoma of the head and neck. Clin Cancer Res 16:65–76

Gotze S, Wolter M, Reifenberger G, Muller O, Sievers S (2010) Frequent promoter hypermethylation of Wnt pathway inhibitor genes in malignant astrocytic gliomas. Int J Cancer 126:2584–2593

Grabsch H, Takeno S, Noguchi T, Hommel G, Gabbert HE, Mueller W (2001) Different patterns of beta-catenin expression in gastric carcinomas: relationship with clinicopathological parameters and prognostic outcome. Histopathology 39:141–149

Gregorieff A, Clevers H (2005) Wnt signaling in the intestinal epithelium: from endoderm to cancer. Genes Dev 19:877–890

Groden J, Thliveris A, Samowitz W, Carlson M, Gelbert L, Albertsen H, Joslyn G, Stevens J, Spirio L, Robertson M, Sargeant L, Krapcho K, Wolff E, Burt R, Hughes J, Warrington J, McPherson J, Wasmuth J, Le Paslier D, Abderrahim H, Cohen D, Leppert M, White R (1991) Identification and characterization of the familial adenomatous polyposis coli gene. Cell 66:589–600

Gruner BA, DeNapoli TS, Andrews W, Tomlinson G, Bowman L, Weitman SD (1998) Hepatocellular carcinoma in children associated with Gardner syndrome or familial adenomatous polyposis. J Pediatr Hematol Oncol 20:274–278

Guo Y, Xie J, Rubin E, Tang YX, Lin F, Zi X, Hoang BH (2008) Frzb, a secreted Wnt antagonist, decreases growth and invasiveness of fibrosarcoma cells associated with inhibition of Met signaling. Cancer Res 68:3350–3360

Guo G, Mao X, Wang P, Liu B, Zhang X, Jiang X, Zhong C, Huo J, Jin J, Zhuo Y (2010) The expression profile of FRAT1 in human gliomas. Brain Res 1320:152–158

Gurbuz AK, Giardiello FM, Petersen GM, Krush AJ, Offerhaus GJ, Booker SV, Kerr MC, Hamilton SR (1994) Desmoid tumours in familial adenomatous polyposis. Gut 35:377–381

Hall CL, Bafico A, Dai J, Aaronson SA, Keller ET (2005) Prostate cancer cells promote osteoblastic bone metastases through Wnts. Cancer Res 65:7554–7560

Hall CL, Daignault SD, Shah RB, Pienta KJ, Keller ET (2008) Dickkopf-1 expression increases early in prostate cancer development and decreases during progression from primary tumor to metastasis. Prostate 68:1396–1404

Hamilton SR, Liu B, Parsons RE, Papadopoulos N, Jen J, Powell SM, Krush AJ, Berk T, Cohen Z, Tetu B et al (1995) The molecular basis of Turcot's syndrome. N Engl J Med 332:839–847

Han JC, Zhang KL, Chen XY, Jiang HF, Kong QY, Sun Y, Wu ML, Huang L, Li H, Liu J (2007) Expression of seven gastric cancer-associated genes and its relevance for Wnt, NF-kappaB and Stat3 signaling. APMIS 115:1331–1343

Hassanein AM, Glanz SM (2004) Beta-catenin expression in benign and malignant pilomatrix neoplasms. Br J Dermatol 150:511–516

Haydon RC, Deyrup A, Ishikawa A, Heck R, Jiang W, Zhou L, Feng T, King D, Cheng H, Breyer B, Peabody T, Simon MA, Montag AG, He TC (2002) Cytoplasmic and/or nuclear accumulation of the beta-catenin protein is a frequent event in human osteosarcoma. Int J Cancer 102:338–342

Hayes MJ, Thomas D, Emmons A, Giordano TJ, Kleer CG (2008) Genetic changes of Wnt pathway genes are common events in metaplastic carcinomas of the breast. Clin Cancer Res 14:4038–4044

Hendrix ND, Wu R, Kuick R, Schwartz DR, Fearon ER, Cho KR (2006) Fibroblast growth factor 9 has oncogenic activity and is a downstream target of Wnt signaling in ovarian endometrioid adenocarcinomas. Cancer Res 66:1354–1362

Henrique R, Ribeiro FR, Fonseca D, Hoque MO, Carvalho AL, Costa VL, Pinto M, Oliveira J, Teixeira MR, Sidransky D, Jeronimo C (2007) High promoter methylation levels of APC predict poor prognosis in sextant biopsies from prostate cancer patients. Clin Cancer Res 13:6122–6129

Hiltunen MO, Alhonen L, Koistinaho J, Myohanen S, Paakkonen M, Marin S, Kosma VM, Janne J (1997) Hypermethylation of the APC (adenomatous polyposis coli) gene promoter region in human colorectal carcinoma. Int J Cancer 70:644–648

Hirata H, Hinoda Y, Nakajima K, Kawamoto K, Kikuno N, Kawakami K, Yamamura S, Ueno K, Majid S, Saini S, Ishii N, Dahiya R (2009) Wnt antagonist gene DKK2 is epigenetically silenced and inhibits renal cancer progression through apoptotic and cell cycle pathways. Clin Cancer Res 15:5678–5687

Hirata H, Hinoda Y, Ueno K, Majid S, Saini S, Dahiya R (2010) Role of secreted frizzled-related protein 3 in human renal cell carcinoma. Cancer Res 70:1896–1905

Ho KY, Kalle WH, Lo TH, Lam WY, Tang CM (1999) Reduced expression of APC and DCC gene protein in breast cancer. Histopathology 35:249–256

Hoang BH, Kubo T, Healey JH, Sowers R, Mazza B, Yang R, Huvos AG, Meyers PA, Gorlick R (2004) Expression of LDL receptor-related protein 5 (LRP5) as a novel marker for disease progression in high-grade osteosarcoma. Int J Cancer 109:106–111

Hoban PR, Cowen RL, Mitchell EL, Evans DG, Kelly M, Howard PJ, Heighway J (1997) Physical localisation of the breakpoints of a constitutional translocation t(5;6)(q21;q21) in a child with bilateral Wilms' tumour. J Med Genet 34:343–345

Holcombe RF, Marsh JL, Waterman ML, Lin F, Milovanovic T, Truong T (2002) Expression of Wnt ligands and Frizzled receptors in colonic mucosa and in colon carcinoma. Mol Pathol 55:220–226

Hommura F, Furuuchi K, Yamazaki K, Ogura S, Kinoshita I, Shimizu M, Moriuchi T, Katoh H, Nishimura M, Dosaka-Akita H (2002) Increased expression of beta-catenin predicts better prognosis in nonsmall cell lung carcinomas. Cancer 94:752–758

Horii A, Nakatsuru S, Miyoshi Y, Ichii S, Nagase H, Kato Y, Yanagisawa A, Nakamura Y (1992) The APC gene, responsible for familial adenomatous polyposis, is mutated in human gastric cancer. Cancer Res 52:3231–3233

Horvath LG, Henshall SM, Kench JG, Saunders DN, Lee CS, Golovsky D, Brenner PC, O'Neill GF, Kooner R, Stricker PD, Grygiel JJ, Sutherland RL (2004) Membranous expression of secreted frizzled-related protein 4 predicts for good prognosis in localized prostate cancer and inhibits PC3 cellular proliferation in vitro. Clin Cancer Res 10:615–625

Horvath LG, Lelliott JE, Kench JG, Lee CS, Williams ED, Saunders DN, Grygiel JJ, Sutherland RL, Henshall SM (2007) Secreted frizzled-related protein 4 inhibits proliferation and metastatic potential in prostate cancer. Prostate 67:1081–1090

Hovanes K, Li TW, Munguia JE, Truong T, Milovanovic T, Lawrence Marsh J, Holcombe RF, Waterman ML (2001) Beta-catenin-sensitive isoforms of lymphoid enhancer factor-1 are selectively expressed in colon cancer. Nat Genet 28:53–57

Howng SL, Wu CH, Cheng TS, Sy WD, Lin PC, Wang C, Hong YR (2002) Differential expression of Wnt genes, beta-catenin and E-cadherin in human brain tumors. Cancer Lett 183:95–101

Hrzenjak A, Tippl M, Kremser ML, Strohmeier B, Guelly C, Neumeister D, Lax S, Moinfar F, Tabrizi AD, Isadi-Moud N, Zatloukal K, Denk H (2004) Inverse correlation of secreted frizzled-related protein 4 and beta-catenin expression in endometrial stromal sarcomas. J Pathol 204:19–27

Huang J, Papadopoulos N, McKinley AJ, Farrington SM, Curtis LJ, Wyllie AH, Zheng S, Willson JK, Markowitz SD, Morin P, Kinzler KW, Vogelstein B, Dunlop MG (1996) APC mutations in colorectal tumors with mismatch repair deficiency. Proc Natl Acad Sci U S A 93:9049–9054

Huang H, Mahler-Araujo BM, Sankila A, Chimelli L, Yonekawa Y, Kleihues P, Ohgaki H (2000) APC mutations in sporadic medulloblastomas. Am J Pathol 156:433–437

Huang CL, Liu D, Nakano J, Ishikawa S, Kontani K, Yokomise H, Ueno M (2005) Wnt5a expression is associated with the tumor proliferation and the stromal vascular endothelial growth factor – an expression in non-small-cell lung cancer. J Clin Oncol 23:8765–8773

Huang L, Zhang KL, Li H, Chen XY, Kong QY, Sun Y, Gao X, Guan HW, Liu J (2006) Infrequent COX-2 expression due to promoter hypermethylation in gastric cancers in Dalian, China. Hum Pathol 37:1557–1567

Huang J, Zhang YL, Teng XM, Lin Y, Zheng DL, Yang PY, Han ZG (2007) Down-regulation of SFRP1 as a putative tumor suppressor gene can contribute to human hepatocellular carcinoma. BMC Cancer 7:126

Huang CL, Liu D, Ishikawa S, Nakashima T, Nakashima N, Yokomise H, Kadota K, Ueno M (2008) Wnt1 overexpression promotes tumour progression in non-small cell lung cancer. Eur J Cancer 44:2680–2688

Hughes LJ, Michels VV (1992) Risk of hepatoblastoma in familial adenomatous polyposis. Am J Med Genet 43:1023–1025

Huguet EL, McMahon JA, McMahon AP, Bicknell R, Harris AL (1994) Differential expression of human Wnt genes 2, 3, 4, and 7B in human breast cell lines and normal and disease states of human breast tissue. Cancer Res 54:2615–2621

Ikeda T, Yoshinaga K, Semba S, Kondo E, Ohmori H, Horii A (2000) Mutational analysis of the CTNNB1 (beta-catenin) gene in human endometrial cancer: frequent mutations at codon 34 that cause nuclear accumulation. Oncol Rep 7:323–326

Iozzo RV, Eichstetter I, Danielson KG (1995) Aberrant expression of the growth factor Wnt-5A in human malignancy. Cancer Res 55:3495–3499

Ishigaki K, Namba H, Nakashima M, Nakayama T, Mitsutake N, Hayashi T, Maeda S, Ichinose M, Kanematsu T, Yamashita S (2002) Aberrant localization of beta-catenin correlates with overexpression of its target gene in human papillary thyroid cancer. J Clin Endocrinol Metab 87:3433–3440

Ishizaki Y, Ikeda S, Fujimori M, Shimizu Y, Kurihara T, Itamoto T, Kikuchi A, Okajima M, Asahara T (2004) Immunohistochemical analysis and mutational analyses of beta-catenin, Axin family and APC genes in hepatocellular carcinomas. Int J Oncol 24:1077–1083

Janssens N, Andries L, Janicot M, Perera T, Bakker A (2004) Alteration of frizzled expression in renal cell carcinoma. Tumour Biol 25:161–171

Jeng YM, Wu MZ, Mao TL, Chang MH, Hsu HC (2000) Somatic mutations of beta-catenin play a crucial role in the tumorigenesis of sporadic hepatoblastoma. Cancer Lett 152:45–51

Jeronimo C, Henrique R, Hoque MO, Mambo E, Ribeiro FR, Varzim G, Oliveira J, Teixeira MR, Lopes C, Sidransky D (2004) A quantitative promoter methylation profile of prostate cancer. Clin Cancer Res 10:8472–8478

Jesse S, Koenig A, Ellenrieder V, Menke A (2010) Lef-1 isoforms regulate different target genes and reduce cellular adhesion. Int J Cancer 126:1109–1120

Jiang Y, Zhou XD, Liu YK, Wu X, Huang XW (2002) Association of hTcf-4 gene expression and mutation with clinicopathological characteristics of hepatocellular carcinoma. World J Gastroenterol 8:804–807

Jin Z, Tamura G, Tsuchiya T, Sakata K, Kashiwaba M, Osakabe M, Motoyama T (2001) Adenomatous polyposis coli (APC) gene promoter hypermethylation in primary breast cancers. Br J Cancer 85:69–73

Joesting MS, Perrin S, Elenbaas B, Fawell SE, Rubin JS, Franco OE, Hayward SW, Cunha GR, Marker PC (2005) Identification of SFRP1 as a candidate mediator of stromal-to-epithelial signaling in prostate cancer. Cancer Res 65:10423–10430

Jonsson M, Borg A, Nilbert M, Andersson T (2000) Involvement of adenomatous polyposis coli (APC)/beta-catenin signalling in human breast cancer. Eur J Cancer 36:242–248

Joslyn G, Carlson M, Thliveris A, Albertsen H, Gelbert L, Samowitz W, Groden J, Stevens J, Spirio L, Robertson M, Krapcho K, Sargeant L, Wolff E, Burt R, Hughes JP, Warrington J, McPherson J, Wasmuth J, Le Paslier D, Abderrahim H, Cohen D, Leppert M, White R (1991) Identification of deletion mutations and three new genes at the familial polyposis locus. Cell 66:601–613

Jozwiak J, Kotulska K, Grajkowska W, Jozwiak S, Zalewski W, Oldak M, Lojek M, Rainko K, Maksym R, Lazarczyk M, Skopinski P, Wlodarski P (2007) Upregulation of the WNT pathway in tuberous sclerosis-associated subependymal giant cell astrocytomas. Brain Dev 29:273–280

Juhlin CC, Haglund F, Villablanca A, Forsberg L, Sandelin K, Branstrom R, Larsson C, Hoog A (2009) Loss of expression for the Wnt pathway components adenomatous polyposis coli and glycogen synthase kinase 3-beta in parathyroid carcinomas. Int J Oncol 34:481–492

Kageshita T, Hamby CV, Ishihara T, Matsumoto K, Saida T, Ono T (2001) Loss of beta-catenin expression associated with disease progression in malignant melanoma. Br J Dermatol 145:210–216

Kanzaki H, Ouchida M, Hanafusa H, Yano M, Suzuki H, Aoe M, Imai K, Shimizu N, Nakachi K, Shimizu K (2006) Single nucleotide polymorphism of the AXIN2 gene is preferentially associated with human lung cancer risk in a Japanese population. Int J Mol Med 18:279–284

Karbova E, Davidson B, Metodiev K, Trope CG, Nesland JM (2002) Adenomatous polyposis coli (APC) protein expression in primary and metastatic serous ovarian carcinoma. Int J Surg Pathol 10:175–180

Kashiwaba M, Tamura G, Ishida M (1994) Aberrations of the APC gene in primary breast carcinoma. J Cancer Res Clin Oncol 120:727–731

Kastritis E, Murray S, Kyriakou F, Horti M, Tamvakis N, Kavantzas N, Patsouris ES, Noni A, Legaki S, Dimopoulos MA, Bamias A (2009) Somatic mutations of adenomatous polyposis coli gene and nuclear b-catenin accumulation have prognostic significance in invasive urothelial carcinomas: evidence for Wnt pathway implication. Int J Cancer 124:103–108

Katoh M (2001) Frequent up-regulation of WNT2 in primary gastric cancer and colorectal cancer. Int J Oncol 19:1003–1007

Kawakami K, Hirata H, Yamamura S, Kikuno N, Saini S, Majid S, Tanaka Y, Kawamoto K, Enokida H, Nakagawa M, Dahiya R (2009) Functional significance of Wnt inhibitory factor-1 gene in kidney cancer. Cancer Res 69:8603–8610

Kawakami K, Yamamura S, Hirata H, Ueno K, Saini S, Majid S, Tanaka Y, Kawamoto K, Enokida H, Nakagawa M, Dahiya R (2011) Secreted frizzled-related protein-5 (sFRP-5) is epigenetically downregulated and functions as a tumor suppressor in kidney cancer. Int J Cancer 128:541–550

Kawano Y, Kitaoka M, Hamada Y, Walker MM, Waxman J, Kypta RM (2006) Regulation of prostate cell growth and morphogenesis by Dickkopf-3. Oncogene 25:6528–6537

Khramtsov AI, Khramtsova GF, Tretiakova M, Huo D, Olopade OI, Goss KH (2010) Wnt/{beta}-catenin pathway activation is enriched in basal-like breast cancers and predicts poor outcome. Am J Pathol 176:2911–2920

Kielhorn E, Provost E, Olsen D, D'Aquila TG, Smith BL, Camp RL, Rimm DL (2003) Tissue microarray-based analysis shows phospho-beta-catenin expression in malignant melanoma is associated with poor outcome. Int J Cancer 103:652–656

Kildal W, Risberg B, Abeler VM, Kristensen GB, Sudbo J, Nesland JM, Danielsen HE (2005) beta-catenin expression, DNA ploidy and clinicopathological features in ovarian cancer: a study in 253 patients. Eur J Cancer 41:1127–1134

Kildal W, Pradhan M, Abeler VM, Kristensen GB, Danielsen HE (2009) Beta-catenin expression in uterine sarcomas and its relation to clinicopathological parameters. Eur J Cancer 45:2412–2417

Kim YS, Kang YK, Kim JB, Han SA, Kim KI, Paik SR (2000) Beta-catenin expression and mutational analysis in renal cell carcinomas. Pathol Int 50:725–730

Kim HS, Hong EK, Park SY, Kim WH, Lee HS (2003) Expression of beta-catenin and E-cadherin in the adenoma-carcinoma sequence of the stomach. Anticancer Res 23:2863–2868

Kim YD, Park CH, Kim HS, Choi SK, Rew JS, Kim DY, Koh YS, Jeung KW, Lee KH, Lee JS, Juhng SW, Lee JH (2008) Genetic alterations of Wnt signaling pathway-associated genes in hepatocellular carcinoma. J Gastroenterol Hepatol 23:110–118

Kim B, Byun SJ, Kim YA, Kim JE, Lee BL, Kim WH, Chang MS (2010) Cell cycle regulators, APC/beta-catenin, NF-kappaB and Epstein-Barr virus in gastric carcinomas. Pathology 42:58–65

Kinzler K, Nilbert MC, Su L-K, Vogelstein B, Bryan TM, Levy DB, Smith KJ, Preisinger AM, Hedge P, McKechnie D, Finniear R, Markham A, Groffen J, Boguski MS, Altschul SF, Horii A, Ando H, Miyoshi Y, Miki Y, Nishisho I, Nakamura Y (1991) Identification of FAP locus genes from chromosome 5q21. Science 253:661–665

Kirikoshi H, Inoue S, Sekihara H, Katoh M (2001a) Expression of WNT10A in human cancer. Int J Oncol 19:997–1001

Kirikoshi H, Sekihara H, Katoh M (2001b) Expression profiles of 10 members of Frizzled gene family in human gastric cancer. Int J Oncol 19:767–771

Kirikoshi H, Sekihara H, Katoh M (2001c) Up-regulation of Frizzled-7 (FZD7) in human gastric cancer. Int J Oncol 19:111–115

Kirikoshi H, Sekihara H, Katoh M (2001d) Up-regulation of WNT10A by tumor necrosis factor alpha and Helicobacter pylori in gastric cancer. Int J Oncol 19:533–536

Kizildag S, Zengel B, Vardar E, Sakizli M (2008) Beta-catenin gene mutation in invasive ductal breast cancer. J BUON 13:533–536

Klopocki E, Kristiansen G, Wild PJ, Klaman I, Castanos-Velez E, Singer G, Stohr R, Simon R, Sauter G, Leibiger H, Essers L, Weber B, Hermann K, Rosenthal A, Hartmann A, Dahl E (2004) Loss of SFRP1 is associated with breast cancer progression and poor prognosis in early stage tumors. Int J Oncol 25:641–649

Kobayashi K, Sagae S, Nishioka Y, Tokino T, Kudo R (1999) Mutations of the beta-catenin gene in endometrial carcinomas. Jpn J Cancer Res 90:55–59

Koch A, Denkhaus D, Albrecht S, Leuschner I, von Schweinitz D, Pietsch T (1999) Childhood hepatoblastomas frequently carry a mutated degradation targeting box of the beta-catenin gene. Cancer Res 59:269–273

Koch A, Waha A, Tonn JC, Sorensen N, Berthold F, Wolter M, Reifenberger J, Hartmann W, Reifenberger G, Wiestler OD, Pietsch T (2001) Somatic mutations of WNT/wingless signaling pathway components in primitive neuroectodermal tumors. Int J Cancer 93:445–449

Koesters R, Ridder R, Kopp-Schneider A, Betts D, Adams V, Niggli F, Briner J, von Knebel DM (1999) Mutational activation of the beta-catenin proto-oncogene is a common event in the development of Wilms' tumors. Cancer Res 59:3880–3882

Koesters R, Niggli F, von Knebel DM, Stallmach T (2003) Nuclear accumulation of beta-catenin protein in Wilms' tumours. J Pathol 199:68–76

Koinuma K, Yamashita Y, Liu W, Hatanaka H, Kurashina K, Wada T, Takada S, Kaneda R, Choi YL, Fujiwara SI, Miyakura Y, Nagai H, Mano H (2006) Epigenetic silencing of AXIN2 in colorectal carcinoma with microsatellite instability. Oncogene 25:139–146

Kongkham PN, Northcott PA, Croul SE, Smith CA, Taylor MD, Rutka JT (2010) The SFRP family of WNT inhibitors function as novel tumor suppressor genes epigenetically silenced in medulloblastoma. Oncogene 29:3017–3024

Konishi M, Kikuchi-Yanoshita R, Tanaka K, Muraoka M, Onda A, Okumura Y, Kishi N, Iwama T, Mori T, Koike M, Ushio K, Chiba M, Nomizu S, Konishi F, Utsunomiya J, Miyaki M (1996) Molecular nature of colon tumors in hereditary nonpolyposis colon cancer, familial polyposis, and sporadic colon cancer. Gastroenterology 111:307–317

Konopka B, Janiec-Jankowska A, Czapczak D, Paszko Z, Bidzinski M, Olszewski W, Goluda C (2007) Molecular genetic defects in endometrial carcinomas: microsatellite instability, PTEN and beta-catenin (CTNNB1) genes mutations. J Cancer Res Clin Oncol 133:361–371

Kool M, Koster J, Bunt J, Hasselt NE, Lakeman A, van Sluis P, Troost D, Meeteren NS, Caron HN, Cloos J, Mrsic A, Ylstra B, Grajkowska W, Hartmann W, Pietsch T, Ellison D, Clifford SC, Versteeg R (2008) Integrated genomics identifies five medulloblastoma subtypes with distinct genetic profiles, pathway signatures and clinicopathological features. PLoS One 3:e3088

Korabiowska M, Schlott T, Siems N, Muller A, Cordon-Cardo C, Fischer G, Brinck U (2004) Analysis of adenomatous polyposis coli gene expression, APC locus-microsatellite instability and APC promoter methylation in the progression of melanocytic tumours. Mod Pathol 17:1539–1544

Kremenevskaja N, von Wasielewski R, Rao AS, Schofl C, Andersson T, Brabant G (2005) Wnt-5a has tumor suppressor activity in thyroid carcinoma. Oncogene 24:2144–2154

Kren L, Hermanova M, Goncharuk VN, Kaur P, Ross JS, Pavlovsky Z, Dvorak K (2003) Downregulation of plasma membrane expression/cytoplasmic accumulation of beta-catenin predicts shortened survival in non-small cell lung cancer. A clinicopathologic study of 100 cases. Cesk Patol 39:17–20

Kuphal S, Lodermeyer S, Bataille F, Schuierer M, Hoang BH, Bosserhoff AK (2006) Expression of Dickkopf genes is strongly reduced in malignant melanoma. Oncogene 25:5027–5036

Kurahashi H, Takami K, Oue T, Kusafuka T, Okada A, Tawa A, Okada S, Nishisho I (1995) Biallelic inactivation of the APC gene in hepatoblastoma. Cancer Res 55:5007–5011

Kurayoshi M, Oue N, Yamamoto H, Kishida M, Inoue A, Asahara T, Yasui W, Kikuchi A (2006) Expression of Wnt-5a is correlated with aggressiveness of gastric cancer by stimulating cell migration and invasion. Cancer Res 66:10439–10448

Kurihara T, Ikeda S, Ishizaki Y, Fujimori M, Tokumoto N, Hirata Y, Ozaki S, Okajima M, Sugino K, Asahara T (2004) Immunohistochemical and sequencing analyses of the Wnt signaling components in Japanese anaplastic thyroid cancers. Thyroid 14:1020–1029

Kurihara S, Oda Y, Ohishi Y, Kaneki E, Kobayashi H, Wake N, Tsuneyoshi M (2010) Coincident expression of beta-catenin and cyclin D1 in endometrial stromal tumors and related high-grade sarcomas. Mod Pathol 23:225–234

Kusafuka T, Miao J, Kuroda S, Udatsu Y, Yoneda A (2002) Codon 45 of the beta-catenin gene, a specific mutational target site of Wilms' tumor. Int J Mol Med 10:395–399

Lamlum H, Ilyas M, Rowan A, Clark S, Johnson V, Bell J, Frayling I, Efstathiou J, Pack K, Payne S, Roylance R, Gorman P, Sheer D, Neale K, Phillips R, Talbot I, Bodmer W, Tomlinson I (1999) The type of somatic mutation at APC in familial adenomatous polyposis is determined by the site of the germline mutation: a new facet to Knudson's "two-hit" hypothesis. Nat Med 5:1071–1075

Lamlum H, Papadopoulou A, Ilyas M, Rowan A, Gillet C, Hanby A, Talbot I, Bodmer W, Tomlinson I (2000) APC mutations are sufficient for the growth of early colorectal adenomas. Proc Natl Acad Sci U S A 97:2225–2228

Lammi L, Arte S, Somer M, Jarvinen H, Lahermo P, Thesleff I, Pirinen S, Nieminen P (2004) Mutations in AXIN2 cause familial tooth agenesis and predispose to colorectal cancer. Am J Hum Genet 74:1043–1050

Landesman-Bollag E, Romieu-Mourez R, Song DH, Sonenshein GE, Cardiff RD, Seldin DC (2001) Protein kinase CK2 in mammary gland tumorigenesis. Oncogene 20:3247–3257

Lantsov D, Meirmanov S, Nakashima M, Kondo H, Saenko V, Naruke Y, Namba H, Ito M, Abrosimov A, Lushnikov E, Sekine I, Yamashita S (2005) Cyclin D1 overexpression in thyroid papillary microcarcinoma: its association with tumour size and aberrant beta-catenin expression. Histopathology 47:248–256

Latchford A, Volikos E, Johnson V, Rogers P, Suraweera N, Tomlinson I, Phillips R, Silver A (2007) APC mutations in FAP-associated desmoid tumours are non-random but not "just right". Hum Mol Genet 16:78–82

Lazar AJ, Calonje E, Grayson W, Dei Tos AP, Mihm MC Jr, Redston M, McKee PH (2005) Pilomatrix carcinomas contain mutations in CTNNB1, the gene encoding beta-catenin. J Cutan Pathol 32:148–157

Lee JH, Abraham SC, Kim HS, Nam JH, Choi C, Lee MC, Park CS, Juhng SW, Rashid A, Hamilton SR, Wu TT (2002) Inverse relationship between APC gene mutation in gastric adenomas and development of adenocarcinoma. Am J Pathol 161:611–618

Lee AY, He B, You L, Dadfarmay S, Xu Z, Mazieres J, Mikami I, McCormick F, Jablons DM (2004) Expression of the secreted frizzled-related protein gene family is downregulated in human mesothelioma. Oncogene 23:6672–6676

Lee EJ, Jo M, Rho SB, Park K, Yoo YN, Park J, Chae M, Zhang W, Lee JH (2009a) Dkk3, downregulated in cervical cancer, functions as a negative regulator of beta-catenin. Int J Cancer 124:287–297

Lee HH, Uen YH, Tian YF, Sun CS, Sheu MJ, Kuo HT, Koay LB, Lin CY, Tzeng CC, Cheng CJ, Tang LY, Tsai SL, Wang AH (2009b) Wnt-1 protein as a prognostic biomarker for hepatitis B-related and hepatitis C-related hepatocellular carcinoma after surgery. Cancer Epidemiol Biomarkers Prev 18:1562–1569

Leethanakul C, Patel V, Gillespie J, Pallente M, Ensley JF, Koontongkaew S, Liotta LA, Emmert-Buck M, Gutkind JS (2000) Distinct pattern of expression of differentiation and growth-related genes in squamous cell carcinomas of the head and neck revealed by the use of laser capture microdissection and cDNA arrays. Oncogene 19:3220–3224

Lejeune S, Huguet EL, Hamby A, Poulsom R, Harris AL (1995) Wnt5a cloning, expression, and up-regulation in human primary breast cancers. Clin Cancer Res 1:215–222

Leppert M, Dobbs M, Scambler P, O'Connell P, Nakamura Y, Stauffer D, Woodward S, Burt RW, Hughes JP, Gardner EJ, Lathrop M, Wasmuth J, Lalouel J-M, White R (1987) The gene for familial polyposis coli maps to the long arm of chromosome 5. Science 238:1411–1413

Li Y, Hively WP, Varmus HE (2000) Use of MMTV-Wnt-1 transgenic mice for studying the genetic basis of breast cancer. Oncogene 19:1002–1009

Li CM, Kim CE, Margolin AA, Guo M, Zhu J, Mason JM, Hensle TW, Murty VV, Grundy PE, Fearon ER, D'Agati V, Licht JD, Tycko B (2004) CTNNB1 mutations and overexpression of Wnt/beta-catenin target genes in WT1-mutant Wilms' tumors. Am J Pathol 165: 1943–1953

Li AF, Hsu PK, Tzao C, Wang YC, Hung IC, Huang MH, Hsu HS (2009) Reduced axin protein expression is associated with a poor prognosis in patients with squamous cell carcinoma of esophagus. Ann Surg Oncol 16:2486–2493

Licchesi JD, Westra WH, Hooker CM, Machida EO, Baylin SB, Herman JG (2008) Epigenetic alteration of Wnt pathway antagonists in progressive glandular neoplasia of the lung. Carcinogenesis 29:895–904

Lin SY, Xia W, Wang JC, Kwong KY, Spohn B, Wen Y, Pestell RG, Hung MC (2000) Beta-catenin, a novel prognostic marker for breast cancer: its roles in cyclin D1 expression and cancer progression. Proc Natl Acad Sci U S A 97:4262–4266

Lin YW, Chung MT, Lai HC, De Yan M, Shih YL, Chang CC, Yu MH (2009) Methylation analysis of SFRP genes family in cervical adenocarcinoma. J Cancer Res Clin Oncol 135:1665–1674

Lind GE, Thorstensen L, Lovig T, Meling GI, Hamelin R, Rognum TO, Esteller M, Lothe RA (2004) A CpG island hypermethylation profile of primary colorectal carcinomas and colon cancer cell lines. Mol Cancer 3:28

Lindvall C, Zylstra CR, Evans N, West RA, Dykema K, Furge KA, Williams BO (2009) The Wnt co-receptor Lrp6 is required for normal mouse mammary gland development. PLoS One 4:e5813

Lips DJ, Barker N, Clevers H, Hennipman A (2009) The role of APC and beta-catenin in the aetiology of aggressive fibromatosis (desmoid tumors). Eur J Surg Oncol 35:3–10

Liu W, Dong X, Mai M, Seelan RS, Taniguchi K, Krishnadath KK, Halling KC, Cunningham JM, Boardman LA, Qian C, Christensen E, Schmidt SS, Roche PC, Smith DI, Thibodeau SN (2000) Mutations in AXIN2 cause colorectal cancer with defective mismatch repair by activating beta-catenin/TCF signalling. Nat Genet 26:146–147

Liu C, Li Y, Semenov M, Han C, Baeg GH, Tan Y, Zhang Z, Lin X, He X (2002) Control of beta-catenin phosphorylation/degradation by a dual-kinase mechanism. Cell 108:837–847

Liu XH, Pan MH, Lu ZF, Wu B, Rao Q, Zhou ZY, Zhou XJ (2008) Expression of Wnt-5a and its clinicopathological significance in hepatocellular carcinoma. Dig Liver Dis 40:560–567

Lo Muzio L, Pannone G, Staibano S, Mignogna MD, Grieco M, Ramires P, Romito AM, De Rosa G, Piattelli A (2002) WNT-1 expression in basal cell carcinoma of head and neck. An immunohistochemical and confocal study with regard to the intracellular distribution of beta-catenin. Anticancer Res 22:565–576

Lo Muzio L, Goteri G, Capretti R, Rubini C, Vinella A, Fumarulo R, Bianchi F, Mastrangelo F, Porfiri E, Mariggio MA (2005) Beta-catenin gene analysis in oral squamous cell carcinoma. Int J Immunopathol Pharmacol 18:33–38

Lodygin D, Epanchintsev A, Menssen A, Diebold J, Hermeking H (2005) Functional epigenomics identifies genes frequently silenced in prostate cancer. Cancer Res 65:4218–4227

Lopez-Knowles E, Zardawi SJ, McNeil CM, Millar EK, Crea P, Musgrove EA, Sutherland RL, O'Toole SA (2010) Cytoplasmic localization of beta-catenin is a marker of poor outcome in breast cancer patients. Cancer Epidemiol Biomarkers Prev 19:301–309

Lowy AM, Fenoglio-Preiser C, Kim OJ, Kordich J, Gomez A, Knight J, James L, Groden J (2003) Dysregulation of beta-catenin expression correlates with tumor differentiation in pancreatic duct adenocarcinoma. Ann Surg Oncol 10:284–290

Luchtenborg M, Weijenberg MP, Wark PA, Saritas AM, Roemen GM, van Muijen GN, de Bruine AP, van den Brandt PA, de Goeij AF (2005) Mutations in APC, CTNNB1 and K-ras genes and expression of hMLH1 in sporadic colorectal carcinomas from the Netherlands Cohort Study. BMC Cancer 5:160

Maelandsmo GM, Holm R, Nesland JM, Fodstad O, Florenes VA (2003) Reduced beta-catenin expression in the cytoplasm of advanced-stage superficial spreading malignant melanoma. Clin Cancer Res 9:3383–3388

Mahomed F, Altini M, Meer S (2007) Altered E-cadherin/beta-catenin expression in oral squamous carcinoma with and without nodal metastasis. Oral Dis 13:386–392

Mai M, Qian C, Yokomizo A, Smith DI, Liu W (1999) Cloning of the human homolog of conductin (AXIN2), a gene mapping to chromosome 17q23-q24. Genomics 55:341–344

Maiti S, Alam R, Amos CI, Huff V (2000) Frequent association of beta-catenin and WT1 mutations in Wilms tumors. Cancer Res 60:6288–6292

Makino T, Yamasaki M, Takemasa I, Takeno A, Nakamura Y, Miyata H, Takiguchi S, Fujiwara Y, Matsuura N, Mori M, Doki Y (2009) Dickkopf-1 expression as a marker for predicting clinical outcome in esophageal squamous cell carcinoma. Ann Surg Oncol 16:2058–2064

Mannens M, Devilee P, Bliek J, Mandjes I, de Kraker J, Heyting C, Slater RM, Westerveld A (1990) Loss of heterozygosity in Wilms' tumors, studied for six putative tumor suppressor regions, is limited to chromosome 11. Cancer Res 50:3279–3283

Marsit CJ, Karagas MR, Andrew A, Liu M, Danaee H, Schned AR, Nelson HH, Kelsey KT (2005) Epigenetic inactivation of SFRP genes and TP53 alteration act jointly as markers of invasive bladder cancer. Cancer Res 65:7081–7085

Marsit CJ, McClean MD, Furniss CS, Kelsey KT (2006) Epigenetic inactivation of the SFRP genes is associated with drinking, smoking and HPV in head and neck squamous cell carcinoma. Int J Cancer 119:1761–1766

Matsui A, Yamaguchi T, Maekawa S, Miyazaki C, Takano S, Uetake T, Inoue T, Otaka M, Otsuka H, Sato T, Yamashita A, Takahashi Y, Enomoto N (2009) DICKKOPF-4 and -2 genes are upregulated in human colorectal cancer. Cancer Sci 100:1923–1930

Matushansky I, Hernando E, Socci ND, Mills JE, Matos TA, Edgar MA, Singer S, Maki RG, Cordon-Cardo C (2007) Derivation of sarcomas from mesenchymal stem cells via inactivation of the Wnt pathway. J Clin Invest 117:3248–3257

Mazieres J, He B, You L, Xu Z, Lee AY, Mikami I, Reguart N, Rosell R, McCormick F, Jablons DM (2004) Wnt inhibitory factor-1 is silenced by promoter hypermethylation in human lung cancer. Cancer Res 64:4717–4720

Mazieres J, You L, He B, Xu Z, Twogood S, Lee AY, Reguart N, Batra S, Mikami I, Jablons DM (2005) Wnt2 as a new therapeutic target in malignant pleural mesothelioma. Int J Cancer 117:326–332

Merle P, de la Monte S, Kim M, Herrmann M, Tanaka S, Von Dem Bussche A, Kew MC, Trepo C, Wands JR (2004) Functional consequences of frizzled-7 receptor overexpression in human hepatocellular carcinoma. Gastroenterology 127:1110–1122

Merle P, Kim M, Herrmann M, Gupte A, Lefrancois L, Califano S, Trepo C, Tanaka S, Vitvitski L, de la Monte S, Wands JR (2005) Oncogenic role of the frizzled-7/beta-catenin pathway in hepatocellular carcinoma. J Hepatol 43:854–862

Miao J, Kusafuka T, Kuroda S, Yoneda A, Zhou Z, Okada A (2003) Mutation of beta-catenin and its protein accumulation in solid and cystic tumor of the pancreas associated with metastasis. Int J Mol Med 11:461–464

Min Kim S, Sun CD, Park KC, Kim HG, Lee WJ, Choi SH (2006) Accumulation of beta-catenin protein, mutations in exon-3 of the beta-catenin gene and a loss of heterozygosity of 5q22 in solid pseudopapillary tumor of the pancreas. J Surg Oncol 94:418–425

Mirabelli-Primdahl L, Gryfe R, Kim H, Millar A, Luceri C, Dale D, Holowaty E, Bapat B, Gallinger S, Redston M (1999) Beta-catenin mutations are specific for colorectal carcinomas with microsatellite instability but occur in endometrial carcinomas irrespective of mutator pathway. Cancer Res 59:3346–3351

Miyaki M, Konishi M, Kikuchi-Yanoshita R, Enomoto M, Igari T, Tanaka K, Muraoka M, Takahashi H, Amada Y, Fukayama M et al (1994) Characteristics of somatic mutation of the adenomatous polyposis coli gene in colorectal tumors. Cancer Res 54:3011–3020

Miyakoshi T, Takei M, Kajiya H, Egashira N, Takekoshi S, Teramoto A, Osamura RY (2008) Expression of Wnt4 in human pituitary adenomas regulates activation of the beta-catenin-independent pathway. Endocr Pathol 19:261–273

Miyoshi Y, Nagase H, Ando H, Horii A, Ichii S, Nakatsuru S, Aoki T, Miki Y, Mori T, Nakamura Y (1992) Somatic mutations of the APC gene in colorectal tumors: mutation cluster region in the APC gene. Hum Mol Genet 1:229–233

Miyoshi K, Shillingford JM, Le Provost F, Gounari F, Bronson R, von Boehmer H, Taketo MM, Cardiff RD, Hennighausen L, Khazaie K (2002) Activation of beta -catenin signaling in differentiated mammary secretory cells induces transdifferentiation into epidermis and squamous metaplasias. Proc Natl Acad Sci U S A 99:219–224

Mizutani K, Miyamoto S, Nagahata T, Konishi N, Emi M, Onda M (2005) Upregulation and overexpression of DVL1, the human counterpart of the Drosophila dishevelled gene, in prostate cancer. Tumori 91:546–551

Moreno CS, Evans CO, Zhan X, Okor M, Desiderio DM, Oyesiku NM (2005) Novel molecular signaling and classification of human clinically nonfunctional pituitary adenomas identified by gene expression profiling and proteomic analyses. Cancer Res 65:10214–10222

Moreno-Bueno G, Gamallo C, Perez-Gallego L, Contreras F, Palacios J (2001a) Beta-catenin expression in pilomatrixomas. Relationship with beta-catenin gene mutations and comparison with beta-catenin expression in normal hair follicles. Br J Dermatol 145:576–581

Moreno-Bueno G, Gamallo C, Perez-Gallego L, de Mora JC, Suarez A, Palacios J (2001b) Beta-catenin expression pattern, beta-catenin gene mutations, and microsatellite instability in endometrioid ovarian carcinomas and synchronous endometrial carcinomas. Diagn Mol Pathol 10:116–122

Nabais S, Machado JC, Lopes C, Seruca R, Carneiro F, Sobrinho-Simoes M (2003) Patterns of beta-catenin expression in gastric carcinoma: clinicopathological relevance and mutation analysis. Int J Surg Pathol 11:1–9

Nakashima T, Liu D, Nakano J, Ishikawa S, Yokomise H, Ueno M, Kadota K, Huang CL (2008) Wnt1 overexpression associated with tumor proliferation and a poor prognosis in non-small cell lung cancer patients. Oncol Rep 19:203–209

Nakatani Y, Masudo K, MiySagi Y, Inayama Y, Kawano N, Tanaka Y, Kato K, Ito T, Kitamura H, Nagashima Y, Yamanaka S, Nakamura N, Sano J, Ogawa N, Ishiwa N, Notohara K, Resl M, Mark EJ (2002) Aberrant nuclear localization and gene mutation of beta-catenin in low-grade adenocarcinoma of fetal lung type: up-regulation of the Wnt signaling pathway may be a common denominator for the development of tumors that form morules. Mod Pathol 15:617–624

Nakopoulou L, Mylona E, Papadaki I, Kavantzas N, Giannopoulou I, Markaki S, Keramopoulos A (2006) Study of phospho-beta-catenin subcellular distribution in invasive breast carcinomas in relation to their phenotype and the clinical outcome. Mod Pathol 19:556–563

Navarro D, Agra N, Pestana A, Alonso J, Gonzalez-Sancho JM (2010) The EWS/FLI1 oncogenic protein inhibits expression of the Wnt inhibitor DICKKOPF-1 gene and antagonizes beta-catenin/TCF-mediated transcription. Carcinogenesis 31:394–401

Nei H, Saito T, Yamasaki H, Mizumoto H, Ito E, Kudo R (1999) Nuclear localization of beta-catenin in normal and carcinogenic endometrium. Mol Carcinog 25:207–218

Nhieu JT, Renard CA, Wei Y, Cherqui D, Zafrani ES, Buendia MA (1999) Nuclear accumulation of mutated beta-catenin in hepatocellular carcinoma is associated with increased cell proliferation. Am J Pathol 155:703–710

Nikuseva Martic T, Pecina-Slaus N, Kusec V, Kokotovic T, Musinovic H, Tomas D, Zeljko M (2010) Changes of AXIN-1 and beta-catenin in neuroepithelial brain tumors. Pathol Oncol Res 16:75–79

Nishimori I, Kohsaki T, Tochika N, Takeuchi T, Minakuchi T, Okabayashi T, Kobayashi M, Hanazaki K, Onishi S (2006) Non-cystic solid-pseudopapillary tumor of the pancreas showing nuclear accumulation and activating gene mutation of beta-catenin. Pathol Int 56:707–711

Nishisho I, Nakamura Y, Miyoshi Y, Miki Y, Ando H, Horii A, Koyama K, Utsunomiya J, Baba S, Hedge P, Markham A, Krush AJ, Peterson G, Hamiltom SR, Nilbert MC, Levy DB, Bryan TM, Preisinger AM, Smith KJ, Su L-K, Kinzler KW, Vogelstein B (1991) Mutations of chromosome 5q21 genes in FAP and colorectal cancer patients. Science 253:665–669

Nojima M, Suzuki H, Toyota M, Watanabe Y, Maruyama R, Sasaki S, Sasaki Y, Mita H, Nishikawa N, Yamaguchi K, Hirata K, Itoh F, Tokino T, Mori M, Imai K, Shinomura Y (2007) Frequent epigenetic inactivation of SFRP genes and constitutive activation of Wnt signaling in gastric cancer. Oncogene 26:4699–4713

Nozaki I, Tsuji T, Iijima O, Ohmura Y, Andou A, Miyazaki M, Shimizu N, Namba M (2001) Reduced expression of REIC/Dkk-3 gene in non-small cell lung cancer. Int J Oncol 19:117–121

Nusse R, Varmus HE (1982) Many tumors induced by the mouse mammary tumor virus contain a provirus integrated in the same region of the host genome. Cell 31:99–109

Nusse R, Brown A, Papkoff J, Scambler P, Shackleford G, McMahon A, Moon R, Varmus H (1991) A new nomenclature for int-1 and related genes: the Wnt gene family. Cell 64:231

Oberwalder M, Zitt M, Wontner C, Fiegl H, Goebel G, Zitt M, Kohle O, Muhlmann G, Ofner D, Margreiter R, Muller HM (2008) SFRP2 methylation in fecal DNA – a marker for colorectal polyps. Int J Colorectal Dis 23:15–19

Oda H, Imai Y, Nakatsuru Y, Hata J, Ishikawa T (1996) Somatic mutations of the APC gene in sporadic hepatoblastomas. Cancer Res 56:3320–3323

Ogasawara N, Tsukamoto T, Mizoshita T, Inada K, Cao X, Takenaka Y, Joh T, Tatematsu M (2006) Mutations and nuclear accumulation of beta-catenin correlate with intestinal phenotypic expression in human gastric cancer. Histopathology 49:612–621

Ohgaki H, Kros JM, Okamoto Y, Gaspert A, Huang H, Kurrer MO (2004) APC mutations are infrequent but present in human lung cancer. Cancer Lett 207:197–203

Okino K, Nagai H, Hatta M, Nagahata T, Yoneyama K, Ohta Y, Jin E, Kawanami O, Araki T, Emi M (2003) Up-regulation and overproduction of DVL-1, the human counterpart of the Drosophila dishevelled gene, in cervical squamous cell carcinoma. Oncol Rep 10:1219–1223

Omholt K, Platz A, Ringborg U, Hansson J (2001) Cytoplasmic and nuclear accumulation of beta-catenin is rarely caused by CTNNB1 exon 3 mutations in cutaneous malignant melanoma. Int J Cancer 92:839–842

Ooi CH, Ivanova T, Wu J, Lee M, Tan IB, Tao J, Ward L, Koo JH, Gopalakrishnan V, Zhu Y, Cheng LL, Lee J, Rha SY, Chung HC, Ganesan K, So J, Soo KC, Lim D, Chan WH, Wong WK, Bowtell D, Yeoh KG, Grabsch H, Boussioutas A, Tan P (2009) Oncogenic pathway combinations predict clinical prognosis in gastric cancer. PLoS Genet 5:e1000676

Ozaki S, Ikeda S, Ishizaki Y, Kurihara T, Tokumoto N, Iseki M, Arihiro K, Kataoka T, Okajima M, Asahara T (2005) Alterations and correlations of the components in the Wnt signaling pathway and its target genes in breast cancer. Oncol Rep 14:1437–1443

Palm T, Figarella-Branger D, Chapon F, Lacroix C, Gray F, Scaravilli F, Ellison DW, Salmon I, Vikkula M, Godfraind C (2009) Expression profiling of ependymomas unravels localization and tumor grade-specific tumorigenesis. Cancer 115:3955–3968

Pan KF, Liu WG, Zhang L, You WC, Lu YY (2008) Mutations in components of the Wnt signaling pathway in gastric cancer. World J Gastroenterol 14:1570–1574

Park SW, Suh KS, Wang HY, Kim ST, Sung HS (2001a) Beta-catenin expression in the transitional cell zone of pilomatricoma. Br J Dermatol 145:624–629

Park WS, Oh RR, Park JY, Kim PJ, Shin MS, Lee JH, Kim HS, Lee SH, Kim SY, Park YG, An WG, Kim HS, Jang JJ, Yoo NJ, Lee JY (2001b) Nuclear localization of beta-catenin is an important prognostic factor in hepatoblastoma. J Pathol 193:483–490

Park JY, Park WS, Nam SW, Kim SY, Lee SH, Yoo NJ, Lee JY, Park CK (2005) Mutations of beta-catenin and AXIN I genes are a late event in human hepatocellular carcinogenesis. Liver Int 25:70–76

Pecina-Slaus N, Zigmund M, Kusec V, Martic TN, Cacic M, Slaus M (2007) E-cadherin and beta-catenin expression patterns in malignant melanoma assessed by image analysis. J Cutan Pathol 34:239–246

Pecina-Slaus N, Nikuseva Martic T, Tomas D, Beros V, Zeljko M, Cupic H (2008) Meningiomas exhibit loss of heterozygosity of the APC gene. J Neurooncol 87:63–70

Peng H, Zhong XY, Liu KP, Li SM (2009) Expression and significance of adenomatous polyposis coli, beta-catenin, E-cadherin and cyclin D1 in esophageal squamous cell carcinoma assessed by tissue microarray. Ai Zheng 28:38–41

Pham K, Milovanovic T, Barr RJ, Truong T, Holcombe RF (2003) Wnt ligand expression in malignant melanoma: pilot study indicating correlation with histopathological features. Mol Pathol 56:280–285

Phillips SM, Morton DG, Lee SJ, Wallace DM, Neoptolemos JP (1994) Loss of heterozygosity of the retinoblastoma and adenomatous polyposis susceptibility gene loci and in chromosomes 10p, 10q and 16q in human prostate cancer. Br J Urol 73:390–395

Pijnenborg JM, Kisters N, van Engeland M, Dunselman GA, de Haan J, de Goeij AF, Groothuis PG (2004) APC, beta-catenin, and E-cadherin and the development of recurrent endometrial carcinoma. Int J Gynecol Cancer 14:947–956

Pilarsky C, Ammerpohl O, Sipos B, Dahl E, Hartmann A, Wellmann A, Braunschweig T, Lohr M, Jesnowski R, Friess H, Wente MN, Kristiansen G, Jahnke B, Denz A, Ruckert F, Schackert HK, Kloppel G, Kalthoff H, Saeger HD, Grutzmann R (2008) Activation of Wnt signalling in stroma from pancreatic cancer identified by gene expression profiling. J Cell Mol Med 12:2823–2835

Porfiri E, Rubinfeld B, Albert I, Hovanes K, Waterman M, Polakis P (1997) Induction of a beta-catenin-LEF-1 complex by wnt-1 and transforming mutants of beta-catenin. Oncogene 15:2833–2839

Powell SM, Zilz N, Beazer-Barclay Y, Bryan TM, Hamilton SR, Thibodeau SN, Vogelstein B, Kinzler KW (1992) APC mutations occur early during colorectal tumorigenesis. Nature 359: 235–237

Prange W, Breuhahn K, Fischer F, Zilkens C, Pietsch T, Petmecky K, Eilers R, Dienes HP, Schirmacher P (2003) Beta-catenin accumulation in the progression of human hepatocarcino-genesis correlates with loss of E-cadherin and accumulation of p53, but not with expression of conventional WNT-1 target genes. J Pathol 201:250–259

Prasad CP, Mirza S, Sharma G, Prashad R, DattaGupta S, Rath G, Ralhan R (2008) Epigenetic alterations of CDH1 and APC genes: relationship with activation of Wnt/beta-catenin pathway in invasive ductal carcinoma of breast. Life Sci 83:318–325

Pretto D, Barco R, Rivera J, Neel N, Gustavson MD, Eid JE (2006) The synovial sarcoma trans-location protein SYT-SSX2 recruits beta-catenin to the nucleus and associates with it in an active complex. Oncogene 25:3661–3669

Prosperi JR, Goss KH (2010) A Wnt-ow of opportunity: Targeting the Wnt/β-catenin pathway in breast cancer. Curr Drug Targets 11:1074–1088

Pu P, Zhang Z, Kang C, Jiang R, Jia Z, Wang G, Jiang H (2009) Downregulation of Wnt2 and beta-catenin by siRNA suppresses malignant glioma cell growth. Cancer Gene Ther 16:351–361

Qi J, Zhu YQ, Luo J, Tao WH (2007) The role of secreted Wnt-antagonist genes hypermethylation in early detection of colorectal tumor. Zhonghua Yi Xue Za Zhi 87:1954–1957

Queimado L, Obeso D, Hatfield MD, Yang Y, Thompson DM, Reis AM (2008) Dysregulation of Wnt pathway components in human salivary gland tumors. Arch Otolaryngol Head Neck Surg 134:94–101

Rask K, Nilsson A, Brannstrom M, Carlsson P, Hellberg P, Janson PO, Hedin L, Sundfeldt K (2003) Wnt-signalling pathway in ovarian epithelial tumours: increased expression of beta-catenin and GSK3beta. Br J Cancer 89:1298–1304

Redston MS, Papadopoulos N, Caldas C, Kinzler KW, Kern SE (1995) Common occurrence of APC and K-ras gene mutations in the spectrum of colitis-associated neoplasias. Gastroenterology 108:383–392

Reifenberger J, Knobbe CB, Wolter M, Blaschke B, Schulte KW, Pietsch T, Ruzicka T, Reifenberger G (2002) Molecular genetic analysis of malignant melanomas for aberrations of the WNT signaling pathway genes CTNNB1, APC, ICAT and BTRC. Int J Cancer 100:549–556

Rezk S, Brynes RK, Nelson V, Thein M, Patwardhan N, Fischer A, Khan A (2004) Beta-catenin expression in thyroid follicular lesions: potential role in nuclear envelope changes in papillary carcinomas. Endocr Pathol 15:329–337

Rijsewijk F, Schuermann M, Wagenaar E, Parren P, Weigel D, Nusse R (1987) The Drosophila homolog of the mouse mammary oncogene int-1 is identical to the segment polarity gene wingless. Cell 50:649–657

Rimm DL, Caca K, Hu G, Harrison FB, Fearon ER (1999) Frequent nuclear/cytoplasmic localization of beta-catenin without exon 3 mutations in malignant melanoma. Am J Pathol 154:325–329

Risinger JI, Maxwell GL, Chandramouli GV, Aprelikova O, Litzi T, Umar A, Berchuck A, Barrett JC (2005) Gene expression profiling of microsatellite unstable and microsatellite stable endometrial cancers indicates distinct pathways of aberrant signaling. Cancer Res 65:5031–5037

Roelink H, Wagenaar E, Lopes da Silva S, Nusse R (1990) Wnt-3, a gene activated by proviral insertion in mouse mammary tumors, is homologous to int-1/Wnt-1 and is normally expressed in mouse embryos and adult brain. Proc Natl Acad Sci U S A 87:4519–4523

Rogers HA, Miller S, Lowe J, Brundler MA, Coyle B, Grundy RG (2009) An investigation of WNT pathway activation and association with survival in central nervous system primitive neuroectodermal tumours (CNS PNET). Br J Cancer 100:1292–1302

Rowan AJ, Lamlum H, Ilyas M, Wheeler J, Straub J, Papadopoulou A, Bicknell D, Bodmer WF, Tomlinson IP (2000) APC mutations in sporadic colorectal tumors: a mutational "hotspot" and interdependence of the "two hits". Proc Natl Acad Sci U S A 97:3352–3357

Ryo A, Nakamura M, Wulf G, Liou YC, Lu KP (2001) Pin1 regulates turnover and subcellular localization of beta-catenin by inhibiting its interaction with APC. Nat Cell Biol 3:793–801

Saegusa M, Okayasu I (2001) Frequent nuclear beta-catenin accumulation and associated mutations in endometrioid-type endometrial and ovarian carcinomas with squamous differentiation. J Pathol 194:59–67

Saegusa M, Hashimura M, Yoshida T, Okayasu I (2001) Beta-catenin mutations and aberrant nuclear expression during endometrial tumorigenesis. Br J Cancer 84:209–217

Saegusa M, Hashimura M, Kuwata T, Hamano M, Okayasu I (2005) Upregulation of TCF4 expression as a transcriptional target of beta-catenin/p300 complexes during trans-differentiation of endometrial carcinoma cells. Lab Invest 85:768–779

Sagae S, Kobayashi K, Nishioka Y, Sugimura M, Ishioka S, Nagata M, Terasawa K, Tokino T, Kudo R (1999) Mutational analysis of beta-catenin gene in Japanese ovarian carcinomas: frequent mutations in endometrioid carcinomas. Jpn J Cancer Res 90:510–515

Saini S, Liu J, Yamamura S, Majid S, Kawakami K, Hirata H, Dahiya R (2009) Functional significance of secreted Frizzled-related protein 1 in metastatic renal cell carcinomas. Cancer Res 69:6815–6822

Saito T, Oda Y, Kawaguchi K, Tanaka K, Matsuda S, Tamiya S, Iwamoto Y, Tsuneyoshi M (2002) Possible association between higher beta-catenin mRNA expression and mutated beta-catenin in sporadic desmoid tumors: real-time semiquantitative assay by TaqMan polymerase chain reaction. Lab Invest 82:97–103

Saitoh T, Mine T, Katoh M (2002a) Frequent up-regulation of WNT5A mRNA in primary gastric cancer. Int J Mol Med 9:515–519

Saitoh T, Mine T, Katoh M (2002b) Up-regulation of WNT8B mRNA in human gastric cancer. Int J Oncol 20:343–348

Sakamoto A, Oda Y, Adachi T, Saito T, Tamiya S, Iwamoto Y, Tsuneyoshi M (2002) Beta-catenin accumulation and gene mutation in exon 3 in dedifferentiated liposarcoma and malignant fibrous histiocytoma. Arch Pathol Lab Med 126:1071–1078

Saldanha G, Ghura V, Potter L, Fletcher A (2004) Nuclear beta-catenin in basal cell carcinoma correlates with increased proliferation. Br J Dermatol 151:157–164

Sareddy GR, Panigrahi M, Challa S, Mahadevan A, Babu PP (2009) Activation of Wnt/beta-catenin/Tcf signaling pathway in human astrocytomas. Neurochem Int 55:307–317

Sarrio D, Moreno-Bueno G, Hardisson D, Sanchez-Estevez C, Guo M, Herman JG, Gamallo C, Esteller M, Palacios J (2003) Epigenetic and genetic alterations of APC and CDH1 genes in lobular breast cancer: relationships with abnormal E-cadherin and catenin expression and microsatellite instability. Int J Cancer 106:208–215

Sarrio D, Moreno-Bueno G, Sanchez-Estevez C, Banon-Rodriguez I, Hernandez-Cortes G, Hardisson D, Palacios J (2006) Expression of cadherins and catenins correlates with distinct histologic types of ovarian carcinomas. Hum Pathol 37:1042–1049

Sato H, Suzuki H, Toyota M, Nojima M, Maruyama R, Sasaki S, Takagi H, Sogabe Y, Sasaki Y, Idogawa M, Sonoda T, Mori M, Imai K, Tokino T, Shinomura Y (2007) Frequent epigenetic inactivation of DICKKOPF family genes in human gastrointestinal tumors. Carcinogenesis 28:2459–2466

Satoh S, Daigo Y, Furukawa Y, Kato T, Miwa N, Nishiwaki T, Kawasoe T, Ishiguro H, Fujita M, Tokino T, Sasaki Y, Imaoka S, Murata M, Shimano T, Yamaoka Y, Nakamura Y (2000) AXIN1 mutations in hepatocellular carcinomas, and growth suppression in cancer cells by virus-mediated transfer of AXIN1. Nat Genet 24:245–250

Schlosshauer PW, Ellenson LH, Soslow RA (2002) Beta-catenin and E-cadherin expression patterns in high-grade endometrial carcinoma are associated with histological subtype. Mod Pathol 15:1032–1037

Schmitt-Graeff A, Ertelt-Heitzmann V, Allgaier HP, Olschewski M, Nitschke R, Haxelmans S, Koelble K, Behrens J, Blum HE (2005) Coordinated expression of cyclin D1 and LEF-1/TCF transcription factor is restricted to a subset of hepatocellular carcinoma. Liver Int 25:839–847

Scholten AN, Creutzberg CL, van den Broek LJ, Noordijk EM, Smit VT (2003) Nuclear beta-catenin is a molecular feature of type I endometrial carcinoma. J Pathol 201:460–465

Segditsas S, Sieber OM, Rowan A, Setien F, Neale K, Phillips RK, Ward R, Esteller M, Tomlinson IP (2008) Promoter hypermethylation leads to decreased APC mRNA expression in familial polyposis and sporadic colorectal tumours, but does not substitute for truncating mutations. Exp Mol Pathol 85:201–206

Semba S, Han SY, Ikeda H, Horii A (2001) Frequent nuclear accumulation of beta-catenin in pituitary adenoma. Cancer 91:42–48

Sheng SL, Huang G, Yu B, Qin WX (2009) Clinical significance and prognostic value of serum Dickkopf-1 concentrations in patients with lung cancer. Clin Chem 55:1656–1664

Shih YL, Shyu RY, Hsieh CB, Lai HC, Liu KY, Chu TY, Lin YW (2006) Promoter methylation of the secreted frizzled-related protein 1 gene SFRP1 is frequent in hepatocellular carcinoma. Cancer 107:579–590

Shih YL, Hsieh CB, Lai HC, Yan MD, Hsieh TY, Chao YC, Lin YW (2007) SFRP1 suppressed hepatoma cells growth through Wnt canonical signaling pathway. Int J Cancer 121:1028–1035

Shiina H, Igawa M, Shigeno K, Terashima M, Deguchi M, Yamanaka M, Ribeiro-Filho L, Kane CJ, Dahiya R (2002) Beta-catenin mutations correlate with over expression of C-myc and cyclin D1 genes in bladder cancer. J Urol 168:2220–2226

Shinohara A, Yokoyama Y, Wan X, Takahashi Y, Mori Y, Takami T, Shimokawa K, Tamaya T (2001) Cytoplasmic/nuclear expression without mutation of exon 3 of the beta-catenin gene is frequent in the development of the neoplasm of the uterine cervix. Gynecol Oncol 82:450–455

Smith TG, Clark SK, Katz DE, Reznek RH, Phillips RK (2000) Adrenal masses are associated with familial adenomatous polyposis. Dis Colon Rectum 43:1739–1742

Sogabe Y, Suzuki H, Toyota M, Ogi K, Imai T, Nojima M, Sasaki Y, Hiratsuka H, Tokino T (2008) Epigenetic inactivation of SFRP genes in oral squamous cell carcinoma. Int J Oncol 32:1253–1261

Steg A, Wang W, Blanquicett C, Grunda JM, Eltoum IA, Wang K, Buchsbaum DJ, Vickers SM, Russo S, Diasio RB, Frost AR, LoBuglio AF, Grizzle WE, Johnson MR (2006) Multiple gene expression analyses in paraffin-embedded tissues by TaqMan low-density array: application to hedgehog and Wnt pathway analysis in ovarian endometrioid adenocarcinoma. J Mol Diagn 8:76–83

Stoehr R, Wissmann C, Suzuki H, Knuechel R, Krieg RC, Klopocki E, Dahl E, Wild P, Blaszyk H, Sauter G, Simon R, Schmitt R, Zaak D, Hofstaedter F, Rosenthal A, Baylin SB, Pilarsky C, Hartmann A (2004) Deletions of chromosome 8p and loss of sFRP1 expression are progression markers of papillary bladder cancer. Lab Invest 84:465–478

Su LK, Abdalla EK, Law CH, Kohlmann W, Rashid A, Vauthey JN (2001) Biallelic inactivation of the APC gene is associated with hepatocellular carcinoma in familial adenomatous polyposis coli. Cancer 92:332–339

Su TH, Chang JG, Yeh KT, Lin TH, Lee TP, Chen JC, Lin CC (2003) Mutation analysis of CTNNB1 (beta-catenin) and AXIN1, the components of Wnt pathway, in cervical carcinomas. Oncol Rep 10:1195–1200

Su MC, Huang WC, Lien HC (2008) Beta-catenin expression and mutation in adult and pediatric Wilms' tumors. APMIS 116:771–778

Su HY, Lai HC, Lin YW, Chou YC, Liu CY, Yu MH (2009) An epigenetic marker panel for screening and prognostic prediction of ovarian cancer. Int J Cancer 124:387–393

Su HY, Lai HC, Lin YW, Liu CY, Chen CK, Chou YC, Lin SP, Lin WC, Lee HY, Yu MH (2010) Epigenetic silencing of SFRP5 is related to malignant phenotype and chemoresistance of ovarian cancer through Wnt signaling pathway. Int J Cancer 127:555–567

Sun C, Yamato T, Kondo E, Furukawa T, Ikeda H, Horii A (2005) Infrequent mutation of APC, AXIN1, and GSK3B in human pituitary adenomas with abnormal accumulation of CTNNB1. J Neurooncol 73:131–134

Sunaga N, Kohno T, Kolligs FT, Fearon ER, Saito R, Yokota J (2001) Constitutive activation of the Wnt signaling pathway by CTNNB1 (beta-catenin) mutations in a subset of human lung adenocarcinoma. Genes Chromosomes Cancer 30:316–321

Suzuki T, Yano H, Nakashima Y, Nakashima O, Kojiro M (2002) Beta-catenin expression in hepatocellular carcinoma: a possible participation of beta-catenin in the dedifferentiation process. J Gastroenterol Hepatol 17:994–1000

Suzuki M, Shigematsu H, Nakajima T, Kubo R, Motohashi S, Sekine Y, Shibuya K, Iizasa T, Hiroshima K, Nakatani Y, Gazdar AF, Fujisawa T (2007) Synchronous alterations of Wnt and epidermal growth factor receptor signaling pathways through aberrant methylation and mutation in non small cell lung cancer. Clin Cancer Res 13:6087–6092

Suzuki H, Toyota M, Carraway H, Gabrielson E, Ohmura T, Fujikane T, Nishikawa N, Sogabe Y, Nojima M, Sonoda T, Mori M, Hirata K, Imai K, Shinomura Y, Baylin SB, Tokino T (2008) Frequent epigenetic inactivation of Wnt antagonist genes in breast cancer. Br J Cancer 98:1147–1156

Tadjine M, Lampron A, Ouadi L, Bourdeau I (2008) Frequent mutations of beta-catenin gene in sporadic secreting adrenocortical adenomas. Clin Endocrinol (Oxf) 68:264–270

Takada T, Yagi Y, Maekita T, Imura M, Nakagawa S, Tsao SW, Miyamoto K, Yoshino O, Yasugi T, Taketani Y, Ushijima T (2004) Methylation-associated silencing of the Wnt antagonist SFRP1 gene in human ovarian cancers. Cancer Sci 95:741–744

Takagi H, Sasaki S, Suzuki H, Toyota M, Maruyama R, Nojima M, Yamamoto H, Omata M, Tokino T, Imai K, Shinomura Y (2008) Frequent epigenetic inactivation of SFRP genes in hepatocellular carcinoma. J Gastroenterol 43:378–389

Takahashi N, Fukushima T, Yorita K, Tanaka H, Chijiiwa K, Kataoka H (2010) Dickkopf-1 is overexpressed in human pancreatic ductal adenocarcinoma cells and is involved in invasive growth. Int J Cancer 126:1611–1620

Takayama T, Ohi M, Hayashi T, Miyanishi K, Nobuoka A, Nakajima T, Satoh T, Takimoto R, Kato J, Sakamaki S, Niitsu Y (2001) Analysis of K-ras, APC, and beta-catenin in aberrant crypt foci in sporadic adenoma, cancer, and familial adenomatous polyposis. Gastroenterology 121:599–611

Takayasu H, Horie H, Hiyama E, Matsunaga T, Hayashi Y, Watanabe Y, Suita S, Kaneko M, Sasaki F, Hashizume K, Ozaki T, Furuuchi K, Tada M, Ohnuma N, Nakagawara A (2001) Frequent deletions and mutations of the beta-catenin gene are associated with overexpression of cyclin D1 and fibronectin and poorly differentiated histology in childhood hepatoblastoma. Clin Cancer Res 7:901–908

Takeda H, Lyle S, Lazar AJ, Zouboulis CC, Smyth I, Watt FM (2006) Human sebaceous tumors harbor inactivating mutations in LEF1. Nat Med 12:395–397

Tang M, Torres-Lanzas J, Lopez-Rios F, Esteller M, Sanchez-Cespedes M (2006) Wnt signaling promoter hypermethylation distinguishes lung primary adenocarcinomas from colorectal metastasis to the lung. Int J Cancer 119:2603–2606

Taniguchi K, Roberts LR, Aderca IN, Dong X, Qian C, Murphy LM, Nagorney DM, Burgart LJ, Roche PC, Smith DI, Ross JA, Liu W (2002) Mutational spectrum of beta-catenin, AXIN1, and AXIN2 in hepatocellular carcinomas and hepatoblastomas. Oncogene 21:4863–4871

Taniguchi H, Yamamoto H, Hirata T, Miyamoto N, Oki M, Nosho K, Adachi Y, Endo T, Imai K, Shinomura Y (2005) Frequent epigenetic inactivation of Wnt inhibitory factor-1 in human gastrointestinal cancers. Oncogene 24:7946–7952

Thompson MC, Fuller C, Hogg TL, Dalton J, Finkelstein D, Lau CC, Chintagumpala M, Adesina A, Ashley DM, Kellie SJ, Taylor MD, Curran T, Gajjar A, Gilbertson RJ (2006) Genomics identifies medulloblastoma subgroups that are enriched for specific genetic alterations. J Clin Oncol 24:1924–1931

Tiemann K, Heitling U, Kosmahl M, Kloppel G (2007) Solid pseudopapillary neoplasms of the pancreas show an interruption of the Wnt-signaling pathway and express gene products of 11q. Mod Pathol 20:955–960

Tien LT, Ito M, Nakao M, Niino D, Serik M, Nakashima M, Wen CY, Yatsuhashi H, Ishibashi H (2005) Expression of beta-catenin in hepatocellular carcinoma. World J Gastroenterol 11:2398–2401

Tissier F, Cavard C, Groussin L, Perlemoine K, Fumey G, Hagnere AM, Rene-Corail F, Jullian E, Gicquel C, Bertagna X, Vacher-Lavenu MC, Perret C, Bertherat J (2005) Mutations of beta-catenin in adrenocortical tumors: activation of the Wnt signaling pathway is a frequent event in both benign and malignant adrenocortical tumors. Cancer Res 65:7622–7627

To KF, Chan MW, Leung WK, Yu J, Tong JH, Lee TL, Chan FK, Sung JJ (2001) Alterations of frizzled (FzE3) and secreted frizzled related protein (hsFRP) expression in gastric cancer. Life Sci 70:483–489

Tsai MH, Yang YC, Chen KH, Jiang JK, Chou SJ, Chiang TC, Jan HS, Lou MA (2002) RER and LOH association with sporadic colorectal cancer in Taiwanese patients. Hepatogastroenterology 49:672–677

Tsukamoto AS, Grosschedl R, Guzman RC, Parslow T, Varmus HE (1988) Expression of the int-1 gene in transgenic mice is associated with mammary gland hyperplasia and adenocarcinomas in male and female mice. Cell 55:619–625

Udatsu Y, Kusafuka T, Kuroda S, Miao J, Okada A (2001) High frequency of beta-catenin mutations in hepatoblastoma. Pediatr Surg Int 17:508–512

Ueda M, Gemmill RM, West J, Winn R, Sugita M, Tanaka N, Ueki M, Drabkin HA (2001) Mutations of the beta- and gamma-catenin genes are uncommon in human lung, breast, kidney, cervical and ovarian carcinomas. Br J Cancer 85:64–68

Ueda G, Sunakawa H, Nakamori K, Shinya T, Tsuhako W, Tamura Y, Kosugi T, Sato N, Ogi K, Hiratsuka H (2006) Aberrant expression of beta- and gamma-catenin is an independent prognostic marker in oral squamous cell carcinoma. Int J Oral Maxillofac Surg 35:356–361

Uematsu K, He B, You L, Xu Z, McCormick F, Jablons DM (2003a) Activation of the Wnt pathway in non small cell lung cancer: evidence of dishevelled overexpression. Oncogene 22:7218–7221

Uematsu K, Kanazawa S, You L, He B, Xu Z, Li K, Peterlin BM, McCormick F, Jablons DM (2003b) Wnt pathway activation in mesothelioma: evidence of Dishevelled overexpression and transcriptional activity of beta-catenin. Cancer Res 63:4547–4551

Ugolini F, Charafe-Jauffret E, Bardou VJ, Geneix J, Adelaide J, Labat-Moleur F, Penault-Llorca F, Longy M, Jacquemier J, Birnbaum D, Pebusque MJ (2001) WNT pathway and mammary carcinogenesis: loss of expression of candidate tumor suppressor gene SFRP1 in most invasive carcinomas except of the medullary type. Oncogene 20:5810–5817

Urakami S, Shiina H, Enokida H, Hirata H, Kawamoto K, Kawakami T, Kikuno N, Tanaka Y, Majid S, Nakagawa M, Igawa M, Dahiya R (2006a) Wnt antagonist family genes as biomarkers for diagnosis, staging, and prognosis of renal cell carcinoma using tumor and serum DNA. Clin Cancer Res 12:6989–6997

Urakami S, Shiina H, Enokida H, Kawakami T, Kawamoto K, Hirata H, Tanaka Y, Kikuno N, Nakagawa M, Igawa M, Dahiya R (2006b) Combination analysis of hypermethylated Wnt-antagonist family genes as a novel epigenetic biomarker panel for bladder cancer detection. Clin Cancer Res 12:2109–2116

Uren A, Wolf V, Sun YF, Azari A, Rubin JS, Toretsky JA (2004) Wnt/Frizzled signaling in Ewing sarcoma. Pediatr Blood Cancer 43:243–249

Usadel H, Brabender J, Danenberg KD, Jeronimo C, Harden S, Engles J, Danenberg PV, Yang S, Sidransky D (2002) Quantitative adenomatous polyposis coli promoter methylation analysis in tumor tissue, serum, and plasma DNA of patients with lung cancer. Cancer Res 62:371–375

Van der Auwera I, Van Laere SJ, Van den Bosch SM, Van den Eynden GG, Trinh BX, van Dam PA, Colpaert CG, van Engeland M, Van Marck EA, Vermeulen PB, Dirix LY (2008) Aberrant methylation of the Adenomatous Polyposis Coli (APC) gene promoter is associated with the inflammatory breast cancer phenotype. Br J Cancer 99:1735–1742

Veeck J, Niederacher D, An H, Klopocki E, Wiesmann F, Betz B, Galm O, Camara O, Durst M, Kristiansen G, Huszka C, Knuchel R, Dahl E (2006) Aberrant methylation of the Wnt antagonist SFRP1 in breast cancer is associated with unfavourable prognosis. Oncogene 25:3479–3488

Veeck J, Geisler C, Noetzel E, Alkaya S, Hartmann A, Knuchel R, Dahl E (2008) Epigenetic inactivation of the secreted frizzled-related protein-5 (SFRP5) gene in human breast cancer is associated with unfavorable prognosis. Carcinogenesis 29:991–998

Vibhakar R, Foltz G, Yoon JG, Field L, Lee H, Ryu GY, Pierson J, Davidson B, Madan A (2007) Dickkopf-1 is an epigenetically silenced candidate tumor suppressor gene in medulloblastoma. Neuro Oncol 9:135–144

Vider BZ, Zimber A, Chastre E, Prevot S, Gespach C, Estlein D, Wolloch Y, Tronick SR, Gazit A, Yaniv A (1996) Evidence for the involvement of the Wnt 2 gene in human colorectal cancer. Oncogene 12:153–158

Virmani AK, Rathi A, Sathyanarayana UG, Padar A, Huang CX, Cunnigham HT, Farinas AJ, Milchgrub S, Euhus DM, Gilcrease M, Herman J, Minna JD, Gazdar AF (2001) Aberrant methylation of the adenomatous polyposis coli (APC) gene promoter 1A in breast and lung carcinomas. Clin Cancer Res 7:1998–2004

Voeller HJ, Truica CI, Gelmann EP (1998) Beta-catenin mutations in human prostate cancer. Cancer Res 58:2520–2523

Wada M, Miller CW, Yokota J, Lee E, Mizoguchi H, Koeffler HP (1997) Molecular analysis of the adenomatous polyposis coli gene in sarcomas, hematological malignancies and noncolonic, neoplastic tissues. J Mol Med 75:139–144

Wang Y, Hewitt SM, Liu S, Zhou X, Zhu H, Zhou C, Zhang G, Quan L, Bai J, Xu N (2006) Tissue microarray analysis of human FRAT1 expression and its correlation with the subcellular localisation of beta-catenin in ovarian tumours. Br J Cancer 94:686–691

Wang Q, Williamson M, Bott S, Brookman-Amissah N, Freeman A, Nariculam J, Hubank MJ, Ahmed A, Masters JR (2007) Hypomethylation of WNT5A, CRIP1 and S100P in prostate cancer. Oncogene 26:6560–6565

Wang L, Heidt DG, Lee CJ, Yang H, Logsdon CD, Zhang L, Fearon ER, Ljungman M, Simeone DM (2009a) Oncogenic function of ATDC in pancreatic cancer through Wnt pathway activation and beta-catenin stabilization. Cancer Cell 15:207–219

Wang M, Xue L, Cao Q, Lin Y, Ding Y, Yang P, Che L (2009b) Expression of Notch1, Jagged1 and beta-catenin and their clinicopathological significance in hepatocellular carcinoma. Neoplasma 56:533–541

Wang W, Xue L, Wang P (2010) Prognostic value of beta-catenin, c-myc, and cyclin D1 expressions in patients with esophageal squamous cell carcinoma. Med Oncol [Epub ahead of print]

Watanabe O, Imamura H, Shimizu T, Kinoshita J, Okabe T, Hirano A, Yoshimatsu K, Konno S, Aiba M, Ogawa K (2004) Expression of twist and wnt in human breast cancer. Anticancer Res 24:3851–3856

Webster MT, Rozycka M, Sara E, Davis E, Smalley M, Young N, Dale TC, Wooster R (2000) Sequence variants of the axin gene in breast, colon, and other cancers: an analysis of mutations that interfere with GSK3 binding. Genes Chromosomes Cancer 28:443–453

Wei Y, Fabre M, Branchereau S, Gauthier F, Perilongo G, Buendia MA (2000) Activation of beta-catenin in epithelial and mesenchymal hepatoblastomas. Oncogene 19:498–504

Wei Q, Zhao Y, Yang ZQ, Dong QZ, Dong XJ, Han Y, Zhao C, Wang EH (2008) Dishevelled family proteins are expressed in non-small cell lung cancer and function differentially on tumor progression. Lung Cancer 62:181–192

Weinberger PM, Adam BL, Gourin CG, Moretz WH 3rd, Bollag RJ, Wang BY, Liu Z, Lee JR, Terris DJ (2007) Association of nuclear, cytoplasmic expression of galectin-3 with beta-catenin/Wnt-pathway activation in thyroid carcinoma. Arch Otolaryngol Head Neck Surg 133:503–510

Whitaker HC, Girling J, Warren AY, Leung H, Mills IG, Neal DE (2008) Alterations in beta-catenin expression and localization in prostate cancer. Prostate 68:1196–1205

Winn RA, Marek L, Han SY, Rodriguez K, Rodriguez N, Hammond M, Van Scoyk M, Acosta H, Mirus J, Barry N, Bren-Mattison Y, Van Raay TJ, Nemenoff RA, Heasley LE (2005) Restoration of Wnt-7a expression reverses non-small cell lung cancer cellular transformation through frizzled-9-mediated growth inhibition and promotion of cell differentiation. J Biol Chem 280:19625–19634

Wirths O, Waha A, Weggen S, Schirmacher P, Kuhne T, Goodyer CG, Albrecht S, Von Schweinitz D, Pietsch T (2003) Overexpression of human Dickkopf-1, an antagonist of wingless/WNT signaling, in human hepatoblastomas and Wilms' tumors. Lab Invest 83:429–434

Wissmann C, Wild PJ, Kaiser S, Roepcke S, Stoehr R, Woenckhaus M, Kristiansen G, Hsieh JC, Hofstaedter F, Hartmann A, Knuechel R, Rosenthal A, Pilarsky C (2003) WIF1, a component of the Wnt pathway, is down-regulated in prostate, breast, lung, and bladder cancer. J Pathol 201:204–212

Wong CM, Fan ST, Ng IO (2001) Beta-catenin mutation and overexpression in hepatocellular carcinoma: clinicopathologic and prognostic significance. Cancer 92:136–145

Woo DK, Kim HS, Lee HS, Kang YH, Yang HK, Kim WH (2001) Altered expression and mutation of beta-catenin gene in gastric carcinomas and cell lines. Int J Cancer 95:108–113

Worm J, Christensen C, Gronbaek K, Tulchinsky E, Guldberg P (2004) Genetic and epigenetic alterations of the APC gene in malignant melanoma. Oncogene 23:5215–5226

Worsham MJ, Chen KM, Meduri V, Nygren AO, Errami A, Schouten JP, Benninger MS (2006) Epigenetic events of disease progression in head and neck squamous cell carcinoma. Arch Otolaryngol Head Neck Surg 132:668–677

Wright K, Wilson P, Morland S, Campbell I, Walsh M, Hurst T, Ward B, Cummings M, Chenevix-Trench G (1999) beta-catenin mutation and expression analysis in ovarian cancer: exon 3 mutations and nuclear translocation in 16% of endometrioid tumours. Int J Cancer 82:625–629

Wu R, Zhai Y, Fearon ER, Cho KR (2001) Diverse mechanisms of beta-catenin deregulation in ovarian endometrioid adenocarcinomas. Cancer Res 61:8247–8255

Wu Q, Lothe RA, Ahlquist T, Silins I, Trope CG, Micci F, Nesland JM, Suo Z, Lind GE (2007a) DNA methylation profiling of ovarian carcinomas and their in vitro models identifies HOXA9, HOXB5, SCGB3A1, and CRABP1 as novel targets. Mol Cancer 6:45

Wu R, Hendrix-Lucas N, Kuick R, Zhai Y, Schwartz DR, Akyol A, Hanash S, Misek DE, Katabuchi H, Williams BO, Fearon ER, Cho KR (2007b) Mouse model of human ovarian endometrioid adenocarcinoma based on somatic defects in the Wnt/beta-catenin and PI3K/Pten signaling pathways. Cancer Cell 11:321–333

Xia J, Urabe K, Moroi Y, Koga T, Duan H, Li Y, Furue M (2006) Beta-catenin mutation and its nuclear localization are confirmed to be frequent causes of Wnt signaling pathway activation in pilomatricomas. J Dermatol Sci 41:67–75

Xu HT, Wei Q, Liu Y, Yang LH, Dai SD, Han Y, Yu JH, Liu N, Wang EH (2007) Overexpression of axin downregulates TCF-4 and inhibits the development of lung cancer. Ann Surg Oncol 14:3251–3259

Yamamoto H, Oue N, Sato A, Hasegawa Y, Yamamoto H, Matsubara A, Yasui W, Kikuchi A (2010) Wnt5a signaling is involved in the aggressiveness of prostate cancer and expression of metalloproteinase. Oncogene 29:2036–2046

Yang TM, Leu SW, Li JM, Hung MS, Lin CH, Lin YC, Huang TJ, Tsai YH, Yang CT (2009) WIF-1 promoter region hypermethylation as an adjuvant diagnostic marker for non-small cell lung cancer-related malignant pleural effusions. J Cancer Res Clin Oncol 135:919–924

Yang Z, Wang Y, Fang J, Chen F, Liu J, Wu J, Wang Y (2010) Expression and aberrant promoter methylation of Wnt inhibitory factor-1 in human astrocytomas. J Exp Clin Cancer Res 29:26

Yardy GW, Bicknell DC, Wilding JL, Bartlett S, Liu Y, Winney B, Turner GD, Brewster SF, Bodmer WF (2009) Mutations in the AXIN1 gene in advanced prostate cancer. Eur Urol 56:486–494

Yashima K, Nakamori S, Murakami Y, Yamaguchi A, Hayashi K, Ishikawa O, Konishi Y, Sekiya T (1994) Mutations of the adenomatous polyposis coli gene in the mutation cluster region: comparison of human pancreatic and colorectal cancers. Int J Cancer 59:43–47

Yegnasubramanian S, Kowalski J, Gonzalgo ML, Zahurak M, Piantadosi S, Walsh PC, Bova GS, De Marzo AM, Isaacs WB, Nelson WG (2004) Hypermethylation of CpG islands in primary and metastatic human prostate cancer. Cancer Res 64:1975–1986

Yi N, Liao QP, Li T, Xiong Y (2009) Novel expression profiles and invasiveness-related biology function of DKK1 in endometrial carcinoma. Oncol Rep 21:1421–1427

Yokota N, Nishizawa S, Ohta S, Date H, Sugimura H, Namba H, Maekawa M (2002) Role of Wnt pathway in medulloblastoma oncogenesis. Int J Cancer 101:198–201

You L, He B, Xu Z, Uematsu K, Mazieres J, Mikami I, Reguart N, Moody TW, Kitajewski J, McCormick F, Jablons DM (2004) Inhibition of Wnt-2-mediated signaling induces programmed cell death in non-small-cell lung cancer cells. Oncogene 23:6170–6174

Yu C, Wang J (1998) Mutation of APC gene in sporadic colorectal tumors. Zhonghua Zhong Liu Za Zhi 20:348–350

Yu JM, Jun ES, Jung JS, Suh SY, Han JY, Kim JY, Kim KW, Jung JS (2007) Role of Wnt5a in the proliferation of human glioblastoma cells. Cancer Lett 257:172–181

Yu J, Tao Q, Cheng YY, Lee KY, Ng SS, Cheung KF, Tian L, Rha SY, Neumann U, Rocken C, Ebert MP, Chan FK, Sung JJ (2009) Promoter methylation of the Wnt/beta-catenin signaling antagonist Dkk-3 is associated with poor survival in gastric cancer. Cancer 115:49–60

Zeng G, Germinaro M, Micsenyi A, Monga NK, Bell A, Sood A, Malhotra V, Sood N, Midda V, Monga DK, Kokkinakis DM, Monga SP (2006) Aberrant Wnt/beta-catenin signaling in pancreatic adenocarcinoma. Neoplasia 8:279–289

Zenzmaier C, Untergasser G, Hermann M, Dirnhofer S, Sampson N, Berger P (2008) Dysregulation of Dkk-3 expression in benign and malignant prostatic tissue. Prostate 68:540–547

Zhang H, Xue Y (2008) Wnt pathway is involved in advanced gastric carcinoma. Hepatogastroenterology 55:1126–1130

Zhang LY, Jiang LN, Li FF, Li H, Liu F, Gu Y, Song Y, Zhang F, Ye J, Li Q (2010) Reduced beta-catenin expression is associated with good prognosis in astrocytoma. Pathol Oncol Res 16:253–257

Zhao CH, Bu XM, Zhang N (2007) Hypermethylation and aberrant expression of Wnt antagonist secreted frizzled-related protein 1 in gastric cancer. World J Gastroenterol 13:2214–2217

Zhao C, Bu X, Zhang N, Wang W (2009) Downregulation of SFRP5 expression and its inverse correlation with those of MMP-7 and MT1-MMP in gastric cancer. BMC Cancer 9:224

Zou H, Molina JR, Harrington JJ, Osborn NK, Klatt KK, Romero Y, Burgart LJ, Ahlquist DA (2005) Aberrant methylation of secreted frizzled-related protein genes in esophageal adenocarcinoma and Barrett's esophagus. Int J Cancer 116:584–591

Zucman-Rossi J, Benhamouche S, Godard C, Boyault S, Grimber G, Balabaud C, Cunha AS, Bioulac-Sage P, Perret C (2007) Differential effects of inactivated Axin1 and activated beta-catenin mutations in human hepatocellular carcinomas. Oncogene 26:774–780

Zurawel RH, Chiappa SA, Allen C, Raffel C (1998) Sporadic medulloblastomas contain oncogenic beta-catenin mutations. Cancer Res 58:896–899

Chapter 6
WNT/β-Catenin Signaling in Leukemia

Markus Müschen

Abstract Leukemia represents the malignant outgrowth of a transformed hematopoietic cell. Normal hematopoiesis develops in a hierarchy with a hematopoietic stem cell at its apex and gives rise to progenitor cells that are committed to multiple hematopoietic lineages. Leukemia can develop from the stem cell compartment (i.e., leading to chronic myeloid leukemia, CML) or committed lymphoid (acute lymphoblastic leukemia, ALL) and myeloid (acute myeloid leukemia, AML) progenitors. WNT/β-catenin signaling is not only critical for stem cell self-renewal and differentiation in normal hematopoiesis, but also affects the natural history of leukemic clones. Interestingly, individual components of the WNT/β-catenin signaling pathway have a lineage-specific role and regulate stem cell self-renewal, proliferation, or differentiation specifically in one leukemia subset. The identification of lineage-specific regulators of WNT/β-catenin signaling will be important in the development of novel therapy approaches to selectively eradicate leukemia stem cells. Leukemia-initiating cells are implicated in relapse of leukemia and drug resistance, which represent two major clinical problems in the treatment of leukemia. At least in CML and AML, leukemia-initiating cells critically depend on active WNT/β-catenin signaling and targeted inhibition of this pathway will likely result in eradication of leukemia stem cells in these leukemia subtypes.

Keywords Leukemia • ALL • CML • AML • Progenitors • Hematopoiesis

Leukemia can be subdivided based on cell of origin and lineage derivation of the malignant clone and the transforming oncogene or cytogenetic lesion. Three major subtypes of leukemia are distinguished. Chronic myeloid leukemia (CML) and most cases of acute myeloid leukemia (AML) are thought to be derived from a transformed hematopoietic stem cell (Fialkow et al. 1980). Some AML and virtually all

M. Müschen (✉)
Department of Laboratory Medicine, Department of Pathology and Department of Medicine,
UCSF School of Medicine, University of California San Francisco, 521 Parnassus Avenue,
San Francisco, CA 94143, USA
e-mail: Markus.muschen@ucsf.edu

K.H. Goss and M. Kahn (eds.), *Targeting the Wnt Pathway in Cancer*,
DOI 10.1007/978-1-4419-8023-6_6, © Springer Science+Business Media, LLC 2011

cases of B- and T-cell lineage acute lymphoblastic leukemia (ALL) originate from committed myeloid or lymphoid progenitor cells. This overview focuses on WNT/β-catenin signaling in these three leukemia types relative to their normal counterparts, i.e., hematopoietic stem cells and myeloid or lymphoid progenitor cells. Chronic lymphocytic leukemia (CLL)/small lymphocytic lymphoma, although associated with leukemic dissemination, is considered as a non-Hodgkin's lymphoma subtype and, therefore, not discussed here.

6.1   WNT/β-Catenin Signaling in Normal Hematopoietic Stem Cells

As a reflection of their mesodermal origin, hematopoietic lineages are regulated by factors that also control mesoderm formation and patterning. Therefore, components of the Notch, Hedgehog, and WNT signaling pathways have a critical role in the regulation of hematopoietic stem cell self-renewal, differentiation, and lineage commitment. The first indication for a central role of WNT/β-catenin signaling in normal hematopoiesis came from an experiment, in which mouse WNT factors induced expansion of hematopoietic multilineage progenitor cells from mouse fetal livers (Austin et al. 1997). Subsequent work identified WNT3A as critical growth factor for hematopoietic stem cells (Willert et al. 2003). In addition, WNT5A increased the repopulating capacity and primitive hematopoietic development of human hematopoietic stem cells in vivo (Murdoch et al. 2003). Besides WNT3A and WNT5A ligands, β-catenin was implicated as a critical mediator of hematopoietic stem cell self-renewal. Retroviral transduction of purified Lin$^-$ Sca-1$^+$ c-Kit$^+$ Thy1.1$^+$ hematopoietic stem cells with a constitutively active β-catenin mutant (S33Y) dramatically increased self-renewal capacity and hematopoietic reconstitution efficiency (Reya et al. 2003). These findings, however, were in contrast to two subsequent studies, in which transgenic expression of S33Y β-catenin mutant results in compromised hematopoietic stem cell maintenance and multilineage defects (Kirstetter et al. 2006). Inducible activation of β-catenin by conditional deletion of exon 3 had essentially the same effect and caused loss of hematopoietic stem cells and profound multilineage hematopoietic defects (Scheller et al. 2006). In contrast to the two other studies, Reya et al. used in vitro transduction of *Bcl2*-transgenic hematopoietic stem cells, which may at least in part account for the differences observed.

While Reya et al. (2003) suggest that canonical WNT signaling plays a fundamental role in self-renewal and maintenance of hematopoietic stem cells, subsequent work demonstrated that at least β-catenin is not required (Cobas et al. 2004). Surprisingly, hematopoietic reconstitution from β-catenin-deficient bone marrow was not significantly different from wildtype bone marrow, demonstrating that β-catenin does not, in fact, play a critical role in hematopoietic stem cell self-renewal. This leaves the possibility that γ-catenin might compensate for β-catenin in canonical WNT signaling. A subsequent study based on β- and γ-catenin double-knockout bone marrow, however, demonstrated that neither β- nor γ-catenin is required or compensates for each other in hematopoietic stem cell maintenance and multilineage differentiation (Koch et al. 2008).

Retroviral expression of constitutively active β-catenin seemed to strongly enhance hematopoietic stem cell self-renewal without compromising the hematopoietic differentiation potential in vitro (Reya et al. 2003), thus suggesting a crucial function for canonical WNT signaling in hematopoiesis. In contrast, subsequent genetic gain- and loss-of-function studies demonstrated that transgenic activation of β-catenin results in hematopoietic stem cell depletion (Scheller et al. 2006; Kirstetter et al. 2006) and conditional deletion of neither β- nor γ-catenin negatively impacts the multilineage potential of hematopoietic stem cells (Koch et al. 2008). While it is likely that canonical WNT signaling contributes to self-renewal of hematopoietic stem cells, it remains unclear which factors may compensate for loss of β-catenin and γ-catenin.

6.2 WNT/β-Catenin Signaling in Lymphopoiesis

Lymphoid-enhancing factor (LEF1) and T-cell factor (TCF) are both HMG-domain carrying coactivators of nuclear β-catenin and initially recognized for their role in early lymphocyte development (Travis et al. 1991; Verbeek et al. 1995). TCF1 expression is restricted to the T-cell lineage, whereas LEF1 is expressed both in early T cells and in pro- and pre-B cells (Bruhn et al. 1997). TCF1$^{-/-}$ mice, which carry a deletion of Tcf1 exon 7, exhibit a profound block in thymocyte development with the DN4/DP transition and failure to maintain early thymocyte progenitor cells (Verbeek et al. 1995). By contrast, Lef1-deficient mice have no abnormalities in T cell development, but defects in the development of the B-cell lineage (Reya et al. 2000). Besides other defects, Lef1$^{-/-}$ mice show a profound reduction of fetal liver and bone marrow pro- and pre-B cells, which is owing to increased cell death and decreased proliferation rate of Lef1$^{-/-}$ B-cell progenitors (Reya et al. 2000). These findings suggest that LEF1/TCF signaling provides important survival and proliferation signals during thymocyte and pro-/pre-B cell development, i.e., stages of lymphocyte development that are susceptible to leukemogenesis. Likewise, transgenic expression of a stabilized β-catenin mutant in the T-cell lineage results in a differentiation block and predisposes to T-cell lineage leukemogenesis (Guo et al. 2007). On the other hand, neither β- nor γ-catenin is required for B and T lymphopoiesis (Cobas et al. 2004; Koch et al. 2008). In addition, WNT5A increases self-renewal capacity of hematopoietic stem cells (Murdoch et al. 2003), but also limits the proliferation of B-cell precursors and functions as tumor suppressor against B-cell lineage leukemia (Liang et al. 2003).

6.3 WNT Signaling in B-Cell Lineage Acute Lymphoblastic Leukemia

B-cell lineage ALL typically arises from pro- and pre-B cell stages of B cell development, in which the V(D)J recombinase is active to rearrange immunoglobulin heavy chain or light chain gene segments. Rearrangement of immunoglobulin heavy and light chain gene segments occurs in developing pro- and pre-B cells, respectively. For this reason, errors of the V(D)J recombinase have been implicated in the generation of chromosomal translocations that define major subtypes of ALL (Tsai et al. 2008). A relatively small number of characteristic cytogenetic lesions define biological and clinical subtypes of ALL. For instance, the *MLL-AF4* [t(4;11) (q21;q23)] rearrangement is found in the vast majority of infant leukemia cases (~3% of all cases) and is associated with poor clinical outcome. *MLL-AF4* is typically derived from pro-B cells and exhibit a characteristic *m*ixed-*l*ineage *l*eukemia (MLL) phenotype and oncogenic activity of the FLT3 receptor-type tyrosine kinase, which is owing to somatic mutations in some cases (Armstrong et al. 2004). While the *MLL-AF9* fusion induces WNT/β-catenin signaling in AML (Wang et al. 2010), this has not been shown for the *MLL-AF4* oncogene in ALL. Likewise, oncogenic mutants of the FLT3 receptor tyrosine kinase induce WNT/β-catenin signaling in AML, but not in B-cell lineage ALL (Tickenbrock et al. 2005; Kajiguchi et al. 2007).

    ALL cells with a hyperdiploid karyotype or with *TEL-AML1* gene rearrangement [t(12;21)(p12;q22)] are most frequently found in childhood ALL and are both associated with a favorable clinical prognosis. Both ALL subtypes develop from a transformed pre-B cell and have a prenatal (i.e., in utero) origin (Greaves and Wiemels 2003). The *AML1-ETO* fusion gene induces WNT/β-catenin signaling in AML (Müller-Tidow et al. 2004), however this is not the case for *TEL-AML1* in B-cell lineage ALL. The finding that *MLL-* and *AML1*-fusion genes induce oncogenic WNT/β-catenin signaling in AML but not B-cell lineage ALL may indicate a lineage-specific role of WNT signaling in leukemogenesis. This hypothesis is supported by the finding that aberrant expression of β-catenin is a frequent characteristic of myeloid lineage AML, but not B-cell lineage ALL cells (Serinsöz et al. 2004). In adults, the oncogenic BCR-ABL1 tyrosine kinase defines the most frequent subtype of B-cell lineage ALL (~27% of the cases). The *BCR-ABL1* fusion results from the Philadelphia chromosome [t(9;22)(q34;q11)] and is associated with poor clinical outcome in ALL (Mancini et al. 2005). Also in the case of the BCR-ABL1-induced leukemia, the available evidence suggests a lineage-specific role of WNT/β-catenin signaling in leukemogenesis: BCR-ABL1 is not only found in adult B-cell lineage ALL, but also in virtually all cases of CML. While WNT/β-catenin signaling is critical for leukemia-initiation and leukemia stem cell self-renewal in BCR-ABL1 myeloid CML, it is dispensable in BCR-ABL1 B-cell lineage ALL (Zhao et al. 2007). While these findings collectively indicate that WNT/β-catenin signaling is not involved in the leukemic transformation in major subtypes of ALL including *MLL-AF4*, hyperdiploid ALL, *TEL-AML1*, and *BCR-ABL1*, there is at least one other subtype of ALL, in which WNT signaling plays a distinctive role (Khan et al. 2007). The *E2A-PBX1* [t(1;19)(q23;p13)] fusion is found in ~4% of cases of childhood ALL and involves a rearrangement of the *TCF3* gene (encoding the E2A transcription factor). TCF3/E2A is not only a critical regulator of B-cell lineage commitment and early B cell development (Müschen et al. 2002; Sigvardsson et al. 2002), but also cooperates with LEF1 to activate canonical WNT/β-catenin signaling (Hovanes et al. 2001; Merrill et al. 2001). Of note, gene expression classification analyses showed that *E2A-PBX1* ALL cells exhibit dramatically increased expression levels of LEF1 (Yeoh et al. 2002; Ross et al. 2003). However, whether or not TCF3-PBX1 and LEF1 indeed cooperate to activate canonical WNT signaling in *E2A-PBX1* ALL has not formally been investigated. The finding of autocrine WNT16 production in this ALL subset further supports the hypothesis of constitutively active WNT signaling in *E2A-PBX1* ALL (McWhirter et al. 1999). Aberrant expression of WNT16 is induced by the *E2A-PBX1* fusion gene (McWhirter et al. 1999) and promotes survival and proliferation of the ALL cells (Mazieres et al. 2005). While WNT16 stimulates proliferation in *E2A-PBX1* ALL cells, WNT5A functions as a tumor suppressor in other ALL subtypes, inhibits proliferation (Liang et al. 2003), and is frequently hypermethylated in primary human ALL cells (Ying et al. 2007). It is currently not clear whether this difference is owing to different signaling pathways that are initiated by WNT16 vs. WNT5A or whether *E2A-PBX1* ALL fundamentally differs from other ALL subtypes with respect to WNT signaling.

6.4 Negative Regulation of WNT/β-Catenin Signaling Through BTK

Of note, *E2A-PBX1* pre-B ALL cells also differ from other ALL subsets in that they exhibit active signaling through the pre-B-cell receptor (Trageser et al. 2009). The pre-B-cell receptor is composed of the μ-heavy chain and a complex of signaling molecules close to the cell membrane, which includes the tyrosine kinase BTK. While the pre-B-cell receptor suppresses proliferation in other pre-B ALL subtypes, this is not the case in *E2A-PBX1* ALL (Nahar and Müschen 2009). Interestingly, recent work identified BTK as a strong negative regulator of WNT/β-catenin signaling in human B cells and B-cell lineage leukemia (James et al. 2009). It is therefore tempting to speculate that WNT16/TCF3/LEF1 signaling is needed in E2A-PBX1 ALL cells to balance negative regulation of WNT/β-catenin signaling through BTK downstream of the pre-B-cell receptor. Interestingly, human B-cell lineage ALL cells often show defective expression of BTK (Feldhahn et al. 2005) and loss of BTK expression in mice predisposes to B-cell lineage ALL (Kersseboom et al. 2003).

6.5 WNT/β-Catenin Signaling Promotes Leukemogenesis in the T-Cell Lineage

While the role of WNT/β-catenin signaling in B-cell lineage ALL is poorly understood, multiple lines of evidence indicate a role of WNT signaling in T-cell lineage leukemogenesis. The most direct evidence comes from transgenic expression of the S33Y β-catenin mutant during early thymopoiesis (Guo et al. 2007). A stabilized form of β-catenin not only induces a differentiation block in double-positive thymocytes, but also predisposes to T-cell lineage ALL (Guo et al. 2007). In addition, in the Pten$^{-/-}$ model for T-cell lineage ALL, β-catenin activation was identified as a cooperating event in leukemogenesis: Conditional ablation of one allele of the β-catenin (*Ctnnb*) gene substantially decreased the incidence of T-ALL and prolonged latency of disease in a mouse model for T-ALL caused by Pten loss (Guo et al. 2008). The authors proposed that activation of the β-catenin pathway has an important contribution to leukemia initiation in the T-cell lineage and, hence the maintenance and expansion of leukemia initiating (or leukemia stem) cells (Guo et al. 2008). In addition, Dan Tenen's group identified a novel mechanism through which PU.1 limits proliferation of T lymphoid cells (Rosenbauer et al. 2006). An upstream regulatory element (URE) of PU.1 had opposite functions in the B-cell and T-cell lineages, respectively, and functions as enhancer in B cells but as repressor in T-cell precursors. TCF transcription factors coordinated the PU.1-repressor function of URE and linked PU.1 to TCF/LEF1/WNT signaling. T cell-specific deletion of URE leads to failure of PU.1 repression in T-cell progenitors and results in a differentiation block and T-cell lineage leukemia (Rosenbauer et al. 2006). Of note, a substantial fraction of T-ALL cases is virally induced. The leukemogenic retrovirus human T-cell leukemia virus type 1 (HTLV-1) induces T-cell precursor transformation in part through the transforming protein Tax. As an indication that WNT/β-catenin signaling is uniformly involved in a broad range of T-ALL subsets, Tax-mediated leukemogenesis is also mediated via aberrant activation of the WNT/β-catenin pathway (Tomita et al. 2006).

6.6 WNT/β-Catenin Signaling is Required for Leukemia-Initiation in Acute Myeloid Leukemia

In AML, leukemia subtypes are defined by a set of oncogenic fusion genes that are the result of chromosomal translocations. The importance of the WNT/β-catenin pathway in AML is highlighted by the finding that these subset-defining oncogenic fusion molecules directly activate WNT signaling in AML cells (e.g., *AML-ETO*, *PML-RARA*; Müller-Tidow et al. 2004). Subsequent work showed that oncogenic fusion transcription factors indeed associate with TCFs and influence LEF1/TCF-dependent transcription in the WNT/β-catenin pathway (Moore et al. 2008). These and other findings led to the concept that WNT/β-catenin signaling plays a crucial role in leukemogenesis and, likely, leukemia-initiation in AML (Mikesch et al. 2007). Indeed, primary human AML cells express β-catenin at the mRNA and the protein level to a significantly higher extent than normal hematopoietic progenitors (Serinsöz et al. 2004). Simon et al. (2005) demonstrated constitutively active β-catenin signaling in a broad array of AML subtypes. This was based on the finding of nuclear accumulation of β-catenin and TCF/LEF1 reporter activity in AML cells. In addition, AML cells showed increased mRNA levels of WNT1, WNT2b, and LEF1 (Simon et al. 2005). Mainly based on AML and T-ALL cell lines, a prior study had already shown that dominant-negative β-catenin and TCF mutants compromise cell adhesion, proliferation, and survival of leukemia cell lines (Chung et al. 2002), suggesting that negative regulators of the WNT/β-catenin pathway are inactivated. There is now broad evidence from multiple groups that this is indeed the case: For instance, the Groucho/TLE1 repressor, which displaces β-catenin from TCF/LEF1 in WNT-mediated transcriptional activation, is frequently silenced by hypermethylation in AML cells (Fraga et al. 2008). Two subsequent studies extended these findings on Groucho/TLE1 to additional negative regulators of WNT signaling including the Frizzled decoy receptors sFRP1, sFRP2, sFRP4, and sFRP5 and the WNT antagonists DKK1 and DKK3 (Valencia et al. 2009; Reins et al. 2010). Collectively, these studies indicate that constitutively active WNT/β-catenin signaling in AML is the consequence of direct interaction of leukemogenic fusion molecules with TCFs and β-catenin and global epigenetic silencing of negative regulators of WNT/β-catenin signaling. In addition, overexpression of γ-catenin and Lef1 accelerates myeloid leukemogenesis and development of AML and increases self-renewal capacity of AML-initiating cells (or leukemia stem cells; Zheng et al. 2004; Petropoulos et al. 2008). Similar observations have been made in a clinical context: high expression levels of β-catenin predict relapse in AML and poor overall clinical outcome (Ysebaert et al. 2006). In addition, increased activity of the WNT/β-catenin signaling pathway is associated with decreased sensitivity to chemotherapy and development of drug resistance (De Toni et al. 2006). Likewise, hypermethylation of the negative WNT signaling regulator WIF1 (Wnt inhibitory factor-1) was identified as an independent prognostic factor of poor clinical outcome (Chim et al. 2006).

Besides leukemogenic fusion transcription factors (e.g., *AML-ETO*; *PML-RARA*), AML cells often carry a characteristic mutation resulting in an oncogenic tyrosine kinase. In AML, internal tandem duplications (ITD) in the juxtamembrane domain of the FLT3 receptor-type tyrosine kinase are found in ~20% of the cases. Importantly, not only leukemogenic fusion transcription factors (e.g., *AML-ETO*; *PML-RARA*; Müller-Tidow et al. 2004) induce activation of WNT signaling, but oncogenic tyrosine kinase activity from FLT3-ITD mutants also enhances WNT/β-catenin signaling activity (Tickenbrock et al. 2005; Kajiguchi et al. 2007).

6.7 Role of Prostaglandin E/β-Catenin Signaling in Leukemia Stem Cell Maintenance in AML

The concept of cancer as a hierarchically organized cell population with so-called cancer stem cells at its apex was initially derived from observations in AML. Dick and colleagues have discovered a stem cell hierarchy in AML (Bonnet and Dick 1997) and defined leukemia stem cells based on phenotype and the ability to initiate heterogeneous leukemia populations in transplant-recipient mice (Lapidot et al. 1994). Of note, the phenotype of leukemia stem cells in AML is strikingly similar to stem cell phenotypes in normal hematopoiesis.

Previous work suggested an involvement of WNT/β-catenin signaling in self-renewal of normal hematopoietic stem cell (Willert et al. 2003; Reya et al. 2003). A recent study now provided evidence that WNT/β-catenin signaling is also critical for self-renewal of leukemia stem cells in AML (Wang et al. 2010). This study used the phenotypic (similar to normal hematopoietic stem cells) and operational (leukemia-initiation in transplant-recipient NOD/SCID mice) definition that was introduced by John Dick's work and demonstrated that conditional deletion of β-catenin resulted in depletion of leukemia stem cell populations and loss of leukemia-initiation capacity (Wang et al. 2010). While this outcome was not surprising, the study by Scott Armstrong's group demonstrated for the first time that pharmacological interference with prostaglandin synthesis through the cyclooxygenase-1 inhibitor indomethacin was sufficient to eradicate leukemia stem cells in AML. Based on previous studies on Prostaglandin E2 (PGE2)-mediated stabilization of nuclear β-catenin in colon cancer (Castellone et al. 2005), embryonic stem cells and Zebrafish hematopoietic stem cells (Goessling et al. 2009), it was inferred that inhibition of PGE2-synthesis will destabilize β-catenin and ultimately lead to eradication of leukemia stem cells in AML. Indeed, long-term exposure to indomethacin resulted in a dramatic reduction of β-catenin levels and indomethacin-treated leukemia cells failed to initiate the disease in secondary transplant recipients. Additional studies are needed to directly prove a contribution of PGE2-synthesis to leukemia stem cell maintenance in AML. Given that cyclooxygenase-1 inhibitors are readily available as adjuvant drugs, these findings are of immediate clinical relevance.

6.8 WNT Signaling in Chronic Myeloid Leukemia

Like AML, CML develops as a heterogeneous leukemia population originating from a transformed hematopoietic stem cell. In virtually all cases, CML cells carry the oncogenic BCR-ABL1 tyrosine kinase, which is also present in a major subset of B-cell lineage ALL. Like FLT3-ITD tyrosine kinase activity in AML, also oncogenic tyrosine kinase activity from BCR-ABL1 results in stabilization of β-catenin in CML cells (Coluccia et al. 2007). In addition, the breakpoint cluster region (*BCR*) gene functions as negative regulator of WNT signaling (Ress and Moelling 2005), but is inactivated as part of the fusion with *ABL1*. Even the wild-type BCR molecule, which is still expressed from the nonrearranged allele, is inactivated in BCR-ABL1-driven CML cells. The BCR-ABL1 kinase phosphorylates the BCR protein, which leads to loss of its ability to interfere with WNT/β-catenin signaling (Ress and Moelling 2005). A previous report suggested that WNT/β-catenin signaling is increased in granulocyte-macrophage progenitor cells during blast crisis progression of CML (Jamieson et al. 2004). Committed granulocyte-macrophage progenitor cells were proposed as leukemia stem cells in blast crisis CML (Jamieson et al. 2004). This proposal, however, is in direct conflict with findings by Huntly and colleagues (2004): Huntly et al. demonstrated that BCR-ABL1 can initiate leukemia from a transformed hematopoietic stem cell but not from a committed progenitor cell (Huntly and Gilliland 2004), such as the committed granulocyte-macrophage progenitor cells proposed by Jamieson et al. (2004). While the phenotypic definition of the leukemia stem cell population(s) in CML remains controversial, two recent studies demonstrated that WNT/β-catenin signaling is critical for leukemia stem cell maintenance in CML (Zhao et al. 2007; Hu et al. 2009).

In addition, gene expression analyses suggested increased activation of the WNT/β-catenin signaling pathway during progression of CML from chronic phase into accelerated phase and ultimate blast crisis (Radich et al. 2006). In analogy to AML, where negative regulators of the WNT/β-catenin signaling pathway are often inactivated by hypermethylation, defective expression of the WNT/β-catenin signaling inhibitor GSK3β was reported (Abrahamsson et al. 2009). This study showed that aberrant splicing of the GSK3β pre-mRNA resulted in loss-of-function variants and increased WNT/β-catenin signaling activity. In seeming contrast to these findings, however, pharmacological inhibition of GSK3β seems to inhibit leukemia cell growth, but not self-renewal signaling of normal hematopoietic stem cells (Holmes et al. 2008).

6.9 Perspective

Pharmacologic inhibition of GSK3β as a potential treatment option for CML remains controversial. Future endeavors to eradicate leukemia stem cells in AML and CML will likely focus on strategies to modulate coactivator usage of β-catenin: While CBP/β-catenin complexes activate a transcriptional program leading to self-renewal and maintenance of stem cell characteristics, p300/β-catenin interactions induce transcriptional activation of differentiation (Takahashi-Yanaga and Kahn 2010). The distinctive role of CBP vs. p300 coactivators in stem cell self-renewal vs. lineage commitment decisions was previously exemplified for hematopoietic differentiation (Rebel et al. 2002). Importantly, small molecule inhibitors to selectively block interactions between CBP and β-catenin (Emami et al. 2004) and p300 and β-catenin (Miyabayashi et al. 2007) have been recently developed. From a therapeutic point of view, selective inhibition of CBP and β-catenin interactions will be a highly attractive approach to eradicate leukemia stem cells, while differentiation processes in normal hematopoiesis will be left intact (Rebel et al. 2002). From a scientific point of view, the concept is attractive, because it would resolve much of the controversial aspects related to WNT signaling in stem cell self-renewal and differentiation discussed in this overview. The concept reflects the ambivalent nature of WNT/β-catenin signaling in that it is critical for both stem cell self-renewal *and* commitment and differentiation decisions.

References

Abrahamsson AE, Geron I, Gotlib J, Dao KH, Barroga CF, Newton IG, Giles FJ, Durocher J, Creusot RS, Karimi M, Jones C, Zehnder JL, Keating A, Negrin RS, Weissman IL, Jamieson CH (2009) Glycogen synthase kinase 3beta missplicing contributes to leukemia stem cell generation. Proc Natl Acad Sci U S A 106:3925–3929

Armstrong SA, Mabon ME, Silverman LB, Li A, Gribben JG, Fox EA, Sallan SE, Korsmeyer SJ (2004) FLT3 mutations in childhood acute lymphoblastic leukemia. Blood 103:3544–3546

Austin TW, Solar GP, Ziegler FC, Liem L, Matthews W (1997) A role for the Wnt gene family in hematopoiesis: expansion of multilineage progenitor cells. Blood 89:3624–3635

Bonnet D, Dick JE (1997) Human acute myeloid leukemia is organized as a hierarchy that originates from a primitive hematopoietic cell. Nat Med 3:730–737

Bruhn L, Munnerlyn A, Grosschedl R (1997) ALY, a context-dependent coactivator of LEF-1 and AML-1, is required for TCRα enhancer function. Genes Dev 11:640–653

Castellone MD, Teramoto H, Williams BO, Druey KM, Gutkind JS (2005) Prostaglandin E2 promotes colon cancer cell growth through a Gs-axin-beta-catenin signaling axis. Science 310:1504–1510

Chim CS, Chan WW, Pang A, Kwong YL (2006) Preferential methylation of Wnt inhibitory factor-1 in acute promyelocytic leukemia: an independent poor prognostic factor. Leukemia 20:907–909

Chung EJ, Hwang SG, Nguyen P, Lee S, Kim JS, Kim JW, Henkart PA, Bottaro DP, Soon L, Bonvini P, Lee SJ, Karp JE, Oh HJ, Rubin JS, Trepel JB (2002) Regulation of leukemic cell adhesion, proliferation, and survival by beta-catenin. Blood 100:982–990

Cobas M, Wilson A, Ernst B, Mancini SJ, MacDonald HR, Kemler R, Radtke F (2004) Beta-catenin is dispensable for hematopoiesis and lymphopoiesis. J Exp Med 199:221–229

Coluccia AM, Vacca A, Duñach M, Mologni L, Redaelli S, Bustos VH, Benati D, Pinna LA, Gambacorti-Passerini C (2007) Bcr-Abl stabilizes beta-catenin in chronicmyeloid leukemia through its tyrosine phosphorylation. EMBO J 26:1456–1466

De Toni F, Racaud-Sultan C, Chicanne G, Mas VM, Cariven C, Mesange F, Salles JP, Demur C, Allouche M, Payrastre B, Manenti S, Ysebaert L (2006) A crosstalk between the Wnt and the adhesion-dependent signaling pathways governs the chemosensitivity of acute myeloid leukemia. Oncogene 25:3113–3122

Emami KH, Nguyen C, Ma H, Kim DH, Jeong KW, Eguchi M, Moon RT, Teo JL, Kim HY, Moon SH, Ha JR, Kahn M (2004) A small molecule inhibitor of beta-catenin/CREB-binding protein transcription. Proc Natl Acad Sci U S A 101:12682–12687

Feldhahn N, Río P, Soh BN, Liedtke S, Sprangers M, Klein F, Wernet P, Jumaa H, Hofmann WK, Hanenberg H, Rowley JD, Müschen M (2005) Deficiency of Bruton's tyrosine kinase in B cell precursor leukemia cells. Proc Natl Acad Sci U S A 102:13266–13271

Fialkow PJ, Jacobson RJ, Singer JW, Sacher RA, McGuffin RW, Neefe JR (1980) Philadelphia chromosome (Ph1) chronic myelogenous leukemia (CML): a clonal disease with origin in a multipotent stem cell. Blood 56:70–73

Fraga MF, Berdasco M, Ballestar E, Ropero S, Lopez-Nieva P, Lopez-Serra L, Martín-Subero JI, Calasanz MJ, Lopez de Silanes I, Setien F, Casado S, Fernandez AF, Siebert R, Stifani S, Esteller M (2008) Epigenetic inactivation of the Groucho homologue gene TLE1 in hematologic malignancies. Cancer Res 68:4116–4122

Goessling W, North TE, Loewer S, Lord AM, Lee S, Stoick-Cooper CL, Weidinger G, Puder M, Daley GQ, Moon RT, Zon LI (2009) Genetic interaction of PGE2 and Wnt signaling regulates developmental specification of stem cells and regeneration. Cell 136:1136–1147

Greaves MF, Wiemels J (2003) Origins of chromosome translocations in childhood leukaemia. Nat Rev Cancer 3:639–649

Guo Z, Dose M, Kovalovsky D, Chang R, O'Neil J, Look AT, von Boehmer H, Khazaie K, Gounari F (2007) Beta-catenin stabilization stalls the transition from double-positive to single-positive stage and predisposes thymocytes to malignant transformation. Blood 109:5463–5472

Guo W, Lasky JL, Chang CJ, Mosessian S, Lewis X, Xiao Y, Yeh JE, Chen JY, Iruela-Arispe ML, Varella-Garcia M, Wu H (2008) Multi-genetic events collaboratively contribute to Pten-null leukaemia stem-cell formation. Nature 453:529–533

Holmes T, O'Brien TA, Knight R, Lindeman R, Shen S, Song E, Symonds G, Dolnikov A (2008) Glycogen synthase kinase-3 beta inhibition preserves hematopoietic stem cell activity and inhibits leukemic cell growth. Stem Cells 26:1288–1297

Hovanes K, Li TW, Munguia JE, Truong T, Milovanovic T, Lawrence Marsh J, Holcombe RF, Waterman ML (2001) Beta-catenin-sensitive isoforms of lymphoid enhancer factor-1 are selectively expressed in colon cancer. Nat Genet 28:53–57

Hu Y, Chen Y, Douglas L, Li S (2009) beta-Catenin is essential for survival of leukemic stem cells insensitive to kinase inhibition in mice with BCR-ABL-induced chronic myeloid leukemia. Leukemia 23:109–116

Huntly BJ, Gilliland DG (2004) Blasts from the past: new lessons in stem cell biology from chronic myelogenous leukemia. Cancer Cell 6:199–201

Huntly BJ, Shigematsu H, Deguchi K, Lee BH, Mizuno S, Duclos N, Rowan R, Amaral S, Curley D, Williams IR, Akashi K, Gilliland DG (2004) MOZ-TIF2, but not BCR-ABL, confers properties of leukemic stem cells to committed murine hematopoietic progenitors. Cancer Cell 6:587–596

James RG, Biechele TL, Conrad WH, Camp ND, Fass DM, Major MB, Sommer K, Yi X, Roberts BS, Cleary MA, Arthur WT, MacCoss M, Rawlings DJ, Haggarty SJ, Moon RT (2009) Bruton's tyrosine kinase revealed as a negative regulator of Wnt-beta-catenin signaling. Sci Signal 2:ra25

Jamieson CH, Ailles LE, Dylla SJ, Muijtjens M, Jones C, Zehnder JL, Gotlib J, Li K, Manz MG, Keating A, Sawyers CL, Weissman IL (2004) Granulocyte-macrophageprogenitors as candidate leukemic stem cells in blast-crisis CML. N Engl J Med 351:657–667

Kajiguchi T, Chung EJ, Lee S, Stine A, Kiyoi H, Naoe T, Levis MJ, Neckers L, Trepel JB (2007) FLT3 regulates beta-catenin tyrosine phosphorylation, nuclear localization, and transcriptional activity in acute myeloid leukemia cells. Leukemia 21:2476–2484

Kersseboom R, Middendorp S, Dingjan GM, Dahlenborg K, Reth M, Jumaa H, Hendriks RW (2003) Bruton's tyrosine kinase cooperates with the B cell linker protein SLP-65 as a tumor suppressor in pre-B cells. J Exp Med 198:91–98

Khan NI, Bradstock KF, Bendall LJ (2007) Activation of Wnt/beta-catenin pathway mediates growth and survival in B-cell progenitor acute lymphoblastic leukaemia. Br J Haematol 138:338–348

Kirstetter P, Anderson K, Porse BT, Jacobsen SE, Nerlov C (2006) Activation of the canonical Wnt pathway leads to loss of hematopoietic stem cell repopulation and multilineage differentiation block. Nat Immunol 7:1048–1056

Koch U, Wilson A, Cobas M, Kemler R, Macdonald HR, Radtke F (2008) Simultaneous loss of beta- and gamma-catenin does not perturb hematopoiesis or lymphopoiesis. Blood 111:160–164

Lapidot T, Sirard C, Vormoor J, Murdoch B, Hoang T, Caceres-Cortes J, Minden M, Paterson B, Caligiuri MA, Dick JE (1994) A cell initiating human acute myeloid leukaemia after transplantation into SCID mice. Nature 367:645–648

Liang H, Chen Q, Coles AH, Anderson SJ, Pihan G, Bradley A, Gerstein R, Jurecic R, Jones SN (2003) Wnt5a inhibits B cell proliferation and functions as a tumor suppressor in hematopoietic tissue. Cancer Cell 4:349–360

Mancini M, Scappaticci D, Cimino G, Nanni M, Derme V, Elia L, Tafuri A, Vignetti M, Vitale A, Cuneo A, Castoldi G, Saglio G, Pane F, Mecucci C, Camera A, Specchia G, Tedeschi A, Di Raimondo F, Fioritoni G, Fabbiano F, Marmont F, Ferrara F, Cascavilla N, Todeschini G, Nobile F, Kropp MG, Leoni P, Tabilio A, Luppi M, Annino L, Mandelli F, Foà R (2005) A comprehensive genetic classification of adult acute lymphoblastic leukemia (ALL): analysis of the GIMEMA 0496 protocol. Blood 105:3434–3441

Mazieres J, You L, He B, Xu Z, Lee AY, Mikami I, McCormick F, Jablons DM (2005) Inhibition of Wnt16 in human acute lymphoblastoid leukemia cells containing thet(1;19) translocation induces apoptosis. Oncogene 24:5396–5400

McWhirter JR, Neuteboom ST, Wancewicz EV, Monia BP, Downing JR, Murre C (1999) Oncogenic homeodomain transcription factor E2A-Pbx1 activates a novel WNT gene in pre-B acute lymphoblastoid leukemia. Proc Natl Acad Sci U S A 96:11464–11469

Merrill BJ, Gat U, DasGupta R, Fuchs E (2001) Tcf3 and Lef1 regulate lineage differentiation of multipotent stem cells in skin. Genes Dev 15:1688–1705

Mikesch JH, Steffen B, Berdel WE, Serve H, Müller-Tidow C (2007) The emerging role of Wnt signaling in the pathogenesis of acute myeloid leukemia. Leukemia 21:1638–1647

Miyabayashi T, Teo JL, Yamamoto M, McMillan M, Nguyen C, Kahn M (2007) Wnt/beta-catenin/CBP signaling maintains long-term murine embryonic stem cell pluripotency. Proc Natl Acad Sci U S A 104:5668–5673

Moore AC, Amann JM, Williams CS, Tahinci E, Farmer TE, Martinez JA, Yang G, Luce KS, Lee E, Hiebert SW (2008) Myeloid translocation gene family members associate with T-cell factors (TCFs) and influence TCF-dependent transcription. Mol Cell Biol 28:977–987

Müller-Tidow C, Steffen B, Cauvet T, Tickenbrock L, Ji P, Diederichs S, Sargin B, Köhler G, Stelljes M, Puccetti E, Ruthardt M, de Vos S, Hiebert SW, Koeffler HP, Berdel WE, Serve H (2004) Translocation products in acute myeloid leukemia activate the Wnt signaling pathway in hematopoietic cells. Mol Cell Biol 24:2890–2904

Murdoch B, Chadwick K, Martin M, Shojaei F, Shah KV, Gallacher L, Moon RT, Bhatia M (2003) Wnt-5A augments repopulating capacity and primitive hematopoietic development of human blood stem cells in vivo. Proc Natl Acad Sci U S A 100:3422–3427

Müschen M, Lee S, Zhou G, Feldhahn N, Barath VS, Chen J, Moers C, Krönke M, Rowley JD, Wang SM (2002) Molecular portraits of B cell lineage commitment. Proc Natl Acad Sci U S A 99:10014–10019

Nahar R, Müschen M (2009) Pre-B cell receptor signaling in acute lymphoblastic leukemia. Cell Cycle 8:3874–3877

Petropoulos K, Arseni N, Schessl C, Stadler CR, Rawat VP, Deshpande AJ, Heilmeier B, Hiddemann W, Quintanilla-Martinez L, Bohlander SK, Feuring-Buske M, Buske C (2008) A novel role for Lef-1, a central transcription mediator of Wnt signaling, in leukemogenesis. J Exp Med 205:515–522

Radich JP, Dai H, Mao M, Oehler V, Schelter J, Druker B, Sawyers C, Shah N, Stock W, Willman CL, Friend S, Linsley PS (2006) Gene expression changes associated with progression and response in chronic myeloid leukemia. Proc Natl Acad Sci U S A 103:2794–2799

Rebel VI, Kung AL, Tanner EA, Yang H, Bronson RT, Livingston DM (2002) Distinct roles for CREB-binding protein and p300 in hematopoietic stem cell self-renewal. Proc Natl Acad Sci U S A 99:14789–14794

Reins J, Mossner M, Neumann M, Platzbecker U, Schumann C, Thiel E, Hofmann WK (2010) Transcriptional down-regulation of the Wnt antagonist SFRP1 in haematopoietic cells of patients with different risk types of MDS. Leuk Res 34:1610–1616

Ress A, Moelling K (2005) Bcr is a negative regulator of the Wnt signaling pathway. EMBO Rep 6:1095–1100

Reya T, O'Riordan M, Okamura R, Devaney E, Willert K, Nusse R, Grosschedl R (2000) Wnt signaling regulates B lymphocyte proliferation through a LEF-1 dependent mechanism. Immunity 13:15–24

Reya T, Duncan AW, Ailles L, Domen J, Scherer DC, Willert K, Hintz L, Nusse R, Weissman IL (2003) A role for Wnt signalling in self-renewal of haematopoietic stem cells. Nature 423:409–414

Rosenbauer F, Owens BM, Yu L, Tumang JR, Steidl U, Kutok JL, Clayton LK, Wagner K, Scheller M, Iwasaki H, Liu C, Hackanson B, Akashi K, Leutz A, Rothstein TL, Plass C, Tenen DG (2006) Lymphoid cell growth and transformation are suppressed by a key regulatory element of the gene encoding PU.1. Nat Genet 38:27–37

Ross ME, Zhou X, Song G, Shurtleff SA, Girtman K, Williams WK, Liu HC, Mahfouz R, Raimondi SC, Lenny N, Patel A, Downing JR (2003) Classification of pediatric acute lymphoblastic leukemia by gene expression profiling. Blood 102:2951–2959

Scheller M, Huelsken J, Rosenbauer F, Taketo MM, Birchmeier W, Tenen DG, Leutz A (2006) Hematopoietic stem cell and multilineage defects generated by constitutive beta-catenin activation. Nat Immunol 7:1037–1047

Serinsöz E, Neusch M, Büsche G, Wasielewski R, Kreipe H, Bock O (2004) Aberrant expression of beta-catenin discriminates acute myeloid leukaemia from acute lymphoblastic leukaemia. Br J Haematol 126:313–319

Sigvardsson M, Clark DR, Fitzsimmons D, Doyle M, Akerblad P, Breslin T, Bilke S, Li R, Yeamans C, Zhang G, Hagman J (2002) Early B-cell factor, E2A, and Pax-5 cooperate to activate the early B cell-specific mb-1 promoter. Mol Cell Biol 22:8539–8551

Simon M, Grandage VL, Linch DC, Khwaja A (2005) Constitutive activation of the Wnt/beta-catenin signalling pathway in acute myeloid leukaemia. Oncogene 24:2410–2420

Takahashi-Yanaga F, Kahn M (2010) Targeting Wnt signaling: can we safely eradicate cancer stem cells? Clin Cancer Res 16:3153–3162

Tickenbrock L, Schwäble J, Wiedehage M, Steffen B, Sargin B, Choudhary C, Brandts C, Berdel WE, Müller-Tidow C, Serve H (2005) Flt3 tandem duplication mutations cooperate with Wnt signaling in leukemic signal transduction. Blood 105:3699–3706

Tomita M, Kikuchi A, Akiyama T, Tanaka Y, Mori N (2006) Human T-cell leukemia virus type 1 tax dysregulates beta-catenin signaling. J Virol 80:10497–10505

Trageser D, Iacobucci I, Nahar R, Duy C, von Levetzow G, Klemm L, Park E, Schuh W, Gruber T, Herzog S, Kim YM, Hofmann WK, Li A, Storlazzi CT, Jäck HM, Groffen J, Heisterkamp N, Jumaa H, Müschen M (2009) Pre-B cell receptor-mediated cell cycle arrest in Philadelphia chromosome-positive acute lymphoblastic leukemia requires IKAROS function. J Exp Med 206:1739–1753

Travis A, Amsterdam A, Belanger C, Grosschedl R (1991) LEF-1, a gene encoding a lymphoid-specific protein with an HMG domain, regulates T-cell receptor alpha enhancer function. Genes Dev 5:880–894

Tsai AG, Lu H, Raghavan SC, Muschen M, Hsieh CL, Lieber MR (2008) Human chromosomal translocations at CpG sites and a theoretical basis for their lineage and stage specificity. Cell 135:1130–1142

Valencia A, Román-Gómez J, Cervera J, Such E, Barragán E, Bolufer P, Moscardó F, Sanz GF, Sanz MA (2009) Wnt signaling pathway is epigenetically regulated by methylation of Wnt antagonists in acute myeloid leukemia. Leukemia 23:1658–1666

Verbeek S, Izon D, Hofhuis F, Robanus-Maandag E, te Riele H, van de Wetering M, Oosterwegel M, Wilson A, MacDonald HR, Clevers H (1995) An HMG-box-containing T-cell factor required for thymocyte differentiation. Nature 374:70–74

Wang Y, Krivtsov AV, Sinha AU, North TE, Goessling W, Feng Z, Zon LI, Armstrong SA (2010) The Wnt/beta-catenin pathway is required for the development of leukemia stem cells in AML. Science 327:1650–1653

Willert K, Brown JD, Danenberg E, Duncan AW, Weissman IL, Reya T, Yates JR III, Nusse R (2003) Wnt proteins are lipid-modified and can act as stem cell growth factors. Nature 423:448–452

Yeoh EJ, Ross ME, Shurtleff SA, Williams WK, Patel D, Mahfouz R, Behm FG, Raimondi SC, Relling MV, Patel A, Cheng C, Campana D, Wilkins D, Zhou X, Li J, Liu H, Pui CH, Evans WE, Naeve C, Wong L, Downing JR (2002) Classification, subtype discovery, and prediction of outcome in pediatric acute lymphoblastic leukemia by gene expression profiling. Cancer Cell 1:133–143

Ying J, Li H, Chen YW, Srivastava G, Gao Z, Tao Q (2007) WNT5A is epigenetically silenced in hematologic malignancies and inhibits leukemia cell growth as a tumor suppressor. Blood 110:4130–4132

Ysebaert L, Chicanne G, Demur C, De Toni F, Prade-Houdellier N, Ruidavets JB, Mansat-De Mas V, Rigal-Huguet F, Laurent G, Payrastre B, Manenti S, Racaud-Sultan C (2006) Expression of beta-catenin by acute myeloid leukemia cells predicts enhanced clonogenic capacities and poor prognosis. Leukemia 20:1211–1216

Zhao C, Blum J, Chen A, Kwon HY, Jung SH, Cook JM, Lagoo A, Reya T (2007) Loss of beta-catenin impairs the renewal of normal and CML stem cells in vivo. Cancer Cell 12:528–541

Zheng X, Beissert T, Kukoc-Zivojnov N, Puccetti E, Altschmied J, Strolz C, Boehrer S, Gul H, Schneider O, Ottmann OG, Hoelzer D, Henschler R, Ruthardt M (2004) Gamma-catenin contributes to leukemogenesis induced by AML-associated translocation products by increasing the self-renewal of very primitive progenitor cells. Blood 103:3535–3543

Chapter 7
Use of Genetically Engineered Mouse Models in Identification and Validation of Therapeutic Targets for Colon Cancer

Masahiro Aoki and Makoto Mark Taketo

Abstract Mice harboring heterozygous mutations in the *Apc* gene develop adenomatous polyps in the intestines as a result of loss of heterozygosity at the *Apc* loci, and serve as mouse models for familial adenomatous polyposis and sporadic adenomas. The *Apc* mutant mice, especially the *Apc*^Min mice, have been extensively used as a preclinical model in testing the effects of drugs or compounds on the intestinal tumors. This chapter focuses on those compounds that significantly reduce the number of intestinal polyps and whose molecular targets are relatively well defined, as well as on the putative therapeutic targets proposed by genetic experiments using the *Apc* mutant mice.

Keywords *Apc* • Colon cancer • Genetically engineered mouse models • Familial adenomatous polyposis (FAP)

7.1 Introduction

Colon cancer is a frequent malignancy, especially in the Western world, causing about 1% of deaths worldwide (Boyle and Levin 2008). Although significant progress has been made recently in the surgical treatment, colon cancer cells are relatively resistant to chemotherapy, resulting in poor prognosis for advanced colon cancer patients who suffer metastasis. There is thus a critical need to identify novel therapeutic targets. Progression of the majority of colon cancer is considered to follow the adenoma-carcinoma sequence, involving various genetic and epigenetic changes, and the aberration in Wnt signaling is believed to represent the earliest step in the sequence. The *Apc* (adenomatous polyposis coli) gene codes for a 2,843 (2,842 in mouse) amino-acid protein, which, together with Axin, provides a

M.M. Taketo (✉)
Department of Pharmacology, Graduate School of Medicine, Kyoto University,
Yoshida-Konoé-cho, Sakyo, Kyoto 606-8501, Japan
e-mail: taketo@mfour.med.kyoto-u.ac.jp

K.H. Goss and M. Kahn (eds.), *Targeting the Wnt Pathway in Cancer*,
DOI 10.1007/978-1-4419-8023-6_7, © Springer Science+Business Media, LLC 2011

scaffold for β-catenin phosphorylation by GSK3-β (Aoki and Taketo 2007). Inactivating mutations in *Apc*, as found in familial adenomatous polyposis patients as well as in sporadic colon cancer patients, result in reduced phosphorylation of β-catenin. The stabilized, unphosphorylated β-catenin then accumulates in the nucleus and induces transcription of Wnt target genes by binding to TCF/LEF transcription factors. Importantly, activation of Wnt signaling appears to play essential roles not only in the early stage of carcinogenesis, but also in the maintenance of the growth of late-stage colon cancer cells (van de Wetering et al. 2002).

7.2   Genetically Engineered Mouse Models for Colonic Adenomas

Mice harboring heterozygous mutations in the *Apc* gene that produce truncated Apc protein are known to develop adenomatous polyps in the intestines as a result of loss of heterozygosity at the *Apc* loci (McCart et al. 2008; Taketo and Edelmann 2009). They serve as mouse models for familial adenomatous polyposis and sporadic adenomas. The *Apc* mutant mouse strain that was generated first and has been used most frequently is called Min (multiple intestinal neoplasia) mouse (Apc^{Min}) (Moser et al. 1990). The Apc^{Min} mouse was identified after random mutagenesis with ethylnitrosourea and carries a truncation mutation at codon 850 of the *Apc* gene (Su et al. 1992). On the other hand, $Apc^{\Delta716}$ and Apc^{1638N} were generated by gene knockout and contain truncating mutation at codon 716 and 1638, respectively (Fodde et al. 1994; Oshima et al. 1995). Several other mutants have also been generated and the histopathology of the intestinal tumors in these models appears to be essentially the same, although tumor multiplicity and distribution appear to differ significantly depending on the truncation type, as reviewed thoroughly earlier (McCart et al. 2008; Taketo and Edelmann 2009). Other types of genetically engineered mice that develop intestinal tumors by Wnt signal activation are conditional *Apc* knockout mice and conditionally stabilizing β-catenin mutant mice. The $Apc^{+/lox\,(ex14)}$ mice develop adenomas in the distal colon only when infected with adenovirus expressing cre (Shibata et al. 1997; Sansom et al. 2004). The $Catnb^{+/lox\,(ex3)}$ mice, on the other hand, develop intestinal polyps when cre recombinase expression is driven by cytokeratin 19 (K19) or fatty acid binding protein (FABP) gene promoter (Harada et al. 1999). Deletion of the exon 3 of β-catenin gene leads to the loss of the GSK3β phosphorylation sites and thereby stabilization of β-catenin.

Importantly, although the mutant mice described here all develop adenomatous polyps in the intestines, they do not develop invasive or metastatic adenocarcinomas at any significant frequency; additional genetic changes are required for progression to malignancy.

Mutations in *Apc* or β-catenin in mice can lead to tumorigenesis in other organs as well, including tumors in mammary gland, skin, stomach, prostate, lung, kidney, and liver, either alone or in combination with other mutations (Aoki and Taketo 2008; Grigoryan et al. 2008). However, they have not been established as reliable preclinical mouse models of the corresponding human diseases and will not be discussed further in this chapter.

7.3   Therapeutic Targets Identified by Pharmacological Experiments Using *Apc* Mutant Mice

Apc mutant mice, especially the Apc^{Min} mice, have been extensively used as a pre-clinical model in testing the effects of drugs or compounds on the intestinal polyps. From a number of reagents that have been tested (Corpet and Pierre 2003) (also nicely summarized in http://www.inra.fr/reseau-nacre/sci-memb/corpet/indexan. html), we focus on those compounds that significantly reduce the number of intestinal polyps and whose molecular targets are relatively well defined (Table 7.1).

7.3.1   Nonsteroidal Anti-Inflammatory Drugs (NSAIDs)

The NSAID *sulindac* was first shown to regress colorectal polyps in a FAP patient in 1983, followed by studies that confirmed its efficacy in many FAP patients, as well as in Apc^{Min} mice (Thun et al. 2002). The major action of NSAIDs is to inhibit the enzymatic activity of cyclooxygenase (COX), which consists of two isozymes, COX-1 and COX-2 (Taketo 1998b; Taketo 1998c). COX-1 is constitutively expressed in most organs, while COX-2 expression is transiently induced by various stimuli including cytokines, mitogens, and endotoxins. Many studies have shown since that other NSAIDs can also efficiently reduce the polyp numbers in *Apc* mutant mice, including aspirin, piroxicam, celecoxib, and rofecoxib (Corpet and Pierre 2003). Although the precise mechanisms of how NSAIDs inhibit the growth of adenoma cells are not fully understood, they are considered to restore normal apoptosis in tumor cells and to inhibit angiogenesis (Thun et al. 2002).

7.3.2   Compounds that Target the Wnt Signaling

7.3.2.1   ICG-001: CBP/β-Catenin

ICG-001 was identified from 5,000 compounds in a screen for ability to inhibit the TOPflash reporter activity in SW480 cells, a colon cancer cell line with Wnt signaling activation by the loss of Apc function (Emami et al. 2004). Subsequent analysis revealed that ICG-001 competed with β-catenin for binding the transcriptional coactivator CBP (Creb-binding protein). ICG-001 suppressed the growth of SW480 and HCT116 colon cancer cells, but not the normal colonic epithelial cells CCD-841Co in culture, and treatment of Apc^{Min} mice with ICG-001 for 9 weeks reduced the polyp formation by 42% with no overt toxicity (Emami et al. 2004).

Table 7.1 Selected compounds with defined targets that suppressed intestinal polyp formation in *Apc* mutant mice

Compound	Category	Targets and actions	Route	Dose/duration	Mice	Effects on polyp number	Reference
Sulindac and other NSAIDs	NSAID	Inhibit COX-1 and COX-2, may also affect Wnt signaling	Oral	Various dose and duration	$Apc^{\Delta 716}$, Apc^{Min}	Significant reduction in many studies	Williams et al. 2004
Various COX-2 inhibitors	NSAID	Inhibit COX-2, may also affect Wnt signaling	Oral	Various dose and duration	$Apc^{\Delta 716}$, Apc^{Min}	Significant reduction in many studies	
NO-ASA	NSAID	Inhibits NF-kB and downregulates PPAR δ as well	Intrarectal	100 mg/kg for 21 days	Apc^{Min}	59% Reduction	Emami et al. 2004
ICG-001	Wnt pathway	Disrupts β-catenin/CBP interaction	i.v.	300 mg/kg/day for 9 weeks	Apc^{Min}	42% Reduction	Kawajiri et al. 2009
I3C and DIM	Wnt pathway	Aryl hydrocarbon receptor (AhR) ligand beta-catenin degradation	Oral	0.1% I3C or 0.01% DIM in diet	Apc^{Min}	80% Reduction	Fujishita et al. 2008
RAD001	Other	mTORC1 inhibitor	Oral	10 mg/kg/day by gavage for 8 weeks (from 6 to 14 weeks)	$Apc^{\Delta 716}$	40% Reduction, prolonged survival	Koehl et al. 2010
Rapamycin	Other	mTORC1 inhibitor	Oral	40 mg/kg in diet for 15 weeks	Apc^{Min}	80% Reduction, prolonged survival	Hung et al. 2010
Rapamycin	Other	mTORC1 inhibitor	i.p.	4 mg/kg for 24 days	$Apc^{+/lox(ex14)}$; Adeno-cre	82% Reduction in tumor size (by colonoscopy). No effect in *Apc/Kras* compound mutant tumors	

Compound	Category	Mechanism	Route	Dose	Model	Result	Reference
MCC-555	Other	PPAR γ/δ dual agonist	Oral	30 mg/kg/day, 5 days/week by gavage for 4 weeks	Apc^{Min}	54.8% Reduction	Yamaguchi et al. 2008
(+)-Catechin	Other	FAK inhibitor	Oral	0.1% in diet by weight for 10 weeks	Apc^{Min}	75% Reduction, distribution unchanged	Weyant et al. 2001
Uroguanylin	Other	Endogenous ligand for guanylate cyclase C	Oral	20 μg/5 g diet with additional doses (20 μg) by gavage twice a week for 17 weeks	Apc^{Min}	50% Reduction	Shailubhai et al. 2000
Sphingadienes	Other	Block Akt translocation to the membrane	Oral	25 mg/kg/day for 10 days	Apc^{Min}	35% Reduction	Fyrst et al. 2009
ZD6474	Other	VEGFR/EGFR inhibitor	Oral	50 mg/kg/day by gavage for 28 days	Apc^{Min}	85% Reduction in early intervention, 65% reduction in late intervention	Alferez et al. 2008
AZD2171	Other	VEGFR2 inhibitor	Oral	5 mg/kg/day by gavage for 28 days	Apc^{Min}	30% Reduction in early intervention; 46% reduction in tumor burden in late intervention	Goodlad et al. 2006
Valproic acid	Other	HDAC2 inhibitor	i.p.	800 mg/kg/day for 4 weeks	Apc^{Min}	65% Reduction	Zhu et al. 2004

(continued)

Table 7.1 (continued)

Compound	Category	Targets and actions	Route	Dose/duration	Mice	Effects on polyp number	Reference
Metformin	Other	AMPK activator	Oral	250 mg/kg/day in diet for 10 weeks	Apc^{Min}	The number of polyps larger than 2 mm in diameter was significantly decreased (total polyp number unchanged)	Tomimoto et al. 2008
Atorvastatin	Other	HMG-CoA reductase inhibitor	Oral	100 ppm in diet for 80 days	Apc^{Min}	30% Reduction	Swamy et al. 2006
CP-31398	Other	Rescues destabilized mutant p53 expression and promotes activity of wild-type p53	Oral	200 ppm in diet for 75 days	Apc^{Min}	75% Reduction	Rao et al. 2008
NO-1886	Other	Increases lipoprotein lipase	Oral	800 ppm in diet for 13 weeks	Apc^{1309}	58% Reduction	Niho et al. 2005
EKB-569	Other	Irreversible EGFR inhibitor, EKI-785 derivative	Oral	20 mg/kg/day in diet for 60 days	Apc^{Min}	87% Reduction	Torrance et al. 2000
EKI-785	Other	EGFR inhibitor	Oral	40 mg/kg/day in diet for 60 days	Apc^{Min}	50% Reduction	Torrance et al. 2000
EKI-785	Other	EGFR inhibitor	i.p.	50 mg/kg/day for 8 weeks	Apc^{Min}	60% Reduction	Roberts et al. 2002
ERRP	Other	Inhibitor of EGFR family	i.p.	50 μg in 100 μl HEPES buffer for 10 days	Apc^{Min}	Regression of 50% of preexisting tumors	
Pioglitazone	Other	PPARγ agonist	Oral	200 ppm in diet for 6 weeks	Apc^{1309}	33% Reduction	Niho et al. 2003

GA (glycyrrhizic acid)	Other	Inhibits 11 βHSD2	i.p.	30 mg/kg/day for 8 weeks	Apc^{Min}	60% Reduction	Zhang et al. 2009
Carnosol	Other	Restores lateral membrane localization of E-cadherin and β-catenin	Oral	0.1% in diet for 10 weeks	Apc^{Min}	46% Reduction	Moran et al. 2005
EGCG	Other	Increases E-caherin and decreases nuclear beta-catenin	Oral	0.16% in drinking water for 6 weeks	Apc^{Min}	47% Reduction	Ju et al. 2005
Snail antisense phosphoro-diamidate morpholino oligomer	Other	Increases E-caherin	i.p.	10 μg/g body weight 5 times a week for 6 weeks	Apc^{Min}	22% Reduction, 54% reduction in the number of tumors larger than 2 mm in diameter	Roy et al. 2004

7.3.2.2 NSAIDs and Other Reagents

Although the primary targets of NSAIDs are considered to be COX activity as described above, recent findings suggest that at least part of the suppressive effects of NSAIDs on polyp formation may be mediated by inhibition of the Wnt signaling itself (Boon et al. 2004; Dihlmann and von Knebel 2005). *Sulindac* and its metabolites have been proposed to induce proteasome-mediated degradation of β-catenin (Rice et al. 2003; Boon et al. 2004), and *indomthacin* has been shown to downregulate aberrant Wnt-β-catenin signaling activity to normal levels by repression of β-catenin gene transcription and by a proteasome-independent degradation of β-catenin (Smith et al. 2000; Hawcroft et al. 2002). *Aspirin* (acetyl salicylic acid) has also been shown to suppress Wnt signaling in colon cancer cells and appears to do so by stabilizing the inactive, phosphorylated form of β-catenin (Dihlmann et al. 2003). Moreover, COX hyperactivation itself has been proposed to enhance Wnt signaling by inhibiting β-catenin degradation (Castellone et al. 2005; Shao et al. 2005). *Nitrate oxide (NO)-donating aspirin* is 2,500–5,000-fold more potent than aspirin in inhibiting colon cancer cell proliferation and has also been shown to reduce the polyp numbers in Apc^{Min} mice (Williams et al. 2004). Recent reports suggest that NO-aspirin disrupts β-catenin /TCF complex in the nucleus, although other mechanisms such as inhibition of NFκB or PPARδ have also been proposed (Nath et al. 2003; Ouyang et al. 2006; Williams et al. 2008; Kawajiri et al. 2009). Aryl hydrocarbon receptor (AhR), also known as dioxin receptor, is a bHLH-PAS (Basic Helix-Loop-Helix-Per-Arnt-Sim) family transcription factor with ligand-dependent E3 ubiquitin ligase activity. Interestingly, it has been recently shown that AhR mediates ligand-dependent ubiquitylation and proteasomal degradation of β-catenin, and that $AhR^{-/-}$ mice developed cecal tumors with β-catenin accumulation (Kawajiri et al. 2009). Furthermore, feeding Apc^{Min} mice with *natural AhR ligands* induced a marked reduction in the number of the intestinal tumors (Mahmoud et al. 2000; Kawajiri et al. 2009). *Caffeic acid phenethyl ester* (CAPE) decreased tumor formation in Apc^{Min} mice by 63%, accompanied by decreased expression of β-catenin (Mahmoud et al. 2000). Expression of 11β-dehydrogenase type II (11βHSD2), which converts active glucocorticoids to inactive keto-forms, is increased in Apc^{Min} mouse intestinal adenomas and is correlated with increased COX-2 expression and activity (Zhang et al. 2009). Pharmacologic inhibition of 11βHSD2 inhibited COX-2–mediated PGE_2 production in tumors and prevented adenoma formation (Zhang et al. 2009).

7.3.3 Compounds that Target Other Signaling Pathways

7.3.3.1 RAD001: mTORC1

Mammalian target of rapamycin complex 1 (mTORC1) consists of the protein kinase mTOR, Raptor, and mLST8 and controls cell growth (increase in cell mass) by regulating mRNA translation in response to growth factor signals, as well as to the environmental cues such as energy or nutrition status. The mTORC1 pathway has been implicated in human cancers; rapamycin (sirolimus), an allosteric inhibitor of mTORC1, and its derivatives such as *RAD001* (everolimus), CCI-779 (temsirolimus), and AP23573 (deforolimus) are under clinical trials for treating various types of cancers. RAD001 and CCI-779 have been approved for treating advanced kidney cancer patients. Recently, Fujishita et al. showed that mTORC1 is activated in intestinal polyp epithelial cells of $Apc^{\Delta716}$ mice (Fujishita et al. 2008). Oral administration of RAD001 for 8 weeks significantly reduced the number of the polyps (~60% reduction), with stronger effects on the tumors in the large size class. RAD001 treatment decreased the proliferation rate of adenoma cells and inhibited angiogenesis (Fujishita et al. 2008). Suppression of tumor growth by rapamycin was also observed in Apc^{Min} mice and in conditional *Apc* mutant mice, but not in *Apc/Kras* compound mutant mice that develop adenocarcinomas in the colon (Hung et al. 2010; Koehl et al. 2010).

7.3.3.2 Other Compounds and Their Target Molecules

CP 31398 is known to stabilize wild-type p53 by inhibiting Mdm2-mediated ubiquitylation and degradation. Addition of CP-31398 in the diet resulted in 75% reduction in the number of intestinal polyps in Apc^{Min} mice (Niho et al. 2003; Rao et al. 2008). *Pioglitazone* is an agonist of PPARγ and has been used as an antidiabetic drug for type 2 diabetes patients. Treatment of Apc^{1309} mice with pioglitazone for 6 weeks reduced the number of intestinal polyps to 67% of the control, and 4-week treatment of Apc^{Min} mice with MCC-555, a PPARγ/δ dual agonist, has also been shown to reduce the number of intestinal polyps to 55% of the control (Niho et al. 2003; Tomimoto et al. 2008; Yamaguchi et al. 2008). *Metformin* is a biguanide derivative widely used for treating type 2 diabetes, and its pharmacologic action is considered to be mediated by activation of adenosine monophosphate-activated protein kinase (AMPK) (Tomimoto et al. 2008). Loss of Apc function has been shown to induce expression of HDAC2, which is required for and sufficient to prevent apoptosis of colon cancer cells. Interference with HDAC2 activity by *valpronic acid* reduced the number of intestinal tumors in Apc^{Min} mice, especially those in the large size class (reduced to ~10% of the control) (Zhu et al. 2004). Crossing of HDAC2 mutant mice with Apc^{Min} mice significantly reduced the number of tumors in the small intestines of female mice by ~60% (Zhu et al. 2004; Zimmermann et al. 2007). Dietary administration of *atorvastatin*, an HMG-CoA reductase inhibitor, suppressed intestinal polyp formation in Apc^{Min} mice by ~30% (Swamy et al. 2006). Feeding Apc^{Min} mice with diet containing *EKB-569*, an irreversible inhibitor of EGFR tyrosine kinase, for 60 days reduced the polyp number to 13% of that of those fed with control diet (Torrance et al. 2000; Goodlad et al. 2006). Administration of *AZD2171*, a selective inhibitor of VEGFR2, for 28 days significantly reduced polyp formation in Apc^{Min} mice to 55% of the control (Goodlad et al. 2006). *EGFR-related protein (ERRP)* was isolated and characterized as a pan-erbB inhibitor and targets multiple members of the EGFR family.

ERRP caused regression of the adenomas by 50% in the small intestine (Schmelz et al. 2007). The size of the small intestinal tumors was also significantly reduced by ERRP.

ZD6474 (vandetanib), a selective inhibitor of VEGR and EGFR tyrosine kinase, markedly reduced the number and the size of polyps in Apc^{Min} mice (Alferez et al. 2008). Dietary administration of *carnasol*, a phenolic diterpene constituent of the herb, reduced the number of intestinal tumors in Apc^{Min} mice by 46% (Moran et al. 2005). Carnasol was further shown to enhance E-cadherin-mediated adhesion and to suppress β-catenin tyrosine phosphorylation. *(+)-Catechin* found in certain fruits was shown to inhibit focal adhesion kinase (FAK) and suppressed polyp formation in Apc^{Min} mice (Weyant et al. 2001; Ju et al. 2005). Administration of *(–)-epigallocatechin-3-gallate (EGCG)*, a major constituent of green tea, in Apc^{Min} mice decreased intestinal tumor formation by 47%, accompanied by increased levels of E-cadherin and decreased levels of nuclear β-catenin in the tumor cells (Ju et al. 2005). Treatment of Apc^{Min} mice with an *antisense phosphorodiamidate morpholino oligomer (AS-PMO) to SNAIL* significantly reduced total polyp number and incidence of tumors larger than 2 mm in diameter (by 22% and 54%, respectively) (Roy et al. 2004). NO-1886 has been shown to increase lipoprotein lipase (LPL) mRNA and protein levels without touching PPARα and PPARγ. Administration of NO-1886 decreased intestinal tumors of Apc^{1309} mice by 58%, accompanied by suppression of COX-2 mRNA levels (Niho et al. 2005). Treatment with *uroguanylin*, an endogenous ligand for guanylyl cyclase C (GCC), was shown to induce apoptosis in colon cancer cells in vitro and to suppress polyp formation in Apc^{Min} mice in vivo (Shailubhai et al. 2000). The role of uroguanlyin is further underscored by a more recent work that showed deletion of Gcc gene increased tumor incidence and multiplicity (Li et al. 2007). Sphingomyelin-ceramides have also been shown to suppress intestinal tumorigenesis in Apc^{Min} mice. A recent report shows that C14 or C18 *sphingadienes* block Akt translocation from the cytosol to the membrane, suppressing the PI 3-kinase/Akt pathway and their oral administration to Apc^{Min} mice for 10 days resulting in 35% reduction in polyp numbers (Fyrst et al. 2009).

7.4   Putative Therapeutic Targets Proposed by Genetic Experiments Using *Apc* Mutant Mice

Apc mutant mice can be used to test the effect of a certain protein on tumor formation by crossing with mutant mice in which the gene encoding that molecule is knocked out. Reduced polyp numbers would suggest that the molecule positively regulates tumor formation and thus can be a potential therapeutic target. As a good example, genetic evidence for the role of COX-2 obtained by crossing COX-2 gene (*Ptgs2*) mutant mice with $Apc^{\Delta716}$ mice provided a rationale for treatment of FAP patients with COX-2 inhibitors (Oshima et al. 1996).

7.5 Wnt Signaling Molecules and Its Modifiers

7.5.1 APC-Stimulated Guanine Nucleotide Exchange Factor (Asef)/Asef2

Asef and *Asef2* are guanine nucleotide exchange factors (GEFs) specific for Rac1 and Cdc42. APC enhances the GEF activity of Asef and Asef2 by binding to their amino-terminal regions. Asef and Asef2 can induce c-Jun amino-terminal kinase (JNK) and upregulate matrix metalloproteinase 9 (Kawasaki et al. 2000; Kawasaki et al. 2007). It was recently reported that expression of Asef and Asef2 is enhanced in intestinal tumors of Apc^{Min} mice, and the deficiency of either Asef or Asef2 reduces both the number and size of intestinal adenomas in Apc^{Min} mice (Kawasaki et al. 2009). Because mice deficient in Asef or Asef2 appear normal, authors suggest that compounds targeting Asef and Asef2 might have few serious side effects.

7.5.2 Smoothened

Smoothened (SMO) is a seven-pass transmembrane protein that plays a pivotal role in transducing the Hedgehog (Hh) signal. Arimura et al. recently showed that expression of Smo was markedly increased in the intestinal adenoma epithelium of $Apc^{\Delta716}$ mice (Arimura et al. 2009). SMO knockdown in human colon cancer cell lines caused growth arrest at the G1/S phase, and $Apc^{+/\Delta716}\ Smo^{+/-}$ mice caused reduction in numbers of polyps in the large size class. Unexpectedly, reduced expression of Smo suppressed β-catenin-dependent transcription, rather than Hh-responsive Gli-dependent transcription, and SMO knockdown reduced protein levels of active β-catenin and induced its nuclear exclusion.

7.5.3 Sirtuin (Silent Mating Type Information Regulation 2 Homolog) 1 (SIRT1)

SIRT1 is a NAD⁺-dependent deacetylase induced by calorie restriction and is implicated in longevity. Ectopic expression of SIRT1 in Apc^{Min} mice has been shown to cause 3–4-fold reduction in the number and size of their intestinal adenomas (Firestein et al. 2008; McConnell et al. 2009). Authors further showed that SIRT1 promotes deacetylation of β-catenin, thereby suppressing its transacti-vation activity.

7.5.4   Krüppel-Like Factor 5 (KLF5)

KLF5, a zinc-finger transcription factor, is a Wnt target gene highly expressed in proliferating intestinal epithelial cells in crypts. Heterozygous mutation in *Klf5* caused 96% reduction in the number of polyps in Apc^{Min} mice, accompanied by reduced levels and nuclear localization of β-catenin (McConnell et al. 2009).

7.6   Wnt Targets

7.6.1   c-Myc, Prox1, Tiam1 CD44, and Mdr1

The proto-oncogene c-*myc*, encoding a basic helix-loop-helix/leucine zipper transcription factor, is a well-known target gene of the Wnt signaling pathway. Heterozygous knockout of c-*myc* caused ~75% reduction in the number of intestinal polyps in Apc^{Min} mice and prolongs their survival (Yekkala and Baudino 2007). *Prox1* is an evolutionarily conserved transcription factor that controls lymphatic endothelial and retinal progenitor cell differentiation as well as development of some organs. Prox1 is highly expressed in the polyps of Apc^{Min} mice and is a direct target of β-catenin /TCF pathway (Petrova et al. 2008). Conditional knockout of Prox1 caused a fivefold reduction in the number of tumors exceeding 2 mm in diameter, while the number of microscopic lesions increased. Consistently, transgenic expression of Prox1 under the control of villin promoter promotes colorectal tumorigenesis in mice (Petrova et al. 2008). *Tiam1*, a selective Rac GTPase activator, is a Wnt target gene and its expression is increased in intestinal tumors of Apc^{Min} mice (Malliri et al. 2006). *Tiam1* knockout caused 50% reduction in the number of polyps in Apc^{Min} mice (Malliri et al. 2006). *Cd44* is a target gene of Wnt signaling and considered a marker of colon cancer stem cell. CD44 expression is dramatically increased in Apc^{Min} mice and its knockout caused 50% reduction in the number of intestinal adenomas (Zeilstra et al. 2008). *Mdr1* (*Abcb1*) gene, encoding P-glycoprotein, contains multiple TCF4 binding elements in its promoter and is considered a direct target of Wnt signaling. *Mdr1* deficiency in Apc^{Min} mice resulted in 50% reduction in the polyp number. Several P-glycoprotein antagonists have been developed (Yamada et al. 2003).

7.7   Epigenetic Regulators

7.7.1   DNA-Methyl Transferase 3b (Dnmt3b) and Dnmt1

Expression of DNMT3A, along with DNMT3B and DNMT1, has been shown to be progressively upregulated in the colorectal adenoma-carcinoma sequence in humans (Schmidt et al. 2007). Introduction of *Dnmt1* hypomorphic alleles caused complete suppression of polyp formation in Apc^{Min} mice, accompanied by reduced CpG island methylation frequency (Eads et al. 2002). On the other hand, while the loss of *Dnmt3b* had impact on microadenoma formation, formation of macroscopic colonic adenomas was significantly decreased (Lin et al. 2006). Furthermore, over-expression of Dnmt3b1 in Apc^{Min} mice enhanced the colonic tumor formation in Apc^{Min} mice both in number and size, accompanied by silencing of *Sfrp* genes (Linhart et al. 2007). These findings support the use of DNA methyltransferase inhibitors for the therapeutic reversion of epigenetic mutations as a potential strategy for cancer therapy.

7.7.2   Methyl-CpG Binding Protein 2 (Mbd2), Kaiso, and Histone Deacetylase 2 (HDAC2)

Mbd2 is a methyl-CpG binding repressor that recruits corepressor complexes to methylated DNA. Upon necropsy, $Mbd2^{-/-}$ mice had ~10 times fewer adenomas than $Mbd2^{+/-}$ controls (Sansom et al. 2003). *Dnmt1* deficiency causes embryonic lethality, while *Mbd2*-null mice appear healthy; it would make an attractive target for therapeutic intervention in cancer. Kaiso protein, encoded by *Zbtb33* (zinc finger and BTB domain containing 33) gene, associates with p120-catenin and binds to the methylated sequences to modulate transcription. Expression of Kaiso is upregulated in murine intestinal tumors. Null-mutation of *Kaiso* significantly increased the survival of Apc^{Min} mice, and the size of polyps was significantly decreased at 180 days in mice lacking Kaiso (Prokhortchouk et al. 2006). *Hdac2*-deficiency caused 10–100% decrease in tumor incidence of Apc^{Min} mice, depending on segment of the gut and sex of the mice (Zimmermann et al. 2007). In the small intestine of female mice that showed the highest tumor incidence, the polyp number was reduced by 60% in HDAC2-deficient animals (Zimmermann et al. 2007).

7.8   Inflammation

7.8.1   Cyclooxygenase 2 (COX-2), COX-1, Prostaglandin E2 Receptors (EP2), Cytoplasmic Phospholipase A2 (cPLA₂), and Membrane-Bound Prostaglandin E Synthetase 1 (mPGES-1)

COX-2 is expressed from an early stage of intestinal polyp formation, and mutations in COX-2 gene (*Ptges*) dramatically decrease the number and size of polyps in *Apc* mutant mice (Oshima et al. 1996; Taketo 1998a). This finding was followed by many studies that showed efficacy of COX-2 inhibitors as described above and provided a rationale for treatment of FAP patients with the COX-2 inhibitors. The constitutively expressed enzyme COX-1 cooperates with COX-2 in polyp formation by providing PGE_2, and its deficiency in Apc^{Min} mice causes similar decrease in the polyp number (Chulada et al. 2000).

7.8.2 Apolipoprotein B mRNA Editing Enzyme, Catalytic Polypeptide 1 (Apobec1), Myeloid Differentiation Primary Response Gene 88 (MyD88), Interleukin 6 (IL-6), and Inducible Nitric Oxide Synthase (iNos)

The RNA-specific cytidine deaminase apobec-1 is an AU-rich RNA binding protein that binds the 3' untranslated region (UTR) of Cox-2 mRNA and stabilizes its turnover in vitro (Anant et al. 2004). Apc^{Min} mice crossed into apobec-1 mutant mice showed a 64% decrease in small intestinal adenoma incidence, accompanied by reduced level of COX-2 mRNA (Blanc et al. 2007). Loss of MyD88 (a signaling adaptor of TLRs), downstream of members of the TLR and IL-1R family, decreased (~80% reduction) the number of small intestinal tumors in Apc^{Min} mice (Rakoff-Nahoum and Medzhitov 2007). IL-6 deficiency resulted in 32% reduction in polyp numbers in Apc^{Min} mice (Baltgalvis et al. 2008). Heterozygous and homozygous mutations in iNOS gene (*Nos2a*) caused 50% and 60% reduction in the number of polyps in Apc^{Min} mice, respectively (Ahn and Oshima 2001), although another report showed that *Nos2a* knockout rather promoted intestinal tumorigenesis in Apc^{Min} mice (Scott et al. 2001).

7.9 Other Signals

7.9.1 c-Jun, Jagged1, Epidermal Growth Factor Receptor (EGFR), Insulin Receptor Substrate 1 (IRS-1), Protein Kinase C λ (PKCλ), Eph Receptor A2 (EphA2), and Wip1/ PPM1D (Protein Phosphatase 1D Magnesium-Dependent)

It was shown that phosphorylated c-Jun interacts with the HMG-box transcription factor TCF4 to form a ternary complex containing c-Jun, TCF4, and β-catenin. JNK-phosphorylated c-Jun interacts with TCF4 on the *c-jun* promoter, and c-Jun and TCF4 can cooperatively activate the c-jun promoter in a β-catenin-dependent manner (Nateri et al. 2005). Genetic abrogation of c-Jun N-terminal phosphorylation or gut-specific conditional c-jun inactivation in Apc^{Min} mice reduced tumor number by ~40% and prolonged lifespan (Nateri et al. 2005). Crossing Apc^{Min} with heterozygous *Jagged1* knockout mice significantly reduces the size of the polyps (60% decrease in the number of tumors larger than 1 mm in diameter), indicating that Notch is an essential modulator of tumorigenesis (Rodilla et al. 2009). Specific inhibitors for Jagged1-mediated Notch activation could therefore become a new strategy for colon cancer therapy, avoiding the side effects caused by direct inhibition of Notch signaling pathway (van Es et al. 2005). The hypomorphic $Egfr^{wa2}$ allele contains a single nucleotide mutation producing a valine to glycine substitution in the kinase domain, resulting in up to a 90% reduction in kinase activity (Luetteke et al. 1994). Transfer of the Apc^{Min} allele onto the homozygous $Egfr^{wa2}$ background resulted in a 90% reduction in intestinal polyp number relative to Apc^{Min} mice (Roberts et al. 2002), supporting the pharmacological evidence described above. IRS-1 deficiency caused 55% reduction in the number of intestinal polyps (Ramocki et al. 2008), and conditional knockout of PKCλ caused ~25% reduction in the small intestinal polyps in Apc^{Min} mice (Murray et al. 2009). Apc^{Min} mice carrying a genetic knockout of the $EphA2$ gene developed ~30% fewer tumors in the intestines (Bogan et al. 2009), and the Wip1 phosphatase deficiency prolongs survival of Apc^{Min} mice, with 88% reduction in polyp number (Demidov et al. 2007).

7.10 Environment

7.10.1 Matrix Metalloproteinase 7 (MMP7), Secreted Protein Acidic, Rich in Cysteine (SPARC), Spermidine/Spermine N1-Acetyltransferase-1 (SSAT)

Apc^{Min} mice that lacked MMP7/matrilysin showed 58% reduction in tumor number (Wilson et al. 1997). The average tumor diameter per animal was also reduced by 20%. Similar effects of MMP7 deficiency were observed in cis-Apc/Smad4 mice that spontaneously develop invasive adenocarcinomas. Namely, the cis-Apc/Smad4/Mmp7 mice had 50% smaller number of tumors at the same age, and the ratio of large polyps (1.0–3.0 mm in diameter) in the cis-Apc/Smad4/Mmp7 mice was significantly lower than that in the cis-Apc/Smad4 mice (Kitamura et al. 2009).

SPARC (secreted protein acidic, rich in cysteine) is a matricellular protein upregulated in human gastric and colorectal cancer. $Sparc$ expression is upregulated in intestinal adenomas of Apc^{Min} mice, and $Sparc$ deficiency strongly suppressed adenoma formation in Apc^{Min} mice with no effect on tumor size (Sansom et al. 2007). SSAT, encoded by the X-linked $Sat1$ gene, is the rate-limiting enzyme of polyamine catabolism and catalyzes acetylation of spermine and spermidine in response to cell stress and to excess polyamines. When Apc^{Min} mice were crossed with SSAT-overproducing transgenic mice, they developed three and sixfold more adenomas in the small intestine and colon, respectively, than Apc^{Min} mice, while SSAT deficiency caused 75% reduction of polyp number in the small intestine (Tucker et al. 2005).

7.11 Perspectives: Towards Establishing Preclinical Colon Cancer Mouse Models that Develop Metastasis

Although the *Apc* mutant mice have been used widely as a preclinical model of colon cancer, the major drawback is that they do not develop invasive or metastatic adenocarcinomas at a significant frequency, as mentioned above. Many efforts have been made to establish a mouse model of colorectal adenocarcinomas by generating compound mutant mice that carry additional mutations.

The mouse *Apc* and *Smad4* genes are both found on chromosome 18, about 30 cM apart. Because LOH found in the polyps in *Apc* mutant mice is caused by the loss of the entire chromosome 18, due to recombination at the ribosomal DNA locus near the centromere, LOH of *Apc* is accompanied by LOH of *Smad4*. Taking advantage of this phenomenon, mice that carried $Apc^{\Delta716}$ and *Smad4* mutations on the same chromatid in the *cis*-configuration (*cis-Apc/Smad4* mice) were generated (Takaku et al. 1998). The intestinal polyps of these mice thus carry homozygous mutations in both *Apc* and *Smad4*, and they turned out to be very invasive adenocarcinomas. Interestingly, however, such adenocarcinomas do not metastasize during the short life span of these mice. Consistently, homozygous disruption of the TGF-β type II receptor of gene (*Tgfbr2*) in Apc^{1638N} mice also resulted in malignant progression of the intestinal adenomas caused by the *Apc* mutation (Munoz et al. 2006).

Some tumors in Apc^{580D} mice, Apc^{1638N}, or $Apc^{\Delta ex14}$ mice carrying oncogenic *Kras* alleles were adenocarcinomas (Janssen et al. 2002; Sansom et al. 2006; Haigis et al. 2008). It has also been reported that heterozygous disruption of *Pten* or homozygous mutation of *Prox1* in Apc^{Min} mice induces progression of intestinal adenomas to adenocarcinomas (Shao et al. 2007; Petrova et al. 2008). However, their tumors appear to be less malignant than those in *cis-Apc/Smad4* mice or $Apc^{580D}/Kras^{Val12}$ mice.

The major goal of the efforts in generating preclinical mouse models for colon cancer is, of course, to establish "metastatic models," which develop remote metastasis in the liver or lungs spontaneously. Such models will be useful in identifying and/or validating therapeutic targets, including signaling components of the Wnt pathway.

References

Ahn B, Oshima H (2001) Suppression of intestinal polyposis in $Apc^{Min/+}$ mice by inhibiting nitric oxide production. Cancer Res 61:8357–8360

Alferez D, Wilkinson RW, Watkins J et al (2008) Dual inhibition of VEGFR and EGFR signaling reduces the incidence and size of intestinal adenomas in $Apc^{Min/+}$ mice. Mol Cancer Ther 7:590–598

Anant S, Murmu N, Houchen CW et al (2004) Apobec-1 protects intestine from radiation injury through posttranscriptional regulation of cyclooxygenase-2 expression. Gastroenterology 127:1139–1149

Aoki K, Taketo MM (2007) Adenomatous polyposis coli (APC): a multi-functional tumor suppressor gene. J Cell Sci 120:3327–3335

Aoki K, Taketo MM (2008) Tissue-specific transgenic, conditional knockout and knock-in mice of genes in the canonical Wnt signaling pathway. Methods Mol Biol 468:307–331

Arimura S, Matsunaga A, Kitamura T et al (2009) Reduced level of Smoothened suppresses intestinal tumorigenesis by down-regulation of Wnt signaling. Gastroenterology 137:629–638

Baltgalvis KA, Berger FG, Pena MM et al (2008) Interleukin-6 and cachexia in $Apc^{Min/+}$ mice. Am J Phys Regul Integr Comp Physiol 294:R393–R401

Blanc V, Henderson JO, Newberry RD et al (2007) Deletion of the AU-rich RNA binding protein Apobec-1 reduces intestinal tumor burden in Apc^{min} mice. Cancer Res 67:8565–8573

Bogan C, Chen J, O'Sullivan MG et al (2009) Loss of EphA2 receptor tyrosine kinase reduces $Apc^{Min/+}$ tumorigenesis. Int J Cancer 124:1366–1371

Boon EM, Keller JJ, Wormhoudt TA et al (2004) Sulindac targets nuclear β-catenin accumulation and Wnt signalling in adenomas of patients with familial adenomatous polyposis and in human colorectal cancer cell lines. Br J Cancer 90:224–229

Boyle P, Levin B (eds) (2008) World cancer report 2008. International Agency of Research Against Cancer, Lyon

Castellone MD, Teramoto H, Williams BO et al (2005) Prostaglandin E2 promotes colon cancer cell growth through a novel Gs-axin-β-catenin signaling axis. Science 310:1504–1510

Chulada PC, Thompson MB, Mahler JF et al (2000) Genetic disruption of $Ptgs-1$, as well as of $Ptgs-2$, reduces intestinal tumorigenesis in Min mice. Cancer Res 60:4705–4708

Corpet DE, Pierre F (2003) Point: From animal models to prevention of colon cancer. Systematic review of chemoprevention in min mice and choice of the model system. Cancer Epidemiol Biomarkers Prev 12:391–400

Demidov ON, Timofeev O, Lwin HN et al (2007) Wip1 phosphatase regulates p53-dependent apoptosis of stem cells and tumorigenesis in the mouse intestine. Cell Stem Cell 1:180–190

Dihlmann S, Klein S, Doeberitz Mv MK (2003) Reduction of β-catenin/T-cell transcription factor signaling by aspirin and indomethacin is caused by an increased stabilization of phosphorylated β-catenin. Mol Cancer Ther 2:509–516

Dihlmann S, von Knebel DM (2005) Wnt/β-catenin-pathway as a molecular target for future anticancer therapeutics. Int J Cancer 113:515–524

Eads CA, Nickel AE, Laird PW (2002) Complete genetic suppression of polyp formation and reduction of CpG-island hypermethylation in $Apc^{Min/+}$ $Dnmt1$-hypomorphic mice. Cancer Res 62:1296–1299

Emami KH, Nguyen C, Ma H et al (2004) A small molecule inhibitor of β-catenin/CREB-binding protein transcription. Proc Natl Acad Sci U S A 101:12682–12687

Firestein R, Blander G, Michan S et al (2008) The SIRT1 deacetylase suppresses intestinal tumorigenesis and colon cancer growth. PLoS One 3:e2020

Fodde R, Edelmann W, Yang K et al (1994) A targeted chain-termination mutation in the mouse Apc gene results in multiple tumors. Proc Natl Acad Sci USA 91:8969–8973

Fujishita T, Aoki K, Lane HA et al (2008) Inhibition of the mTORC1 pathway suppresses intestinal polyp formation and reduces mortality in $Apc^{\Delta716}$ mice. Proc Natl Acad Sci USA 105:13544–13549

Fyrst H, Oskouian B, Bandhuvula P et al (2009) Natural sphingadienes inhibit Akt-dependent signaling and prevent intestinal tumorigenesis. Cancer Res 69:9457–9464

Goodlad RA, Ryan AJ, Wedge SR et al (2006) Inhibiting vascular endothelial growth factor receptor-2 signaling reduces tumor burden in the $Apc^{Min/+}$ mouse model of early intestinal cancer. Carcinogenesis 27:2133–2139

Grigoryan T, Wend P, Klaus A et al (2008) Deciphering the function of canonical Wnt signals in development and disease: conditional loss- and gain-of-function mutations of β-catenin in mice. Genes Dev 22:2308–2341

Haigis KM, Kendall KR, Wang Y et al (2008) Differential effects of oncogenic K-Ras and N-Ras on proliferation, differentiation and tumor progression in the colon. Nat Genet 40:600–608

Harada N, Tamai Y, Ishikawa T et al (1999) Intestinal polyposis in mice with a dominant stable mutation of the β-catenin gene. EMBO J 18:5931–5942

Hawcroft G, D'Amico M, Albanese C et al (2002) Indomethacin induces differential expression of β-catenin, γ-catenin and T-cell factor target genes in human colorectal cancer cells. Carcinogenesis 23:107–114

Hung KE, Maricevich MA, Richard LG et al (2010) Development of a mouse model for sporadic and metastatic colon tumors and its use in assessing drug treatment. Proc Natl Acad Sci U S A 107:1565–1570

Janssen K-P, el Marjou F, Pinto D et al (2002) Targeted expression of oncogenic K-ras in intestinal epithelium causes spontaneous tumorigenesis in mice. Gastroenterology 123:492–504

Ju J, Hong J, Zhou JN et al (2005) Inhibition of intestinal tumorigenesis in $Apc^{min/+}$ mice by (-)-epigallocatechin-3-gallate, the major catechin in green tea. Cancer Res 65:10623–10631

Kawajiri K, Kobayashi Y, Ohtake F et al (2009) Aryl hydrocarbon receptor suppresses intestinal carcinogenesis in $Apc^{Min/+}$ mice with natural ligands. Proc Natl Acad Sci USA 106:13481–13486

Kawasaki Y, Sagara M, Shibata Y et al (2007) Identification and characterization of Asef2, a guanine-nucleotide exchange factor specific for Rac1 and Cdc42. Oncogene 26:7620–7627

Kawasaki Y, Senda T, Ishidate T et al (2000) Asef, a link between the tumor suppressor APC and G-protein signaling. Science 289:1194–1197

Kawasaki Y, Tsuji S, Muroya K et al (2009) The adenomatous polyposis coli-associated exchange factors Asef and Asef2 are required for adenoma formation in $Apc^{Min/+}$ mice. EMBO Rep 10:1355–1362

Kitamura T, Biyajima K, Aoki M et al (2009) Matrix metalloproteinase 7 is required for tumor formation, but dispensable for invasion and fibrosis in SMAD4-deficient intestinal adenocarcinomas. Lab Invest 89:98–105

Koehl GE, Spitzner M, Ousingsawat J et al (2010) Rapamycin inhibits oncogenic intestinal ion channels and neoplasia in $Apc^{Min/+}$ mice. Oncogene 29:1553–1560

Li P, Schulz S, Bombonati A et al (2007) Guanylyl cyclase C suppresses intestinal tumorigenesis by restricting proliferation and maintaining genomic integrity. Gastroenterology 133:599–607

Lin H, Yamada Y, Nguyen S et al (2006) Suppression of intestinal neoplasia by deletion of Dnmt3b. Mol Cell Biol 26:2976–2983

Linhart HG, Lin H, Yamada Y et al (2007) Dnmt3b promotes tumorigenesis in vivo by gene-specific de novo methylation and transcriptional silencing. Genes Dev 21:3110–3122

Luetteke NC, Phillips HK, Qiu TH et al (1994) The mouse waved-2 phenotype results from a point mutation in the EGF receptor tyrosine kinase. Genes Dev 8:399–413

Mahmoud NN, Carothers AM, Grunberger D et al (2000) Plant phenolics decrease intestinal tumors in an animal model of familial adenomatous polyposis. Carcinogenesis 21:921–927

Malliri A, RT P, van der Kammen RA et al (2006) The rac activator Tiam1 is a Wnt-responsive gene that modifies intestinal tumor development. J Biol Chem 281:543–548

McCart AE, Vickaryous NK, Silver A (2008) Apc mice: models, modifiers and mutants. Pathol Res Pract 204:479–490

McConnell BB, Bialkowska AB, Nandan MO et al (2009) Haploinsufficiency of Kruppel-like factor 5 rescues the tumor-initiating effect of the $Apc^{Min/+}$ mutation in the intestine. Cancer Res 69:4125–4133

Moran AE, Carothers AM, Weyant MJ et al (2005) Carnosol inhibits β-catenin tyrosine phosphorylation and prevents adenoma formation in the C57BL/6J/Min/+ (Min/+) mouse. Cancer Res 65:1097–1104

Moser AR, Pitot HC, Dove WF (1990) A dominant mutation that predisposes to multiple intestinal neoplasia in the mouse. Science 247:322–324

Munoz NM, Upton M, Rojas A et al (2006) Transforming growth factor β receptor type II inactivation induces the malignant transformation of intestinal neoplasms initiated by Apc mutation. Cancer Res 66:9837–9844

Murray NR, Weems J, Braun U et al (2009) Protein kinase C βII and PKCι/λ: collaborating partners in colon cancer promotion and progression. Cancer Res 69:656–662

Nateri AS, Spencer-Dene B, Behrens A (2005) Interaction of phosphorylated c-Jun with TCF4 regulates intestinal cancer devolopment. Nature 437:281–285

Nath N, Kashfi K, Chen J et al (2003) Nitric oxide-donating aspirin inhibits β-catenin/T cell factor (TCF) signaling in SW480 colon cancer cells by disrupting the nuclear β-catenin-TCF association. Proc Natl Acad Sci U S A 100:12584–12589

Niho N, Mutoh M, Takahashi M et al (2005) Concurrent suppression of hyperlipidemia and intestinal polyp formation by NO-1886, increasing lipoprotein lipase activity in Min mice. Proc Natl Acad Sci U S A 102:2970–2974

Niho N, Takahashi M, Kitamura T et al (2003) Concomitant suppression of hyperlipidemia and intestinal polyp formation in Apc-deficient mice by peroxisome proliferator-activated receptor ligands. Cancer Res 63:6090–6095

Oshima M, Dinchuk JE, Kargman SL et al (1996) Suppression of intestinal polyposis in $Apc^{\Delta716}$ knockout mice by inhibition of cyclooxygenase 2 (COX-2). Cell 87:803–809

Oshima M, Oshima H, Kitagawa K et al (1995) Loss of Apc heterozygosity and abnormal tissue building in nascent intestinal polyps in mice carrying a truncated Apc gene. Proc Natl Acad Sci USA 92:4482–4486

Ouyang N, Williams JL, Rigas B (2006) NO-donating aspirin isomers downregulate peroxisome proliferator-activated receptor (PPAR)δ expression in $Apc^{Min/+}$ mice proportionally to their tumor inhibitory effect: Implications for the role of PPARδ in carcinogenesis. Carcinogenesis 27:232–239

Petrova TV, Nykänen A, Norrimén C et al (2008) Transcription factor PROX1 induces colon cancer progression by promoting the transition from benign to highly dysplastic phenotype. Cancer Cell 13:407–419

Prokhortchouk A, Sansom O, Selfridge J et al (2006) Kaiso-deficient mice show resistance to intestinal cancer. Mol Cell Biol 26:199–208

Rakoff-Nahoum S, Medzhitov R (2007) Regulation of spontaneous intestinal tumorigenesis through the adaptor protein MyD88. Science 317:124–127

Ramocki NM, Wilkins HR, Magness ST et al (2008) Insulin receptor substrate-1 deficiency promotes apoptosis in the putative intestinal crypt stem cell region, limits $Apc^{Min/+}$ tumors, and regulates Sox9. Endocrinology 149:261–267

Rao CV, Swamy MV, Patlolla JM et al (2008) Suppression of familial adenomatous polyposis by CP-31398, a TP53 modulator, in $Apc^{Min/+}$ mice. Cancer Res 68:7670–7675

Rice PL, Kelloff J, Sullivan H et al (2003) Sulindac metabolites induce caspase- and proteasome-dependent degradation of β-catenin protein in human colon cancer cells. Mol Cancer Ther 2:885–892

Roberts RB, Min L, Washington MK et al (2002) Importance of epidermal growth factor receptor signaling in establishment of adenomas and maintenance of carcinomas during intestinal tumorigenesis. Proc Natl Acad Sci U S A 99:1521–1526

Rodilla V, Villanueva A, Obrador-Hevia A et al (2009) Jagged1 is the pathological link between Wnt and Notch pathways in colorectal cancer. Proc Natl Acad Sci U S A 106:6315–6320

Roy HK, Iversen P, Hart J et al (2004) Down-regulation of SNAIL suppresses MIN mouse tumorigenesis: modulation of apoptosis, proliferation, and fractal dimension. Mol Cancer Ther 3:1159–1165

Sansom OJ, Mansergh FC, Evans MJ et al (2007) Deficiency of SPARC suppresses intestinal tumorigenesis in $Apc^{Min/+}$ mice. Gut 56:1410–1414

Sansom OJ, Meniel V, Wilkins JA et al (2006) Loss of Apc allows phenotypic manifestation of the transforming properties of an endogenous K-ras oncogene in vivo. Proc Natl Acad Sci U S A 103:14122–14127

Sansom OJ, Reed KR, Hayes AJ et al (2004) Loss of Apc in vivo immediately perturbs Wnt signaling, differentiation, and migration. Genes Dev 18:1385–1390

Sansom WJ, Berger J, Bishop SM et al (2003) Deficiency of Mbd2 suppresses intestinal tumorigenesis. Nat Genet 34:145–147

Schmelz EM, Xu H, Sengupta R et al (2007) Regression of early and intermediate stages of colon cancer by targeting multiple members of the EGFR family with EGFR-related protein. Cancer Res 67:5389–5396

Schmidt WM, Sedivy R, Forstner B et al (2007) Progressive up-regulation of genes encoding DNA methyltransferases in the colorectal adenoma-carcinoma sequence. Mol Carcinog 46:766–772

Scott DJ, Hull MA, Cartwright EJ et al (2001) Lack of inducible nitric oxide synthase promotes intestinal tumorigenesis in the $Apc^{Min/+}$ mouse. Gastroenterology 121:889–899

Shailubhai K, Yu HH, Karunanandaa K et al (2000) Uroguanylin treatment suppresses polyp formation in the $Apc^{Min/+}$ mouse and induces apoptosis in human colon adenocarcinoma cells via cyclic GMP. Cancer Res 60:5151–5157

Shao J, Jung C, Liu C et al (2005) Prostaglandin E2 Stimulates the β-catenin/T cell factor-dependent transcription in colon cancer. J Biol Chem 280:26565–26572

Shao J, Washington MK, Saxena R et al (2007) Heterozygous disruption of the PTEN promotes intestinal neoplasia in APCmin/+ mouse: roles of osteopontin. Carcinogenesis 28:2476–2483

Shibata H, Toyama K, Shioya H et al (1997) Rapid colorectal adenoma formation initiated by conditional targeting of the Apc gene. Science 278:120–123

Smith ML, Hawcroft G, Hull MA (2000) The effect of non-steroidal anti-inflammatory drugs on human colorectal cancer cells: evidence of different mechanisms of action. Eur J Cancer 36:664–674

Su LK, Kinzler KW, Vogelstein B et al (1992) Multiple intestinal neoplasia caused by a mutation in the murine homolog of the APC gene. Science 256:668–670

Swamy MV, Patlolla JM, Steele VE et al (2006) Chemoprevention of familial adenomatous polyposis by low doses of atorvastatin and celecoxib given individually and in combination to $Apc^{Min/+}$ mice. Cancer Res 66:7370–7377

Takaku K, Oshima M, Miyoshi H et al (1998) Intestinal tumorigenesis in compound mutant mice of both $Dpc4$ ($Smad4$) and Apc genes. Cell 92:645–656

Taketo MM (1998a) COX-2 and colon cancer. Inflamm Res 47:S112–S116

Taketo MM (1998b) Cyclooxygenase-2 inhibitors in tumorigenesis (Part I). J Natl Cancer Inst 90:1529–1536

Taketo MM (1998c) Cyclooxygenase-2 inhibitors in tumorigenesis (Part II). J Natl Cancer Inst 90:1609–1620

Taketo MM, Edelmann W (2009) Mouse models of colon cancer. Gastroenterology 136:780–798

Thun MJ, Henley SJ, Patrono C (2002) Nonsteroidal anti-inflammatory drugs as anticancer agents: mechanistic, pharmacologic, and clinical issues. J Natl Cancer Inst 94:252–266

Tomimoto A, Endo H, Sugiyama M et al (2008) Metformin suppresses intestinal polyp growth in $Apc^{Min/+}$ mice. Cancer Sci 99:2136–2141

Torrance CJ, Jackson PE, Montgomery E et al (2000) Combinatorial chemoprevention of intestinal neoplasia. Nat Med 6:1024–1028

Tucker JM, Murphy JT, Kisiel N et al (2005) Potent modulation of intestinal tumorigenesis in $Apc^{Min/+}$ mice by the polyamine catabolic enzyme spermidine/spermine N1-acetyltransferase. Cancer Res 65:5390–5398

van de Wetering M, Sancho E, Verweij C et al (2002) The β-catenin/TCF-4 complex imposes a crypt progenitor phenotype on colorectal cancer cells. Cell 111:241–250

van Es JH, van Gijn ME, Riccio O et al (2005) Notch/γ-secretase inhibition turns proliferative cells in intestinal crypts and adenomas into goblet cells. Nature 435:959–963

Weyant MJ, Carothers AM, Dannenberg AJ et al (2001) (+)-Catechin inhibits intestinal tumor formation and suppresses focal adhesion kinase activation in the Min/+ mouse. Cancer Res 61:118–125

Williams JL, Ji P, Ouyang N et al (2008) NO-donating aspirin inhibits the activation of NF-κB in human cancer cell lines and Min mice. Carcinogenesis 29:390–397

Williams JL, Kashfi K, Ouyang N et al (2004) NO-donating aspirin inhibits intestinal carcinogenesis in Min ($Apc^{Min/+}$) mice. Biochem Biophys Res Commun 313:784–788

Wilson CL, Heppner KJ, Labosky PA et al (1997) Intestinal tumorigenesis is suppressed in mice lacking the metalloproteinase matrilysin. Proc Natl Acad Sci USA 94:1402–1407

Yamada T, Mori Y, Hayashi R et al (2003) Suppression of intestinal polyposis in $Mdr1$-deficient $Apc^{Min/+}$ mice. Cancer Res 63:895–901

Yamaguchi K, Cekanova M, McEntee MF et al (2008) Peroxisome proliferator-activated receptor ligand MCC-555 suppresses intestinal polyps in *Apc*^Min/+ mice via extracellular signal-regulated kinase and peroxisome proliferator-activated receptor-dependent pathways. Mol Cancer Ther 7:2779–2787

Yekkala K, Baudino TA (2007) Inhibition of intestinal polyposis with reduced angiogenesis in ApcMin/+ mice due to decreases in c-Myc expression. Mol Cancer Res 5:1296–1303

Zeilstra J, Joosten SP, Dokter M et al (2008) Deletion of the WNT target and cancer stem cell marker CD44 in Apc(Min/+) mice attenuates intestinal tumorigenesis. Cancer Res 68:3655–3661

Zhang MZ, Xu J, Yao B et al (2009) Inhibition of 11β-hydroxysteroid dehydrogenase type II selectively blocks the tumor COX-2 pathway and suppresses colon carcinogenesis in mice and humans. J Clin Invest 119:876–885

Zhu P, Martin E, Mengwasser J et al (2004) Induction of HDAC2 expression upon loss of APC in colorectal tumorigenesis. Cancer Cell 5:455–463

Zimmermann S, Kiefer F, Prudenziati M et al (2007) Reduced body size and decreased intestinal tumor rates in HDAC2-mutant mice. Cancer Res 67:9047–9054

Chapter 8
Targeting Wnt Signalling in Cancer

Aliaksei Holik and Alan R. Clarke

Abstract The modular nature of the Wnt pathway provides multiple potential points of intervention to alter its activity. In this chapter we review potential opportunities to inhibit Wnt signalling at various levels, including the synthesis and secretion of Wnt ligands, activation of the Wnt receptor complex, degradation of cytoplasmic β-catenin and finally the nuclear complex between β-catenin and other transcription factors and co-activators. We also discuss the possibility of therapies targeting downstream Wnt target genes and a number of approaches with less defined mechanisms, whose anti-oncogenic properties may be mediated by Wnt pathway suppression. This review mainly focusses on canonical Wnt-β-catenin signalling, although a number of non-canonical Wnt pathways are also discussed, mainly in relation to their role in canonical Wnt pathway inhibition.

Keywords Wnt • β-catenin • cancer • therapy

8.1 Targeting the Wnt Pathway at the Level of Wnt Ligands

One of the major factors hindering the development of drugs targeting the Wnt pathway is the high degree of complexity at the level of ligand/receptor interaction. The Wnt ligand family in humans is represented by at least 19 members, each with differing affinities to the 10 Frizzled family receptors. This results in varied effects upon Wnt signalling. While many Wnt ligands (Wnt1, Wnt3a and Wnt16) act as Wnt activators and thus exhibit oncogenic effects, others (Wnt5a and Wnt7a) may inhibit the canonical Wnt pathway via the activation non-canonical pathways and thus act as tumour suppressors (Moon et al. 2004). Some also have dual roles by activating or inhibiting the pathway, depending on the receptor they bind to (Mikels and Nusse 2006).

A.R. Clarke (✉)
Cardiff School of Biosciences, Cardiff University, Museum Avenue, Cardiff, UK
e-mail: ClarkeAR@cf.ac.uk

K.H. Goss and M. Kahn (eds.), *Targeting the Wnt Pathway in Cancer*,
DOI 10.1007/978-1-4419-8023-6_8, © Springer Science+Business Media, LLC 2011

Aberrant expression of Wnt ligands has been shown to facilitate proliferation in a number of cancer cell lines and human tumours (reviewed in Ewan and Dale (2008)). Therefore, targeting the production of Wnt ligands may have therapeutic potential in these cancers. As a partial proof of this concept, disruption of WNT-1 synthesis using siRNA has been shown to increase apoptosis in a range of cancer cell lines expressing WNT-1 (He et al. 2004).

Other stages of Wnt ligand synthesis may also serve as targets for potential therapies. A study by Chen et al. (2009) showed that a class of small molecules is able to abrogate the function of the acetyltransferase Porcupine, which is involved in the synthesis of a number of Wnt ligands. Disrupted Wnt ligand synthesis led to a number of predicted responses in the treated cells, such as a decrease in phosphorylation of LRP6 receptor and DVL2 as well as depletion of transcriptionally active β-catenin accumulation. These small molecule compounds were, however, unable to manifest their Wnt-inhibitory activity *in vivo* as they did not prevent tissue regeneration in zebrafish (Chen et al. 2009).

Antibodies targeting Wnt ligands have been shown to inhibit Wnt signalling, both *in vitro* and *in vivo*. A monoclonal antibody raised against WNT-1 has been shown to induce apoptosis in lung and breast cancer cell lines overexpressing WNT-1, as well as suppress tumour growth in xenografts (He et al. 2004). The same monoclonal antibody was also able to induce apoptosis in colorectal cancer cell lines and primary cancer cells with elevated expression of WNT-1. Notably, the cell lines tested bore oncogenic mutations in downstream components of the Wnt pathway, namely APC and β-catenin, indicating that ligand depletion may inhibit the pathway even when aberrantly activated downstream of the receptor (He et al. 2005). A similar approach using an antibody against WNT-2 also demonstrated its ability to induce apoptosis in mesothelioma cell lines and primary cancer cells (Mazieres et al. 2005).

Some Wnt ligands display tumour suppressor qualities in a set of cancers. For example, WNT5A has been shown to suppress canonical Wnt/β-catenin signalling via the activation of the Wnt5a-Ca^{2+} pathway. WNT5A loss in breast carcinomas has been linked to increased cell motility and a higher risk of metastasis (Jonsson et al. 2002). Similarly, it has been found that low levels of WNT5A expression are a characteristic of high-risk neuroblastomas (Blanc et al. 2005). Furthermore, hexapeptides that mimic WNT5A have been demonstrated to impair migration and invasion of breast cancer cells *in vitro* as well as inhibiting metastasis in mice inoculated with the same breast cancer cells (Säfholm et al. 2008). Contrary to these findings, overexpression of WNT5A in human metastatic melanoma cells has been associated with increased motility and invasion (Weeraratna et al. 2002). Therefore, therapeutic applicability of WNT5A agonists is likely to be tissue specific.

A number of studies have proposed the use of soluble Wnt inhibitors as putative therapeutic targets. These inhibitors are able to bind to Wnt ligands so preventing the ligand/receptor interaction. Secreted frizzled-related proteins (SFRPs) have been found to be silenced in a variety of human cancers via promoter hypermethylation. Overexpression of SFRP proteins in colorectal cancer cell lines with oncogenic mutations in either APC or β-catenin resulted in inhibition of Wnt signalling, decreased colony formation and induced apoptosis (Suzuki et al. 2004). A similar study demonstrated that ectopic expression of Wnt inhibitory factor-1 (WIF-1) had a similar effect on colorectal cancer cell lines (He et al. 2005).

Protein family members of another Wnt inhibitor, Dickkopf (DKK), have been found to be lost or downregulated in a range of human malignancies. Restoration of their function affected a wide range of cellular processes such as proliferation, apoptosis, colony formation, cell adhesion and migration in melanoma, colorectal and breast cancer cell lines *in vitro* as well as inducing cell death in xenografts (Mikheev et al. 2007, 2008; Sato et al. 2007). It is worth noting however, that some of these effects were independent of Wnt/β-catenin signalling. In addition, since all the mentioned studies used endogenous overexpression of Wnt inhibitors in the very cancer cells they were targeted at, it is not clear whether treatment with exogenous recombinant SFRP, DKK or WIF-1 proteins would have caused the same effect.

Targeting the Wnt pathway at the ligand level raises some concerns about potential toxicity, as well as possible limited effectiveness in cancers with downstream mutations. Nonetheless, multiple strands of evidence now suggest that this approach may prove valuable in cancers characterised by overexpression of Wnt ligands.

8.2   Targeting the Wnt Pathway at the Receptor Level

The binding of a Wnt ligand to its respective receptor triggers a succession of interactions with other proteins in order to activate the pathway. Due to their crucial role in the pathway activation, components of the receptor complex may serve as therapeutic targets. Increased expression of Frizzled receptors has been detected in a range of tumours, such as colorectal and hepatocellular carcinomas (Holcombe et al. 2002; Merle et al. 2004). A neutralising antibody against the extracellular domain of Frizzled homologue 10 (FZD10) showed cytotoxic activity on synovial sarcoma cells overexpressing FZD10. It has also been found to attenuate tumour growth and induce apoptosis in a xenograft mouse model (Nagayama et al. 2005). Another Frizzled family member, FZD7, has been found to be frequently overexpressed in hepatocellular carcinoma cell lines and primary tumours. Overexpression of a dominant negative form of FZD7 in these cells reduced cell motility as well as preventing accumulation of nuclear β-catenin in cells with wild type, but not mutant β-catenin (Merle et al. 2004).

Upon binding to a ligand the receptor complex interacts with a number of proteins, including Dishevelled (DVL). Once bound to the receptor and self-multimerised, DVL recruits components of the β-catenin turnover complex (reviewed in Cadigan and Liu (2006)). In addition, the overexpression of DVL per se has been known to activate Wnt signalling. In accordance with this, elevated DVL3 has been observed in a subset of hepatocellular and lung malignancies (Uematsu et al. 2003a, b; Chan et al. 2006). Transfection of a truncated DVL3 lacking the PDZ domain, which interacts with Frizzled, inhibited Wnt signalling and suppressed tumourigenesis in pleural mesothelioma cells *in vitro* and in xenografts (Uematsu et al. 2003b). Similarly, a small molecule compound, FJ9, that targets the interaction between FZD7 receptor and the PZD domain of DVL has been shown to induce apoptosis in melanoma and non-small cell lung cancer cell lines, and has inhibited growth of lung cancer cell lines in mouse xenografts (Fujii et al. 2007).

8.3 Targeting β-Catenin Degradation

Two distinct classes of oncogenic events at the level of the β-catenin turnover complex may lead to the accumulation of nuclear β-catenin and as a result aberrant activation of the Wnt pathway. Oncogenic mutations in the N-terminal phosphorylation sites of β-catenin prevent its phosphorylation and thus render it resistant to degradation by the proteasome. The second class of mutations involves a loss of function in one of the β-catenin destruction complex components, such as APC or Axin. Either event would result in β-catenin accumulation and an aberrant activation of Wnt signalling (reviewed in Clevers (2006b) and MacDonald et al. (2009)). This section discusses the putative therapies targeted at β-catenin degradation, including a number of pathways alternative to the canonical β-catenin turnover complex.

8.3.1 Targeting the β-Catenin Turnover Complex

Targeting oncogenic β-catenin poses certain difficulties, as this approach would require specific inactivation of the oncogenic protein in favour of the functional one. Specific deletion of the oncogenic β-catenin allele in HCT116 cells has led to a substantial suppression of Wnt signalling and reduced colony forming ability of the cells plated at low density (Chan et al. 2002). However, cells lacking oncogenic β-catenin were still able to grow in anchorage-independent conditions and form tumours in mouse xenografts. Chan et al. therefore argue that simple depletion of oncogenic β-catenin or even complete abolishment of Wnt signalling, may not be sufficient for the tumour suppression. A similar study by Kim et al. (2002) has confirmed that activated β-catenin was not an essential oncogene in the HCT116 cell line used by Chan et al. However, two other cancer cell lines have been shown to rely on the presence of oncogenic β-catenin (Kim et al. 2002). These findings suggest that at least in a subset of cancers the requirement for oncogenic activation of the Wnt pathway may be overcome, possibly via acquirement of additional oncogenic mutations. This should be accounted for during future trials of drugs targeting this aspect of the Wnt pathway.

Therapeutic approaches targeting members of the destruction complex are logistically challenging because of the loss-of-function nature of the mutations. In order to counteract aberrant pathway activation in tumours with a deficiency in the turnover complex, a functional version of the protein needs to be delivered into every cell within the tumour. Although this is unlikely to be achieved in a living organism, a number of studies have provided "proof of concept" evidence that reintroduction of functional APC into colon carcinoma cell lines inhibits cell growth and induces apoptosis, while suppressing the Wnt target gene *C-MYC* (He et al. 1998). As an indication that this approach might be viable *in vivo*, it has been demonstrated that an Apc-expressing construct delivered via liposomes reduces the incidence of tumours in *Apc*[Min] mice (Arenas et al. 1996).

Two recently discovered compounds have suggested a novel approach to surmount the deficiency of the destruction complex. High-throughput screening for Wnt/β-catenin inhibitors in mouse L cells yielded a number of small molecules, including IWR-1 (Chen et al. 2009). A similar screening by Huang et al. (2009) in HEK293 cell line produced a structurally unrelated compound XAV939. Both compounds have been found to target the same enzyme, a poly-ADP-ribose polymerase Tankyrase. In its physiological state, Tankyrase post-translationally modifies Axin with an ADP-ribose polymer thus targeting Axin for ubiquitination and subsequent degradation. Tankyrase inhibition by IWR-1 and XAV939 stabilises Axin so promoting β-catenin phosphorylation and effectively inhibiting Wnt signalling (Huang et al. 2009). Importantly, both IWR-1 and XAV939 have been found to inhibit the Wnt pathway in cells with APC mutations and hence a defective destruction complex. Wnt signalling inhibition via Axin stabilisation has also proven effective *in vivo* where IWR-1 has been shown to inhibit processes where Wnt signalling plays a central role, such as tailfin regeneration and intestinal homeostasis in zebrafish (Chen et al. 2009). These observations indicate the potential for a substantial toxic effect, as Axin stabilisation inhibits physiological levels of Wnt signalling. Further pharmacological assays are required to establish the therapeutic index of these compounds, but encouragingly zebrafish tissues were able to almost fully regenerate after the compound was removed (Chen et al. 2009).

Upon recruitment to the turnover complex, β-catenin is phosphorylated by two kinases, glycogen synthase kinase 3β (GSK3β) and casein kinase 1α (CK1α) and thus is targeted for the degradation by the proteasome (MacDonald et al. 2009). A family of differentiation-inducing factors (DIFs) from *Dictyostelium discoideum* has been found to inhibit the Wnt pathway *in vitro* (Takahashi-Yanaga and Sasaguri 2009). DIF-1 and DIF-3 activate GSK3β via an unknown mechanism, which facilitates β-catenin degradation and leads to the repression of β-catenin/TCF-mediated transcription, in particular, cyclin D1 expression. The repressive effect on cyclin D1 transcription is enhanced by GSK3β-mediated phosphorylation of cyclin D1, that targets it for proteasomal degradation. As a result of Wnt pathway inhibition, DIFs exhibit a potent cyclin D1-dependent anti-proliferative effect in a range of cell lines, including HCT116, which bears a mutated β-catenin (Takahashi-Yanaga and Sasaguri 2009).

8.3.2 Alternative Pathways Contributing to β-Catenin Degradation

A number of alternative pathways involved in the degradation of β-catenin might provide valuable therapeutic targets for Wnt pathway inhibition. A ubiquitin-ligase binding protein, Siah-1, has been shown to interact with APC and promote β-catenin degradation in a GSK3β and βTrCP-independent manner. Reduction in β-catenin levels upon overexpression of Siah-1 coincided with the suppression of TCF/LEF-dependent transcription. Notably, Siah-1-mediated degradation of β-catenin does not require phosphorylation at the GSK3β-specific sites and thus can destroy mutant β-catenin refractory to GSK3β-dependent proteasomal degradation (Liu et al. 2001). In concordance with this, a small molecule compound hexachlorophene has been demonstrated to induce expression of Siah-1 and consequently decrease the levels of β-catenin and inhibit proliferation of human colorectal cancer cells expressing wild type APC and mutant β-catenin (Park et al. 2006).

While Siah-1-mediated degradation of β-catenin relies on a functional copy of APC, another small molecule Wnt pathway inhibitor, Murrayafoline A, has been shown to induce the proteasomal degradation of β-catenin via a novel pathway independent of GSK3β, APC and Siah-1-mediated degradation. Treatment with Murrayafoline A suppressed cyclin D1 and C-MYC expression as well as inhibited growth of a range of colorectal cancer cells, with both functional and deficient APC (Choi et al. 2010).

One more pathway with an as yet undefined mechanism appears to contribute to β-catenin degradation. Engrailed-1 (EN-1) is a transcription factor known to associate with the co-repressors of LEF/TCF transcription Groucho and transducin-like enhancer of split (GRO/TLE) (Courey and Jia 2001). In addition to its role in transcription regulation, EN-1 has also been shown to destabilise β-catenin via proteasomal degradation independent of GSK3β, Siah-1 or APC activity (Bachar-Dahan et al. 2006).

While all previously mentioned pathways require the proteasome for β-catenin degradation, activation of the G protein pathway, G_q, and subsequent Ca^{2+} release from intracellular stores leads to μ-calpain-dependent β-catenin degradation and inhibition of TCF/LEF transcriptional activity independent of the proteasome activity (Li and Iyengar 2002). Stabilisation of μ-calpain by overexpression of a dominant negative form of the μ-calpain inhibitor GAS2 (GAS2DN) has been shown to significantly reduce β-catenin levels. As a result, transient expression of GAS2DN in colorectal cancer cell lines with impaired proteasomal degradation of β-catenin inhibited cell proliferation and anchorage-independent growth (Benetti et al. 2005).

8.4   Targeting Wnt Signalling at the Nuclear Level

At the final stages of Wnt pathway activation, stabilised β-catenin is translocated into the nucleus, where it binds to TCF factors and displaces repressor proteins, whilst also recruiting transcriptional co-activators (MacDonald et al. 2009). The interaction between β-catenin and TCF as well as the interactions with their respective co-repressors and co-activators may provide potential targets for therapeutic intervention of Wnt signalling.

8.4.1 Targeting the β-Catenin/TCF Interaction

In support of the notion that the β-catenin/TCF interaction may represent a valuable therapeutic target, overexpression of the dominant negative forms of TCF1 and TCF4, lacking a β-catenin-binding domain, induced a potent cell cycle arrest in colorectal cancer cell lines (van de Wetering et al. 2002). A screening performed by Lepourcelet et al. (2004) identified a number of low molecular weight compounds that targeted the interaction between β-catenin and TCF4. Disruption of this interaction predictably led to the suppression of Wnt target genes and manifested substantial cytotoxicity towards colon cancer cells with either mutated β-catenin or APC. Although some of the compounds demonstrated selectively higher cytotoxicity towards colon carcinoma cell lines compared to prostate cancer cells with intact Wnt signalling, their cytotoxic effect is unlikely to be solely based on the disruption of β-catenin/TCF interaction, as the targeted deletion of mutant β-catenin made the cells more sensitive to some of the compounds. Indeed, a number of the compounds tested have been shown to impair β-catenin/APC and TCF/DNA interactions in addition to the disruption of the β-catenin/TCF complex. Notably, some of these compounds were also able to suppress the dorsal axis duplication in Xenopus embryos induced by ectopic injection of β-catenin mRNA with minimal toxic effects (Lepourcelet et al. 2004). However, it is difficult to predict the adverse developmental effects of these compounds in humans.

Similarly, the flavonoid quercetin has been found to disrupt β-catenin/TCF and TCF/DNA interactions in colorectal cancer cell lines and suppress TCF-mediated transcription (Park et al. 2005). As a result of this inhibition, quercetin is able to suppress proliferation and induce apoptosis in cancer cells in a dose-dependent manner, while repressing crucial Wnt downstream target genes including cyclin D1 and survivin (Shan et al. 2009). In agreement with these observations quercetin has been previously found to be effective in decreasing the number of chemically induced aberrant crypt foci in rat intestine (Matsukawa et al. 1997).

8.4.2 Targeting Transcriptional Co-Activators of the Wnt Pathway

TCF proteins do not possess an intrinsic ability to modulate transcription, but rather serve as a docking platform for other proteins, β-catenin being one of them, which in turn can activate or repress the transcriptional activity of the promoter they are recruited to (Eastman and Grosschedl 1999). Among the known co-activators of TCF/β-catenin-mediated transcription are the histone acetyltransferases p300 and CREB-binding protein (CBP). The p300/CBP complex has been shown to synergise with β-catenin in activating TCF-regulated reporters, as well as genuine Wnt target genes *in vitro*. Furthermore, expression of the E1A oncoprotein, a known p300/CBP inhibitor, negated the effects of activated Wnt signalling in cultured cells and in Xenopus embryos (Hecht et al. 2000). A small molecule compound ICG-001 that binds to CBP and abrogates its interaction with β-catenin has been shown to induce apoptosis in colorectal carcinoma cells *in vitro*, while normal colonic cells remained unaffected. Notably, the treatment with ICG-001 was successful in suppressing polyp formation in *Apc*[Min] mice and substantially delayed tumour growth in a xenograft model (Emami et al. 2004).

Transducin β-like protein 1 (TBL1), involved in the aforementioned Siah1-mediated β-catenin degradation, and TBL1-related protein (TBLR1), have both been found to play a crucial role in the binding of β-catenin to the promoters of Wnt target genes and their subsequent transcriptional activation (Li and Wang 2008). shRNA knock-down of either TBL1 or TBLR1 impaired the recruitment of β-catenin to Wnt-controlled promoters without affecting nuclear accumulation of β-catenin. As a result, cells transfected with TBL1 or TBLR1 shRNA had reduced expression levels of Wnt target genes, elevated apoptosis levels and completely abolished cell growth in anchorage-independent conditions. Furthermore, TBL1 and TBLR1 knock-down potently inhibited the invasive ability of the cells *in vitro* and tumour growth in xenograft model (Li and Wang 2008).

8.4.3   Targeting Transcriptional Co-Repressors of the Wnt Pathway

A range of transcriptional co-repressors has been shown to interact with TCF and inhibit Wnt signalling. Among these are Groucho or its human homologue transducin-like enhancer of split (TLE), CtBP and nemo-like kinase (NLK) (MacDonald et al. 2009). Therapeutic approaches that would increase activity of these negative regulators of the pathway might prove useful in suppressing Wnt signalling. An obvious benefit of targeting the Wnt pathway at such a late stage is that it would allow manipulation of the pathway even if it was activated by upstream mutations.

Both loss and epigenetic silencing of TLE proteins have been implicated in the development of a range of haematologic malignancies, such as acute myeloid leukaemia and B-cell lymphoma (Dayyani et al. 2008; Fraga et al. 2008). Restoration of TLE1 function in hypermethylated leukaemia and lymphoma cells resulted in significant suppression of cell growth, colony formation and tumour growth when the cells were injected into nude mice (Fraga et al. 2008). It is worth noting however, that although functional TLE1 repressed the expression of Wnt target genes C-MYC and Cyclin D1, it also inhibited the transcriptional activity of the other pathways, such as Notch and AML. It is likely therefore that TLE1 tumour suppressor activity reaches beyond its role in Wnt signalling repression.

TCF-dependent transcription has also been found to be subject to inhibition by non-canonical Wnt pathways. Wnt5a-Ca²⁺ pathway stimulation has been shown to activate the mitogen-activated protein kinase (MAPK) pathway, leading to the activation of NLK/MAPK (Ishitani et al. 2003a). Activated NLK is then able to phosphorylate TCF and thus target it for ubiquitylation and subsequent degradation, effectively inhibiting TCF-mediated transcription (Ishitani et al. 2003b; Yamada et al. 2006). Specific activation of the Wnt5a-Ca^{2+}-NLK pathway may therefore offer some therapeutic potential. However, as yet no cytotoxic assays have been published to validate the feasibility of this approach.

Another non-canonical Wnt pathway that has been demonstrated to inhibit Wnt signalling downstream of β-catenin involves Wnt5a-mediated activation of tyrosine kinase receptor Ror2 (Mikels and Nusse 2006). Although the precise mechanism of this inhibition is still unknown, it has been shown to take place *in vivo* as Ror2 loss in transgenic mice resulted in the increased activity of the Wnt reported construct *Axin2^{LacZ}* (Mikels et al. 2009).

Canonical Wnt signalling is known to modulate a range of nuclear hormone receptors. In turn, some nuclear receptors have been shown to inhibit Wnt signalling (reviewed in Mulholland et al. (2005)). In particular, activation of retinoic acid and vitamin D receptors with their respective ligands have been suggested to inhibit Wnt signalling via depletion of TCF sites available for β-catenin binding in a range of cancer cell lines. Unexpectedly, despite its broadly acknowledged anticancer effects, retinoic acid dietary supplementation to *Apc^{Min}* mice increased both tumour incidence and growth (Møllersen et al. 2004). Vitamin D treatment, on the other hand, has proven potent in decreasing tumour burden in the same model system, but only at doses that had a negative effect on calcium homeostasis. The latter, however, might be alleviated with a use of synthetic, less toxic analogues (Harris and Go 2004).

8.5 Targeting Downstream Wnt Targets

Due to the critical role Wnt signalling plays in the homeostasis of adult tissues, such as the intestinal epithelium and the bone marrow, any drug that abolishes Wnt signalling is likely to display a substantial toxicity in normal tissues. With this in mind, targeting the proteins downstream of the pathway may help to attenuate the toxic effects. In addition, since most of the oncogenic mutations occur within the elements of the pathway, targeting the function of the pathway effector genes may offer the additional advantage of overcoming single or multiple upstream mutations. Targeting genes downstream of the Wnt pathway may therefore offer a more universal approach by inactivating the oncogenic effects of the pathway, rather than the pathway itself. A set of downstream Wnt target genes has shown encouraging results in the ability to repress Wnt-driven tumourigenesis.

The proto-oncogene C-MYC is a well known Wnt target gene both in normal intestinal epithelium and colorectal cancer cells (He et al. 1998; van de Wetering et al. 2002) and is commonly used as a readout of the Wnt pathway activity. c-Myc has been found to be upregulated in response to Apc inactivation in murine small intestinal epithelium, suggesting its importance in the mediation of aberrant Wnt activation (Sansom et al. 2004). In support of this observation, simultaneous inactivation of c-Myc and Apc in the murine small intestinal epithelium reversed the characteristic effects of Apc loss, such as disturbed proliferation, migration and differentiation as well as elevated levels of apoptosis (Sansom et al. 2007b). A number of studies have demonstrated that targeting C-MYC with an anti-sense morpholino oligomer suppresses the growth of prostate and lung cancer cells in xenograft models, while demonstrating good tolerance in healthy individuals and high bioavailability in solid tumours (Iversen et al. 2003; Sekhon et al. 2008). A similar approach might also prove useful in colorectal cancer, however, no assessment of the drug has been performed in colorectal cancer models.

Simultaneous deletion of c-Myc and Apc has revealed a subset of Wnt target genes that are downregulated upon c-Myc inactivation, thus displaying c-Myc-dependent transcription (Sansom et al. 2007b). Among those genes was a guanine nucleotide exchange factor Tiam1 (T-cell lymphoma invasion and metastasis 1) that has been previously found driven by Wnt signalling and uniformly expressed in benign polyps arising in Apc^{Min} mice. However, while $Tiam1$ knock-out reduced the incidence and growth of the polyps in Apc^{Min} mice, it promoted tumour invasiveness, which might make it unfavourble as a therapeutic target (Malliri et al. 2006).

Proteins involved in the interaction with the extracellular matrix play a pivotal role in cancer progression, particularly its late stages. The matricellular protein SPARC, is known for its overexpression in numerous cancers (Framson and Sage 2004). Adenomas from Apc^{Min} mice have been found to display elevated levels of the matricellular protein Sparc, which implicated Sparc in Wnt-mediated tumourigenesis (Sansom et al. 2007a). Accordingly, Sparc deficiency potently inhibited tumour initiation in Apc^{Min} mice, while accelerating physiological migration of normal intestinal epithelium, which may contribute to the anti-oncogenic effects of Sparc deletion.

Cyclin D1 is commonly recognised as a Wnt target gene and numerous experiments implicate it in tumourigenesis (Kim and Diehl 2009). Surprisingly, Apc^{Min} mice with constitutive $Cyclin D1$, knock-out are still prone to neoplastic transformation of the small intestinal epithelium, albeit at a lower frequency. Their ability to develop adenomas in the absence of $Cyclin D1$ indicates that $Cyclin D1$ is dispensable for Wnt-induced tumourigenesis, although it may act as a Wnt-signal modifier (Wilding et al. 2002). Supporting this notion, $Cyclin D1$ deficiency in a range of breast cancer mouse models has been shown to suppress the development of tumours driven by the Neu and Ras oncogenes, but not by c-Myc or Wnt-1 (Yu et al. 2001). Taking these observations into account, the use of therapies targeted at $Cyclin D1$ has a limited potential in Wnt-driven malignancies.

In contrast to the examples cited above, all of which are effectors of Wnt activation, another Wnt target gene, Lect2 (leukocyte cell-derived chemotaxin 2), has been shown to inhibit Wnt-mediated transcription (Phesse et al. 2008). Conditional inactivation of methyl-CpG binding protein 2 (Mbd2) in the context of activated Wnt signalling relieves Mbd2-imposed repression of Lect2, which in turn is suggested to suppress a range of Wnt target genes. As a result, Mbd2 deficiency has been demonstrated to reduce tumour burden and promote animal survival both in Apc^{Min} and conditional Apc knock-out mice (Sansom et al. 2003; Phesse et al. 2008).

Additional unattributed effects of Mbd2 deficiency may, however, contribute to the observed anticarcinogenic effect.

In a similar manner, the family of EphrinB receptors (EphB) and EphrinB ligands, expressed under β-catenin/TCF control, act as key regulators of cell positioning and ordered migration along the crypt–villus axis. The loss of EphB2 and EphB3 in tumours is strongly associated with cancer progression towards invasiveness and metastasis (Clevers and Batlle 2006). In support of this notion, EphB3 overexpression in colorectal cancer cells impairs cell growth *in vitro* and in xenograft models, while shifting cell appearance and physiology towards a more differentiated, epithelial state (Chiu et al. 2009).

8.5.1 Targeting the Wnt Pathway in Cancer Stem Cells

The idea that a specific cell subpopulation termed cancer stem cells (CSC) is responsible for the propagation of the tumour growth and therapy resistance, is gaining strong support (reviewed in Wicha et al. (2006)). One of the implications of the CSC hypothesis is the concept that oncogenic mutations in somatic stem cells pose a higher risk of cancer initiation and progression compared to non-stem cells. This is evidently true in murine small intestinal epithelium, where aberrant activation of Wnt signalling in putative intestinal stem cell leads to the development of more aggressive adenomas than those originating from progenitor cells (Barker et al. 2009). An alternative hypothesis assumes that the cancer stem cell may originate from differentiated cells via de-differentiation and reacquisition of stem cell-like features. Either way, CSCs share many properties with normal stem cells, including a specific gene expression pattern.

A set of genes, which mark specific cell subpopulations within a crypt, have been associated with the putative intestinal stem cell. A subset of these genes, such as Lgr5 (leucine-rich-repeat-containing G-protein-coupled receptor 5), Ascl2 (Achaete Scute-Like 2) and Olfm4 (Olfactomedin-4) mark actively cycling columnar base cells at the bottom of the crypt (Barker et al. 2007; van der Flier et al. 2009a, b), while the expression of genes such as Bmi1 and Dcamkl-1 (Doublecortin and CaM Kinase-Like-1) is mainly confined to cells around position +4 that correspond to the hypothetical label retaining stem cell (May et al. 2008; Sangiorgi and Capecchi 2008). In concordance with the role Wnt signalling plays in intestinal homeostasis (Ireland et al. 2004), Lgr5 and Ascl2 have been found expressed under the control of the Wnt pathway, whereas involvement of Wnt signalling in the regulation of the other genes is ambiguous. Both genes marking the columnar base stem cell and the position +4 stem cell have been found to be expressed in a proportion of the cells within a tumour, which may represent the CSC compartment. These stem cell markers may therefore be exploited to target the CSC population within a tumour.

Notably, conditional deletion of *Ascl2* in the murine intestine led to the elimination of intestinal stem cells marked by Lgr5 expression and gradual epithelium repopulation with wild type cells, indicating the requirement of a functional copy of *Ascl2* in intestinal stem cell maintenance (van der Flier et al. 2009b). Furthermore, ASCL2 knockdown in human colorectal cancer cell lines with elevated levels of the protein have been shown to induce G2/M checkpoint arrest, indicating the possible therapeutic benefit of an ASCL2 inhibitor (Jubb et al. 2006). Similarly to ASCL2, OLMF4 has been found upregulated in human intestinal neoplasia suggesting that its expression may provide the tumour with a selective growth advantage and thus serve as a putative therapeutic target (van der Flier et al. 2009a).

Conditional inactivation of *Lrg5* in the mouse intestine exhibits a mild effect on Paneth cell differentiation, but otherwise does not seem to affect gut development. Moreover, elevated levels of Wnt target genes in Lgr5-deficient intestine have suggested that Lgr5 acts as a negative Wnt-regulator (Garcia et al. 2009). Therefore, Lgr5 and other genes may act merely as markers of the stem cell, rather than facilitators of a stem cell-like state and are unlikely to serve as promising targets for the pharmacological inhibitors or activators. Nonetheless, their specific expression in CSCs may prove useful in the development of the therapeutic approaches based on oncolytic viruses.

8.6   Generic Approaches to Targeting Wnt-Mediated Tumourigenesis

A number of therapeutic approaches not specifically targeted at Wnt signalling may be beneficial in Wnt-driven cancers. This section briefly reviews the possible use of drugs targeted at epigenetic changes as well as non-steroidal anti-inflammatory drugs in Wnt-driven cancers.

8.6.1   Targeting DNA Methylation

Silencing of Wnt negative regulators mediated by promoter hypermethylation has been shown to contribute towards abnormal activation of Wnt signalling. In particular, a range of soluble Wnt inhibitors, such as DKKs, SFRPs or WIF, have been found to be silenced by promoter hypermethylation (reviewed in Ewan and Dale (2008)). The use of DNA-methylation inhibitors may, therefore, have a beneficial effect on suppressing Wnt signalling. The overall effect of such a therapy, however, is likely to involve pathways and processes beyond the Wnt cascade, such as activation of other silenced tumour suppressors, which may facilitate the anti-oncogenic effect. Inhibition of the DNA methyl transferases (DNMT) is a common approach used in the reversion of the aberrant DNA methylation. The prototype DNMT1 inhibitors 5-azacytidine and 5-aza-2'-deoxycytidine have been approved for use in myelodysplastic syndromes, however, their use in solid tumours is limited due to poor bioavailability (reviewed in Sharma et al. (2010)).

8.6.2 Targeting Mediators of Histone Modifications

The repressive effects of CpG island hypermethylation are mediated by chromatin modifications. Methyl-CpG-binding domain (MBD) proteins and a related protein Kaiso are able to recognise methylated CpG islands and recruit mediators of repression such as histone methyl transferases (HAT) and histone deacetylases (HDAC) (reviewed in Klose and Bird (2006)). Since MBD proteins mediate repression caused by promoter hypermethylation, targeting their function provides an attractive opportunity to relieve transcriptional repression and restore the function of the silenced tumour suppressors. Indeed, inactivation of Mbd2 in Apc^{Min} mice substantially suppressed tumour development both in terms of incidence and growth rate (Sansom et al. 2003). Similar results have been observed in Apc^{Min} mice lacking the expression of Kaiso protein (Prokhortchouk et al. 2006). Importantly, both *Mbd2* and *Kaiso* null mice developed subtle or no abnormalities, which makes them very attractive non-toxic targets.

Acetylation of the specific lysine residues within the histone tails is commonly associated with active transcription. HDAC enzymes recruited to the chromatin may therefore establish the repressive signature by the deacetylation of histone tails (Klose and Bird 2006). Groucho/TLE co-repressors of the Wnt pathway are known to act via recruitment of histone deacetylases and thus establish repressive chromatin modifications (reviewed in Gasperowicz and Otto (2005)). Consistent with this hypothesis, the treatment of colorectal cancer cell lines with HDAC inhibitors, such as sodium butyrate (NaB), led to further activation of Wnt signalling. Surprisingly, this effect was not solely mediated by Groucho/TLE as the treatment with NaB also resulted in decreased phosphorylation of β-catenin and thus increased levels of transcriptionally active β-catenin. Counterintuitively, hyperactivation of Wnt signalling induced by HDAC inhibitors led to a potent apoptotic response in a set of colorectal cancer cell lines. At the same time HDAC inhibitor treatment of the cell lines with lower levels of active β-catenin resulted in reversible cell cycle arrest (Bordonaro et al. 2007). This observation indicates that a specific level of Wnt activation might be required for the manifestation of the oncogenic effects. Furthermore, a study by Gaspar et al. (2009) suggests that this requirement for the specific dosage of Wnt activation is tissue specific. They have shown that mice bearing a specific truncating mutation in one of the *Apc* alleles displayed a moderate increase in Wnt activity, compared with other mutations. These mice developed aggressive mammary adenocarcinomas, but did not exhibit any signs of intestinal tumourigenesis (Gaspar et al. 2009).

8.6.3 Non-Steroidal Anti-Inflammatory Drugs

An extensive body of data has accumulated that suggests a potent therapeutic effect of non-steroidal anti-inflammatory drugs (NSAIDs) in various human cancers and particularly in the patients with hereditary forms of colorectal cancer, where Wnt activation plays a central role (reviewed in Barker and Clevers (2006)). One of the disadvantages of traditional NSAIDs is the damaging effect to the gastrointestinal tract and kidneys in a significant proportion of patients. These adverse effects have stimulated development of new generation NSAIDs in order to enhance their anti-cancer effects while diminishing the toxicity. Two major groups of NSAID deriva-tives, cyclooxigenase 2 inhibitors and nitric oxide-releasing NSAIDs (NO-NSAIDs) have demonstrated a potent anticancer activity, while imposing limited toxic side effects (Williams et al. 2001, 2004; Phillips et al. 2002; Solomon et al. 2006). Several studies have linked both old and new generation NSAIDs to the inhibition of various components of Wnt signalling (reviewed in Clevers (2006a)). However it still remains to be decisively proven that anticancer effects of NSAIDs rely on the inhibition of the Wnt pathway.

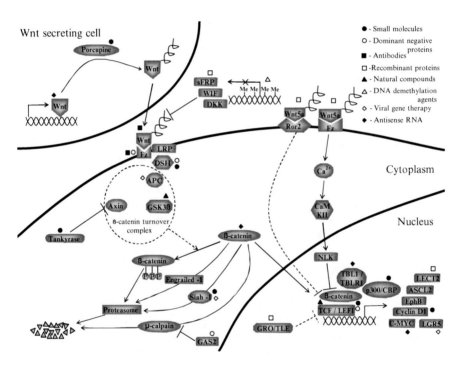

Fig. 8.1 Summary of possible targets and example approaches for therapeutic intervention into the activated Wnt/β-catenin pathway. *APC* adenomatous polyposis coli, *ASCL2* achaete scute-Like 2, *CaMKII* Ca^{2+}/calmodulin-dependent protein kinase II, *CBP* CREB-binding protein, *DKK* Dickkopf, *DSH* Dishevelled, *EphB* Ephrin B receptor, *Fz* Frizzled, *GAS2* growth arrest specific gene 2, *GRO/TLE* Groucho/transducin-like enhancer of split, *GSK3β* glycogen synthase kinase 3 beta, *LECT2* leukocyte cell-derived chemotaxin 2, *LGR5* leucine-rich-repeat-containing G-protein-coupled receptor 5, *LRP* low-density lipoprotein receptor-related protein, *NLK* nemo-like kinase, *P* phosphorylation, *Ror2* tyrosine kinase Ror2, *sFRP* secreted frizzled related protein, *Siah-1* human homolog of Drosophila seven in absentia 1, *TBL1/TBLR1* transducin β-like protein 1/ TBL1-related protein, *TCF/LEF1* T-cell factor/lymphoid enhancer-binding factor 1, *WIF* WNT inhibitory factor

8.7 Summary

Overall, this review has summarised many possible different approaches to target the Wnt pathway therapeutically. These include the use of various classes of therapeutic agents, such as small molecule inhibitors and activators, monoclonal antibodies, anti-sense oligonucleotides and others at different levels of the pathway (Fig. 8.1). Of these, perhaps the most promising are those for which there is already good clinical or preclinical data, such as C-MYC-targeting anti-sense oligonucleotides and the new generation NSAIDs.

Taken together it appears that the Wnt pathway offers a multitude of potential points for therapeutic intervention, and the hope is that these will rapidly translate into urgently needed novel therapies.

References

Arenas RB, Fichera A, Mok P, Blanco MC, Michelassi F (1996) Introduction of human adenomatous polyposis coli gene into Min mice via cationic liposomes. Surgery 120(4):712

Bachar-Dahan L, Goltzmann J, Yaniv A, Gazit A (2006) Engrailed-1 negatively regulates beta-Catenin transcriptional activity by destabilizing beta-Catenin via a glycogen synthase kinase-3independent pathway. Mol Biol Cell 17(6):2572

Barker N, Clevers H (2006) Mining the Wnt pathway for cancer therapeutics. Nat Rev Drug Discov 5(12):997

Barker N et al (2007) Identification of stem cells in small intestine and colon by marker gene Lgr5. Nature 449(7165):1003

Barker N et al (2009) Crypt stem cells as the cells-of-origin of intestinal cancer. Nature 457(7229):608

Benetti R et al (2005) The calpain system is involved in the constitutive regulation of beta-catenin signaling functions. J Biol Chem 280(23):22070

Blanc E, Goldschneider D, Douc-Rasy S, Bénard J, Raguénez G (2005) Wnt-5a gene expression in malignant human neuroblasts. Cancer Lett 228(1–2):117

Bordonaro M, Lazarova DL, Sartorelli AC (2007) The activation of beta-catenin by Wnt signaling mediates the effects of histone deacetylase inhibitors. Exp Cell Res 313(8):1652

Cadigan KM, Liu YI (2006) Wnt signaling: complexity at the surface. J Cell Sci 119(3):395

Chan TA, Wang Z, Dang LH, Vogelstein B, Kinzler KW (2002) Targeted inactivation of CTNNB1 reveals unexpected effects of β-catenin mutation. Proc Natl Acad Sci USA 99(12):8265

Chan DW, Chan C, Yam JW, Ching Y, Ng IO (2006) Prickle-1 negatively regulates Wnt/β-Catenin pathway by promoting dishevelled Ubiquitination/Degradation in liver cancer. Gastroenterology 131(4):1218

Chen B et al (2009) Small molecule-mediated disruption of Wnt-dependent signaling in tissue regeneration and cancer. Nat Chem Biol 5(2):100

Chiu S et al (2009) Over-expression of EphB3 enhances cell-cell contacts and suppresses tumor growth in HT-29 human colon cancer cells. Carcinogenesis 30(9):1475

Choi H et al (2010) Murrayafoline A attenuates the Wnt/β-catenin pathway by promoting the degradation of intracellular β-catenin proteins. Biochem Biophys Res Commun 391(1):915

Clevers H (2006a) Colon cancer – understanding how NSAIDs work. N Engl J Med 354(7):761

Clevers H (2006b) Wnt/β-Catenin signaling in development and disease. Cell 127(3):469

Clevers H, Batlle E (2006) EphB/EphrinB receptors and Wnt signaling in colorectal cancer. Cancer Res 66(1):2

Courey AJ, Jia S (2001) Transcriptional repression: the long and the short of it. Genes Dev 15(21):2786

Dayyani F et al (2008) Loss of TLE1 and TLE4 from the del(9q) commonly deleted region in AML cooperates with AML1-ETO to affect myeloid cell proliferation and survival. Blood 111(8):4338

Eastman Q, Grosschedl R (1999) Regulation of LEF-1/TCF transcription factors by Wnt and other signals. Curr Opin Cell Biol 11(2):233

Emami KH et al (2004) A small molecule inhibitor of beta-catenin/CREB-binding protein transcription. Proc Natl Acad Sci USA 101(34):12682

Ewan KBR, Dale TC (2008) The potential for targeting oncogenic WNT/beta- catenin signaling in therapy. Curr Drug Targets 9(7):532

Fraga MF et al (2008) Epigenetic inactivation of the Groucho homologue gene TLE1 in hematologic malignancies. Cancer Res 68(11):4116

Framson PE, Sage EH (2004) SPARC and tumor growth: Where the seed meets the soil? J Cell Biochem 92(4):679

Fujii N et al (2007) An antagonist of dishevelled protein-protein interaction suppresses beta-catenin-dependent tumor cell growth. Cancer Res 67(2):573

Garcia MI et al (2009) LGR5 deficiency deregulates Wnt signaling and leads to precocious paneth cell differentiation in the fetal intestine. Dev Biol 331(1):58

Gaspar C et al (2009) A targeted constitutive mutation in the Apc tumor suppressor gene underlies mammary but not intestinal tumorigenesis. PLoS Genet 5(7):e1000547

Gasperowicz M, Otto F (2005) Mammalian Groucho homologs: redundancy or specificity? J Cell Biochem 95(4):670

Harris DM, Go VLW (2004) Vitamin D and colon carcinogenesis. J Nutr 134(12):3463S

He T et al (1998) Identification of c-MYC as a target of the APC pathway. Science 281(5382):1509

He B et al (2004) A monoclonal antibody against Wnt-1 induces apoptosis in human cancer cells. Neoplasia 6(1):7

He B et al (2005) Blockade of Wnt-1 signaling induces apoptosis in human colorectal cancer cells containing downstream mutations. Oncogene 24(18):3054

Hecht A, Vleminckx K, Stemmler MP, van Roy F, Kemler R (2000) The p300/CBP acetyltransferases function as transcriptional coactivators of β-catenin in vertebrates. EMBO J 19(8):1839

Holcombe RF et al (2002) Expression of Wnt ligands and Frizzled receptors in colonic mucosa and in colon carcinoma. Mol Pathol 55(4):220

Huang SA et al (2009) Tankyrase inhibition stabilizes axin and antagonizes Wnt signalling. Nature 461(7264):614

Ireland H et al (2004) Inducible cre-mediated control of gene expression in the murine gastrointestinal tract: effect of loss of β-catenin. Gastroenterology 126(5):1236

Ishitani T et al (2003a) The TAK1-NLK Mitogen-Activated protein kinase cascade functions in the Wnt-5a/Ca2+ pathway to antagonize Wnt/beta-Catenin signaling. Mol Cell Biol 23(1):131

Ishitani T, Ninomiya-Tsuji J, Matsumoto K (2003b) Regulation of lymphoid enhancer factor 1/T-cell factor by mitogen-activated protein kinase-related nemo-like kinase-dependent phosphorylation in Wnt/β-catenin signaling. Mol Cell Biol 23(4):1379

Iversen PL, Arora V, Acker AJ, Mason DH, Devi GR (2003) Efficacy of antisense morpholino oligomer targeted to C-MYC in prostate cancer xenograft murine model and a phase I safety study in humans. Clin Cancer Res 9(7):2510

Jonsson M, Dejmek J, Bendahl P, Andersson T (2002) Loss of WNT-5A protein is associated with early relapse in invasive ductal breast carcinomas. Cancer Res 62(2):409

Jubb AM et al (2006) Achaete-scute like 2 (ascl2) is a target of wnt signaling and is upregulated in intestinal neoplasia. Oncogene 25(24):3445

Kim JK, Diehl JA (2009) Nuclear Cyclin D1: an oncogenic driver in human cancer. J Cell Physiol 220(2):292

Kim J, Crooks H, Foxworth A, Waldman T (2002) Proof-of-principle: oncogenic beta-catenin is a valid molecular target for the development of pharmacological inhibitors. Mol Cancer Ther 1(14):1355

Klose RJ, Bird AP (2006) Genomic DNA methylation: the mark and its mediators. Trends Biochem Sci 31(2):89

Lepourcelet M et al (2004) Small-molecule antagonists of the oncogenic TCF/β-catenin protein complex. Cancer Cell 5(1):91

Li G, Iyengar R (2002) Calpain as an effector of the G_q signaling pathway for inhibition of Wnt/β-catenin-regulated cell proliferation. Proc Natl Acad Sci USA 99(20):13254

Li J, Wang C (2008) TBL1-TBLR1 and β-catenin recruit each other to Wnt target-gene promoter for transcription activation and oncogenesis. Nat Cell Biol 10(2):160

Liu J et al (2001) Siah-1 mediates a novel β-Catenin degradation pathway linking p53 to the adenomatous polyposis coli protein. Mol Cell 7(5):927

MacDonald BT, Tamai K, He X (2009) Wnt/β-catenin signaling: components, mechanisms, and diseases. Dev Cell 17(1):9

Malliri A et al (2006) The Rac activator Tiam1 is a Wnt-responsive gene that modifies intestinal tumor development. J Biol Chem 281(1):543

Matsukawa Y et al (1997) Effects of quercetin and/or restraint stress on formation of aberrant crypt foci induced by azoxymethane in rat colons. Oncology 54(2):118

May R et al (2008) Identification of a novel putative gastrointestinal stem cell and adenoma stem cell marker, doublecortin and CaM Kinase-Like-1, following radiation injury and in adenomatous polyposis Coli/Multiple intestinal neoplasia mice. Stem Cells 26(3):630

Mazieres J et al (2005) Wnt2 as a new therapeutic target in malignant pleural mesothelioma. Int J Cancer 117(2):326

Merle P et al (2004) Functional consequences of Frizzled-7 receptor overexpression in human hepatocellular carcinoma. Gastroenterology 127(4):1110

Mikels AJ, Nusse R (2006) Purified WNT5A protein activates or inhibits β-Catenin/TCF signaling depending on receptor context. PLoS Biol 4(4):e115

Mikels A, Minami Y, Nusse R (2009) Ror2 receptor requires tyrosine kinase activity to mediate Wnt5A signaling. J Biol Chem 284(44):30167

Mikheev AM, Mikheeva SA, Rostomily R, Zarbl H (2007) Dickkopf-1 activates cell death in MDA-MB435 melanoma cells. Biochem Biophys Res Commun 352(3):675

Mikheev A et al (2008) Dickkopf-1 mediated tumor suppression in human breast carcinoma cells. Breast Cancer Res Treat 112(2):263

Møllersen L, Paulsen JE, Olstorn HB, Knutsen HK, Alexander J (2004) Dietary retinoic acid supplementation stimulates intestinal tumour formation and growth in multiple intestinal neoplasia (Min)/+ mice. Carcinogenesis 25(1):149

Moon RT, Kohn AD, Ferrari GVD, Kaykas A (2004) WNT and β-catenin signalling: diseases and therapies. Nat Rev Genet 5(9):691

Mulholland DJ, Dedhar S, Coetzee GA, Nelson CC (2005) Interaction of nuclear receptors with the Wnt/beta-Catenin/TCF signaling axis: Wnt you like to know? Endocr Rev 26(7):898

Nagayama S et al (2005) Therapeutic potential of antibodies against FZD10, a cell-surface protein, for synovial sarcomas. Oncogene 24(41):6201

Park CH et al (2005) Quercetin, a potent inhibitor against β-catenin/TCF signaling in SW480 colon cancer cells. Biochem Biophys Res Commun 328(1):227

Park S et al (2006) Hexachlorophene inhibits Wnt/beta-catenin pathway by promoting siah-mediated beta-catenin degradation. Mol Pharmacol 70(3):960

Phesse TJ et al (2008) Deficiency of Mbd2 attenuates Wnt signaling. Mol Cell Biol 28(19):6094

Phillips RKS et al (2002) A randomised, double blind, placebo controlled study of celecoxib, a selective cyclooxygenase 2 inhibitor, on duodenal polyposis in familial adenomatous polyposis. Gut 50(6):857

Prokhortchouk A et al (2006) Kaiso-Deficient mice show resistance to intestinal cancer. Mol Cell Biol 26(1):199

Säfholm A et al (2008) The Wnt-5a-derived hexapeptide foxy-5 inhibits breast cancer metastasis in vivo by targeting cell motility. Clin Cancer Res 14(20):6556

Sangiorgi E, Capecchi MR (2008) Bmi1 is expressed in vivo in intestinal stem cells. Nat Genet 40(7):915

Sansom OJ et al (2003) Deficiency of Mbd2 suppresses intestinal tumorigenesis. Nat Genet 34(2):145

Sansom OJ et al (2004) Loss of Apc in vivo immediately perturbs Wnt signaling, differentiation, and migration. Genes Dev 18(12):1385

Sansom OJ et al (2007a) Myc deletion rescues Apc deficiency in the small intestine. Nature 446(7136):676

Sansom OJ, Mansergh FC, Evans MJ, Wilkins JA, Clarke AR (2007b) Deficiency of SPARC suppresses intestinal tumorigenesis in APCMin/+ mice. Gut 56(10):1410

Sato H et al (2007) Frequent epigenetic inactivation of DICKKOPF family genes in human gastrointestinal tumors. Carcinogenesis 28(12):2459

Sekhon HS, London CA, Sekhon M, Iversen PL, Devi GR (2008) c-MYC antisense phosphosphorodiamidate morpholino oligomer inhibits lung metastasis in a murine tumor model. Lung Cancer 60(3):347

Shan B, Wang MX, Li RQ (2009) Quercetin inhibit human SW480 colon cancer growth in association with inhibition of Cyclin D1 and surviving expression through Wnt/beta-catenin signaling pathway. Cancer Investig 27(6):604

Sharma S, Kelly TK, Jones PA (2010) Epigenetics in cancer. Carcinogenesis 31(1):27

Solomon DH et al (2006) Cardiovascular outcomes in new users of coxibs and non-steroidal anti-inflammatory drugs: high-risk subgroups and time course of risk. Arthritis Rheum 54(5):1378

Suzuki H et al (2004) Epigenetic inactivation of SFRP genes allows constitutive WNT signaling in colorectal cancer. Nat Genet 36(4):417

Takahashi-Yanaga F, Sasaguri T (2009) Drug development targeting the glycogen synthase kinase-3beta (GSK-3beta)-mediated signal transduction pathway: inhibitors of the wnt/beta-catenin signaling pathway as novel anticancer drugs. J Pharmacol Sci 109(2):179

Uematsu K et al (2003a) Activation of the Wnt pathway in non small cell lung cancer: evidence of dishevelled overexpression. Oncogene 22(46):7218

Uematsu K et al (2003b) Wnt pathway activation in mesothelioma: Evidence of dishevelled overexpression and transcriptional activity of beta-Catenin. Cancer Res 63(15):4547

van de Wetering M et al (2002) The β-Catenin/TCF-4 complex imposes a crypt progenitor phenotype on colorectal cancer cells. Cell 111(2):241

van der Flier LG et al (2009a) Transcription factor Achaete Scute-Like 2 controls intestinal stem cell fate. Cell 136(5):903

van der Flier LG, Haegebarth A, Stange DE, van de Wetering M, Clevers H (2009b) OLFM4 is a robust marker for stem cells in human intestine and marks a subset of colorectal cancer cells. Gastroenterology 137(1):15

Weeraratna AT et al (2002) Wnt5a signaling directly affects cell motility and invasion of metastatic melanoma. Cancer Cell 1(3):279

Wicha MS, Liu S, Dontu G (2006) Cancer stem cells: an old idea–a paradigm shift. Cancer Res 66(4):1883

Wilding J et al (2002) Cyclin D1 is not an essential target of beta-Catenin signaling during intestinal tumorigenesis, but it may act as a modifier of disease severity in multiple intestinal neoplasia (Min) mice. Cancer Res 62(16):4562

Williams JL et al (2001) Nitric oxide-releasing nonsteroidal antiinflammatory drugs (NSAIDs) alter the kinetics of human colon cancer cell lines more effectively than traditional NSAIDs: implications for colon cancer chemoprevention. Cancer Res 61(8):3285

Williams JL et al (2004) NO-donating aspirin inhibits intestinal carcinogenesis in min (APC(Min/+)) mice. Biochem Biophys Res Commun 313(3):784

Yamada M et al (2006) NARF, an nemo-like kinase (NLK)-associated ring finger protein regulates the ubiquitylation and degradation of T cell factor/lymphoid enhancer factor (TCF/LEF). J Biol Chem 281(30):20749

Yu Q, Geng Y, Sicinski P (2001) Specific protection against breast cancers by Cyclin D1 ablation. Nature 411(6841):1017

Chapter 9
Inhibiting the Wnt Signaling Pathway with Small Molecules

Ho-Jin Lee, Xinxin Zhang, and Jie J. Zheng

Abstract Wnt signaling plays important roles in embryonic development and in maintenance of adult tissues. Mutation, loss, or overexpression of key Wnt pathway components has been linked to various types of cancer. Therefore, inhibition of Wnt signaling is of interest for the development of novel anticancer agents. The results of recent structure-based screening, high-throughput screening (HTS), and chemical genomics studies demonstrate that small molecules, including synthetic and natural compounds, can inhibit Wnt signaling in various cancers by blocking specific protein–protein interactions or the activity of specific enzymes. In biological studies, these compounds appear promising as potential anticancer agents; however, their efficacy and toxicity have yet to be investigated. Small molecule inhibitors of Wnt signaling also have wide-ranging potential as tools for elucidating disease and basic biology. Indubitably, in the near future, these compounds will yield agents that are clinically useful against malignant diseases.

Abbreviations

APC	Adenomatous polyposis coli
CK1	Casein kinase 1
CLL	Chronic lymphocytic leukemia
COX	Cyclooxygenase
CRC	Colon carcinoma
DEP	Dishevelled Egl-10, and pleckstrin
DIX	Dishevelled and axin

J.J. Zheng (✉)
Department of Structural Biology, St. Jude Children's Research Hospital,
262 Danny Thomas Place, MS 311, Memphis, TN 38105-3678, USA
e-mail: jie.zheng@stjude.org

K.H. Goss and M. Kahn (eds.), *Targeting the Wnt Pathway in Cancer*,
DOI 10.1007/978-1-4419-8023-6_9, © Springer Science+Business Media, LLC 2011

Dvl/Dsh	Dishevelled
EA	Ethacrynic acid
Fz	Frizzled
GSK-3β	Glycogen synthase kinase-3
HTS	High-throughput screening
LRP	Low-density lipoprotein receptor (LDLR)-related protein
MM	Multiple myeloma
NMR	Nuclear magnetic resonance
NSAIDs	Nonsteroidal anti-inflammatory drugs
NSCLC	Nonsmall cell lung cancer
PPAR-γ	Peroxisome proliferator-activated receptor γ

9.1   Introduction

Deregulation of Wnt/β-catenin signaling has been linked to malignancy (Logan and Nusse 2004; Moon et al. 2004; Herbst and Kolligs 2007). Therefore, disruption of this signaling pathway by small molecule inhibitors holds potential as a cancer therapy approach (Clevers 2006; Takahashi-Yanaga and Sasaguri 2007; Ewan and Dale 2008). During the development of Wnt pathway inhibitors, a number of existing drugs and natural compounds were found to target Wnt signaling in various cancers (Figs. 9.1 and 9.2, Table 9.1). One prominent example is nonsteroidal anti-inflammatory drugs (NSAIDs), which inhibit the cyclooxygenase-1 (COX-1) and cyclooxygenase-2 (COX-2) isoenzymes and can also inhibit β-catenin signaling in cancer in a COX-dependent or COX-independent manner (Barker and Clevers 2006; Han et al. 2008; Lee et al. 2009a). In recent years, dozens of additional existing drugs and natural compounds have been identified as Wnt antagonists (Fig. 9.1a, b; Sect. 9.2). Their anticancer effects hold promise for the development of cancer treatment or chemopreventive agents, but determining their efficacy and safety remains challenging because of our poor understanding of their molecular mechanisms (Barker and Clevers 2006).

Advanced technologies and new strategies such as structure-based drug development and chemical genomics have allowed the identification of novel compounds that are specific Wnt signaling inhibitors (Fig. 9.1c–e). Most such compounds developed to date target specific protein–protein interactions in Wnt signaling, such as β-catenin/TCF(LEF) interaction or Dishevelled/Frizzled interaction (Fig. 9.2, Sect. 9.3). Emerging evidence shows that some compounds (Fig. 9.1e) also target specific enzymes in the Wnt pathway. Two enzymes, tankyrase (TNKS) and porcupine, were proved to be potential anticancer targets (Fig. 9.1e, Sect. 9.4). These findings offer the opportunity to develop anticancer

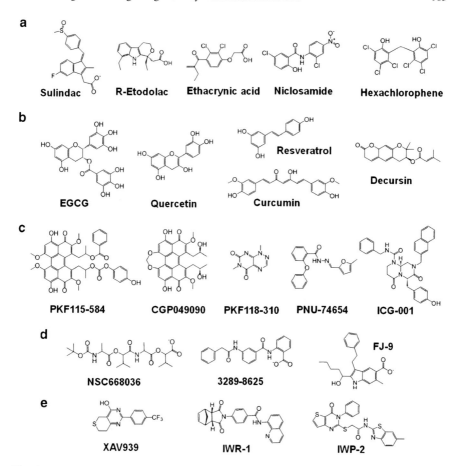

Fig. 9.1 Small-molecule inhibitors that target Wnt signaling at different levels. (**a**) Existing drugs reported to be Wnt signaling antagonists. Recent drug repurposing efforts have discovered additional drugs that antagonize Wnt signaling at different levels. (**b**) Natural compounds reported to be antagonists of Wnt/β-catenin signaling in cancer. (**c**) Natural compounds that target β-catenin/TCF(LEF) interaction, identified by HTS and chemical genomics approaches. (**d**) Inhibitors that target Dishevelled-Fz interaction, identified by HTS and structure-based approaches. (**e**) Inhibitors that target enzyme activity, identified by cell-based HTS and chemical genomics approaches

agents by using a mechanics-based approach. Here we (1) summarize the effects of existing drugs and natural compounds on Wnt signaling in cancer, (2) describe the discovery of new small-molecule inhibitors of relevant protein targets and their effects on cancer cells, and (3) discuss the progress and current challenges of targeting Wnt signaling in cancer.

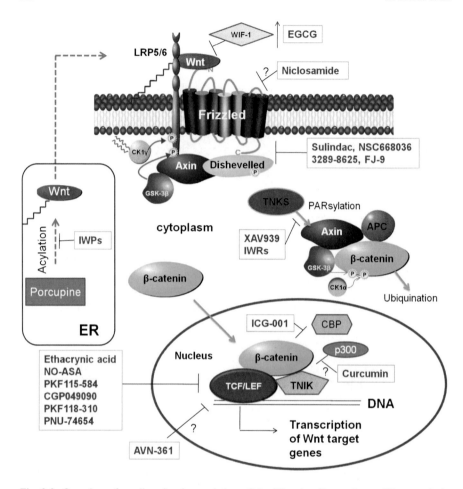

Fig. 9.2 Overview of small-molecule regulation of the Wnt signaling pathway. Wnt protein is acylated by Porcupine in the ER and secreted into the periplasm. The binding of Wnt ligand to the Frizzled-LRP5/6 receptor complex activates the phosphoprotein Dishevelled, which then binds to the cytoplasmic C-terminus of Frizzled. Activated Dishevelled also recruits axin from the β-catenin destruction complex containing axin, GSK-3β, and APC. Thereby, LRP5/6 protein is phosphorylated by CK1γ and GSK-3β and forms a complex with axin. TNKS destroys axin through PARsylation, thereby stabilizing β-catenin. Accumulated β-catenin translocates into the nucleus and induces gene transcription by binding to TCF/LEF transcription factor, Creb-binding protein, or p300 protein. TNIK interacts with both TCF and β-catenin, promoting Wnt target gene transcription. The kinase TNIK binds to transcription factor TCF4 and β-catenin, activating Wnt target genes. WIF-1 antagonizes Wnt signaling by directly binding to Wnt protein. In the absence of Wnt signaling, the destruction complex mediates proteasomal degradation of β-catenin. Small molecules (*boxed*) interrupt Wnt signals by inhibiting Wnt signaling steps or by promoting repression of Wnt signaling (see Table 9.1). *WIF-1* Wnt inhibitory factor-1; *TNKS* tankyrase; *TNIK* TRAF2- and NCK-interacting kinase. The figure was generated by using Pathway Builder (http://www.proteinlounge.com)

Table 9.1 Selected small-molecule inhibitors of Wnt signaling

Small molecule inhibitor	Target	Cancer	Comments; phase of development	References
Sulindac	Dishevelled	CRC, prostate cancer, lung cancer, NSCLC	NSAID, COX-1/2 inhibitor; multiple phases. Chemoprevention agent, COX-1/2 inhibitors	Labayle et al. (1991); Nugent et al. (1993); Winde et al. (1993); Pasricha et al. (1995); Piazza et al. (1997); Han et al. (1998); Rahman et al. (2000); Liu et al. (2002); Nikitakis et al. (2002); Esaki et al. (2002); Boon et al. (2004); Koornstra et al. (2005); Lim et al. (2006); Han et al. (2008); Lu et al. (2009c); Lee et al. (2009a)
R-etodolac	N/D	CLL, MM, HCC	NSAID, non-COX inhibitor; biological studies	Lu et al. (2004); Yasui et al. (2005); Behari et al. (2007)
Ethacrynic acid	LEF-1	CLL	A loop diuretic, biological study	Lu et al. (2009a); Chen et al. (2009b)
Niclosamide	Frizzled1?	N/D	Teniacide; biological study	Chen et al. (2009b)
EGCG	WIF-1?	Breast cancer, lung cancer	Natural compound; biological study, cancer prevention	Dashwood et al. (2002); Kim et al. (2006); Gao et al. (2009)
Quercetin	β-catenin?	CRC	Natural compound; biological studies	Park et al. (2005); Shan et al. (2009)
Resveratrol	N/D	CRC	Natural compound; biological studies	Hope et al. (2008); Roccaro et al. (2008)
Curcumin	N/D	Breast cancer, CRC, osteosarcoma	Natural compound; biological studies, cancer prevention	Aggarwal et al. (2003); Duvoix et al. (2005); Ryu et al. (2008); Prasad et al. (2009); Leow et al. (2010b)
PKF115-584	β-catenin	CRC, MM	Lead compound; biological studies	Lepourcelet et al. (2004); Lu et al. (2009a); Minke et al. (2009)
CGP049090	β-catenin	CRC	Lead compound; biological studies	Lepourcelet et al. (2004)
PKF118-310	β-catenin	CRC, prostate cancer, osteosarcoma	Lead compound; biological studies	Lepourcelet et al. (2004); Lu et al. (2009a); Leow et al. (2010b)

(continued)

Table 9.1 (continued)

Small molecule inhibitor	Target	Cancer	Comments; phase of development	References
ICG-001	β-catenin/ CBP	CRC, breast cancer, prostate cancer	Lead compound; biological studies	Ma et al. (2005)
AVN-361	N/D	CRC	Preclinical I study	Edelson (2009)
3289-8625	Dishevelled	Prostate cancer	Lead compound; biological study	Grandy et al. (2009)
FJ-9	Dishevelled	NSCLC	Lead compound; biological studies	Fujii et al. (2007); You et al. (2008)
XAV939	Tankyrase	CRC	Lead compound; biological studies	Huang et al. (2009)
IWR-1	Tankyrase	N/D	Lead compound; biological studies	Chen et al. (2009a)
IWPs	Porcupine	CRC	Lead compound; biological studies	Chen et al. (2009a)

CLL chronic lymphocytic leukemia; *HCC* hepatocellular carcinoma; *CRC* colon carcinoma; *MM* multiple myeloma; *NSCLC* nonsmall cell lung cancer; *N/D* not determined; "?" indicates mechanisms involved is not clear

9.2   Existing Drugs and Natural Compounds

9.2.1   Effect of Existing Drugs on Wnt Signaling and Anticancer Drug Development

9.2.1.1   Nonsteroidal Anti-Inflammatory Drugs (NSAIDs)

Mounting evidence from epidemiological and clinical studies has shown that NSAIDs such as aspirin (Bos et al. 2006), indomethacin (Sakoguchi-Okada et al. 2007), and sulindac (Piazza et al. 1997; Patten and DeLong 1999; Esaki et al. 2002; Boon et al. 2004; Koornstra et al. 2005; Han et al. 2008; Lee et al. 2009a; Lu et al. 2009c) and specific COX-2 inhibitors such as celecoxib (Sakoguchi-Okada et al. 2007; Takahashi-Yanaga et al. 2008; Lu et al. 2009c) kill cancer cells through inhibition of Wnt/β-catenin signaling (Kelloff et al. 1996; Thun et al. 2002; Barker and Clevers 2006). These drugs are currently being investigated as cancer chemopreventive or treatment agents (Kelloff et al. 1996; Fournier and Gordon 2000; Thun et al. 2002; Barker and Clevers 2006). The molecular mechanism of NSAIDs' action has been extensively explored (Dihlmann and von Knebel 2005; Barker and Clevers 2006; Clevers 2006; Takahashi-Yanaga and Sasaguri 2007). For example, sulindac (Clinoril), an inhibitor of COX-1/2, can suppress canonical β-catenin-related Wnt signaling in breast cancer, lung cancer, and colon cancer cell lines and in adenomas of patients with familial adenomatous polyposis (Fig. 9.1a and Table 9.1) (Labayle et al. 1991; Nugent et al. 1993; Winde et al. 1993; Pasricha et al. 1995; Piazza et al. 1997; Han et al. 1998, 2008; Rahman et al. 2000; Liu et al. 2002; Nikitakis et al. 2002; Esaki et al. 2002; Boon et al. 2004; Koornstra et al. 2005; Lim et al. 2006; Lu et al. 2009c). Lee et al. (2009a) discovered that the binding of sulindac to Dishevelled protein could block Wnt/β-catenin signaling. This finding suggested that at least one of the chemopreventive mechanisms of NSAIDs is the blockade of canonical Wnt signaling downstream of Dishevelled (see also Sect. 9.4.2). However, NSAIDs' effects on Wnt signaling are not simple. For example, R-etodolac (Fig. 9.1a) lacks a COX-inhibitory effect (Demerson et al. 1983), yet exerts cytotoxicity against various cancer cell lines (Lu et al. 2004; Yasui et al. 2005; Behari et al. 2007). R-etodolac treatment diminished the in vitro survival of CLL cells in which Wnt/β-catenin signaling is activated (Lu et al. 2004). In multiple myeloma (MM) cells, including drug-resistant lines and primary cells obtained from patients, R-etodolac treatment induces down-regulation of the Wnt target gene cyclin D1 (Yasui et al. 2005). R-etodolac treatment of Hep3B and HepG2 hepatoma cell lines downregulated TOPflash reporter activity, without affecting FOPflash activity, at 400 μM for 24 h. In hepatocellular carcinoma (HCC) cell lines, R-etodolac treatment reduced the expression of total and activated β-catenin, the activity of a Tcf binding site reporter, and protein expression of the Wnt target genes GS and cyclinD1 (Behari et al. 2007). Lu et al. (2005) reported that the inhibition of β-catenin function by R-etodolac was found only in cells that coexpressed PPAR-γ and its coreceptor RXR-α, suggesting that the inhibitory effect of R-etodolac in HEK293 cells treated with Wnt activators is indirect. Given that R-etodolac does not inhibit COX-2, its therapeutic use might offer the additional advantage of minimizing COX-dependent side effects (Lu et al. 2005).

9.2.1.2 Derivatives of NSAIDs

Because NSAIDs and their metabolites can induce apoptosis of cancer cells through inhibition of Wnt signaling, NSAID derivatives have been developed and tested in various cancer cells. These derivatives include nitric oxide (NO)-donating aspirin (NO-ASA) (Nath et al. 2003, 2009; Gao et al. 2005; Lu et al. 2009c), NO-donating NSAIDs (Yeh et al. 2004; Rigas and Kashfi 2004; Rigas 2007), and the etodolac analogs SDX-308 (CEP-18082) and SDX-309 (Yasui et al. 2007; Feng and Lentzsch 2007; Lentzsch et al. 2007; Lindhagen et al. 2007a, b; Feng et al. 2007). These derivatives hold promise for safe, effective cancer treatment (Rigas 2007; Rigas and Williams 2008).

These studies revealed that existing drugs can be reexamined for potential use as Wnt signaling modulators, using our increasing knowledge of cell signaling and the expanding capacity of drug development. These drugs may provide a crucial "shortcut" between long-term drug development and immediate clinical application.

9.2.1.3 Drug Repurposing to Target Wnt Signaling

The development of novel uses for existing drugs is considered an important alternative to traditional drug discovery, because it may bypass the need for drug safety testing, decrease early costs, and hence make agents more accessible for therapeutic application (Toney et al. 2009; Boguski et al. 2009). To identify Wnt signaling inhibitors, several groups screened libraries containing 960 or 1,200 FDA-approved drugs (Park et al. 2006; Lu et al. 2009a; Jin et al. 2009; Gwak et al. 2009; Chen et al. 2009b). Some drugs, including ethacrynic acid (EA) (Lu et al. 2009a; Jin et al. 2009), hexachlorophene (Park et al. 2006), isoreserpine (Gwak et al. 2009), and niclosamide (Chen et al. 2009b), were discovered to be Wnt signaling inhibitors (Fig. 9.1a and Table 9.1). Although their effects on Wnt signaling are likely to be similar, their mechanisms of interfering Wnt signaling differ. Ethacrynic acid (EA) and niclosamide are excellent examples.

Ethacrynic acid (EA) (Fig. 9.1a) is a loop diuretic. EA treatment of CLL cells decreased the expression of Wnt target genes, including LEF-1, cyclin D1, and fibronectin, indicating that Wnt signaling had been inhibited (Lu et al. 2009a). Co-immunoprecipitation experiments indicated that EA can directly bind to LEF-1 protein, thereby destabilizing the β-catenin/LEF-1 complex (Lu et al. 2009a). In contrast, niclosamide (Fig. 9.1a) modulates Wnt-mediated receptor trafficking. Chen et al. (2009b) showed that niclosamide treatment inhibits Wnt3a-stimulated LEF/TCF(TOPflash) reporter activity and β-catenin stabilization by promoting endocytosis of Frizzled-1 and down-regulation of Dishevelled-2 protein (Fig. 9.2). They also showed that the Frizzled-1 receptor colocalizes in vesicles containing transferrin and agonist-activated β2-adrenergic receptor (Chen et al. 2009b). While the molecular mechanism by which niclosamide stimulates Frizzled-1 internalization remains largely unknown, the function of niclosamide as a Frizzled internalization modulator may offer a valuable tool for further study of cancer and regeneration at the molecular level (Chen et al. 2009b). The effect of niclosamide on cancer cells warrants study and may confirm the proposed mechanism of Wnt signaling.

EA and other existing drugs may bypass the need for drug toxicity and safety testing and become available for therapeutic use more quickly than newly identified compounds that target Wnt signaling. In addition, modification of these existing drugs may increase their efficacy for specific cancer treatment. For example, because of the low efficacy of EA for CLL treatment, approximately 40 EA derivatives were synthesized and evaluated for their inhibitory effect on Wnt signaling (Jin et al. 2009). Some of these compounds effectively decreased CLL cell survival and antagonized Wnt signaling at low micromolar (μM) concentrations (Jin et al. 2009).

9.2.2 Effect of Natural Compounds on Wnt Signaling and Anticancer Drug Development

Accumulating evidence has demonstrated that some natural compounds, including EGCG ((−1)-epigallocatechin-3-gallate, from green tea), quercine (from resveratrol [3,5,4′-trihydroxystilbene, from red wine and grapes]), fisetin (from onions and apples), and curcumin (from turmeric), have anticancer activity (Fig. 9.1b) (Sarkar et al. 2009; Leow et al. 2010a). Because these compounds reduce the risk of several types of cancers in humans and animals, their preventive effects have attracted significant attention (Sarkar et al. 2009). Many studies have sought to elucidate the molecular mechanisms and identify the targets of action of these nontoxic natural products. We will summarize the biological effects of some natural compounds on Wnt signaling in various cancer cells.

9.2.2.1 (−1)-Epigallocatechin-3-Gallate (EGCG)

EGCG is derived from green tea (Fig. 9.1b) and is reported to inhibit Wnt signaling in various cancer cells (Dashwood et al. 2002; Kim et al. 2006; Gao et al. 2009). Kim et al. (2006) reported that EGCG treatment induced transcription of HBP-1, which is known to be a suppressor of Wnt signaling, and reduced the proliferation and invasiveness of breast cancer cells in an HBP1-dependent manner. In the lung cancer cell lines H460 and A549, Wnt inhibitory factor-1 (WIF-1) is frequently silenced due to promoter hypermethylation, but EGCG treatment restored its expression (Gao et al. 2009). Because WIF-1 is a secreted antagonist of Wnt signaling that acts by direct binding of Wnt ligand, EGCG treatment decreases the level of cytosolic β-catenin and inhibits T-cell factor (TCF)/lymphoid enhancer-binding factor (LEF) reporter activity in a dose-dependent manner. These results suggested that EGCG might be useful for reversal of WIF-1 promoter methylation and restoration of

WIF-1 expression. Given that WIF-1 is silenced by promoter hypermethylation in a number of cancers, including nonsmall cell lung cancer (NSCLC), gastrointestinal cancer, Barrett's esophagus, mesothelioma, and nasopharyngeal cancer (Reguart et al. 2004; Mazieres et al. 2004; Lin et al. 2006; Batra et al. 2006; Clement et al. 2008; Yang et al. 2009), the biological effects of EGCG treatment in these cancers will be of great interest.

9.2.2.2 Quercetin

Quercetin (Fig. 9.1b) is an integral part of the average human dietary intake. Studies in vitro and in vivo have demonstrated that quercetin exerts significant activity against colon cancer (Deschner et al. 1993; Kuo 1996). Park et al. (2005) reported that in SW480 colon cancer cells and in HEK293 cells transiently transfected with constitutively active mutant β-catenin, quercetin treatment inhibited β-catenin/TCF transcriptional activity by disrupting the interaction of β-catenin and TCF and resulted in decreased nuclear β-catenin and TCF-4 protein. Shan et al. (2009) reported that quercetin treatment arrested the cell cycle of SW480 cells and clone 26 cells at G2/M-phase and induced apoptosis in a concentration-dependent manner. They showed that quercetin treatment of colon cancer cells inhibited the transcriptional activity of β-catenin/TCF, thereby reducing the expression of the Wnt target genes cyclin D1 and survivin.

9.2.2.3 Resveratrol

Resveratrol (Fig. 9.1b) is known to inhibit proliferation and induce apoptosis in cancer cell lines (Hope et al. 2008; Roccaro et al. 2008). The effect of resveratrol on Wnt signaling is likely to be concentration-dependent, as a low concentration of resveratrol that did not affect cell proliferation (≤40 μM for HT29 colon cancer cells and normal mucosa-derived NCM460 cells; 20 μM for RKO colon cancer cells) still inhibited Wnt signaling (Hope et al. 2008). Resveratrol treatment decreased the nuclear localization of β-catenin by reducing the expression of Legless (BCL9) and pygnols, which are regulators of β-catenin localization (Hope et al. 2008).

9.2.2.4 Curcumin

Curcumin and its derivatives (Fig. 9.1b) have been reported to inhibit the proliferation of several types of cancer cells (Aggarwal et al. 2003; Duvoix et al. 2005; Ryu et al. 2008; Leow et al. 2010b; Teiten et al. 2010). A novel mechanism was proposed in which curcumin and its derivatives, including demethoxycurcumin (DMC) and bisdemethoxycurcumin (BDMC), attenuate Wnt signaling through down-regulation of the transcriptional coactivator p300, a positive Wnt signaling regulator (Fig. 9.2). Consistent with such a mechanism, curcumin derivatives suppressed the proliferative activity of SW480, HCT116, DLD-1, and HCT115 colon cancer cells (Ryu et al. 2008). In U2OS osteosarcoma cells, curcumin treatment dramatically reduced the level of nuclear β-catenin, but not of cytosolic β-catenin, and induced apoptosis and G2/M-phase arrest (Leow et al. 2010b).

9.2.2.5   Other Natural Compounds

Recent cell-based assays of food and plant extracts have shown that several other bioactive dietary agents inhibit Wnt/β-catenin signaling in cancer cells (Song et al. 2007; Sharma et al. 2009; Choi et al. 2010; Suh et al. 2009). For example, decursin (Fig. 9.1b), a pyranocoumarin isolated from the Korean *Angelica gigas* root, exerts activity against human prostate cancer cells (Song et al. 2007). Using a cell-based screening system, Song et al. (2007) demonstrated that about 80% of β-catenin response transcript was blocked at a concentration of 200 μM decursin. Murrayafoline A is a carbazole alkaloid isolated from *Glycosmis stenocarpar* that can repress expression of the Wnt target genes cyclin D1 and c-myc (Choi et al. 2010). The effects of eleutherinoside B and isoeleutherine (isolated from extracts of *Eleutherine palmifolia* plants) were evaluated in DLD1, HCT116, and SW480 colon cancer cell lines, and both compounds were cytotoxic to the cell lines (Li et al. 2009). Treatment with isoeleutherine significantly reduced nuclear β-catenin but not cytoplasmic β-catenin, and also inhibited TCF/β-catenin transcriptional activity in SW480 colon cancer cells in a dose-dependent manner with high cell viability. While nontoxic natural compounds appear to be potentially useful in treating or preventing cancer, insufficient knowledge about their targets limits our ability to modify these compounds to improve their efficacy and safety.

9.3   Targeting Protein–Protein Interactions in Wnt Signaling

Although a number of existing drugs and natural compounds are reported to be antagonists of Wnt signaling (Sect. 9.2), their molecular mechanisms of action and their targets are largely unknown, and therefore their applications in anticancer treatment and drug development are limited. A mechanism-based approach targeting the specific interaction might help to overcome these challenges. Because Wnt signaling is triggered by protein–protein interactions, small molecules that block specific protein–protein interactions in this pathway are of significant interest. Recent studies showed that two proteins, β-catenin and Dishevelled (Dvl/Dsh), may be potentially druggable targets for development of small-molecule inhibitors. High-resolution X-ray and/or NMR structures of both proteins alone or in complex with their binding partners are available to guide rational anticancer drug discovery (Huber et al. 1997; Graham et al. 2000, 2001, 2002; Huber and Weis 2001; Cheyette et al. 2002; Sampietro et al. 2006; Zhang et al. 2009; Lee et al. 2009a, b). Below we summarize the successful discovery of small-molecule inhibitors that specifically target the interactions of the Dvl/Fz, β-catenin/TCF(LEF), and β-catenin/CBP proteins.

9.3.1   Targeting of β-Catenin Activity

The multifunctional protein β-catenin regulates many biological processes essential for embryonic development and adult homeostasis; however, abnormal activation of β-catenin can lead to tumorigenesis and promote tumor growth. Accumulation of nuclear β-catenin, frequently observed in cancer cells, is the hallmark of activated canonical Wnt signaling (Fig. 9.2) (Takemaru et al. 2008). Nuclear β-catenin forms a complex with members of the T-cell factor (TCF)/lymphoid enhancer-binding factor 1 (LEF1) transcription factor family (Cavallo et al. 1997; Roose and Clevers 1999) and recruits their cofactors, such as CBP, p300, and Bcl9, to activate Wnt target genes (gene lists: http://www.stanford.edu/~rnusse/pathways/targets.html). Several strategies have been proposed to block β-catenin protein–protein interactions with small molecules, which are believed to offer a promising route to affect cancer therapy (Dorfman et al. 2003; Arce et al. 2006; Petropoulos et al. 2008; Bengochea et al. 2008; Ravindranath et al. 2008; Nguyen et al. 2009; Chen et al. 2009c; Hale et al. 2009).

9.3.1.1   Targeting β-Catenin/TCF (LEF) Interaction

Abnormal activation of Wnt signaling in cancer, regardless of mutation of APC or β-catenin protein, induces the nuclear translocation of β-catenin, which forms a complex with members of the TCF/LEF1 transcription factor family (Cavallo et al. 1997; Roose and Clevers 1999) (Fig. 9.2). LEF1 regulates the expression of a variety of Wnt target genes, including c-myc, cyclin D1, survivin, and LEF1 itself (Clevers and van de Wetering 1997).

The first small molecules that may disrupt the formation of TCF4/β-catenin complex (Fig. 9.1c) were discovered by conducting high-throughput ELISA-based screening of 7,000 purified natural compounds (Lepourcelet et al. 2004). Among them, two compounds, PKF118-310 and CGP049090, inhibited colon cancer cell proliferation and killed prostate cancer cells (Lepourcelet et al. 2004). Interestingly, the two compounds showed different efficacy in the two cancer cell lines, although the exact mechanism of their action is not yet known.

The effects of these lead compounds have also been examined in several cancer cell lines, in which they inhibited the transcriptional activity of the β-catenin/TCF complex and downregulated Wnt target genes (Sukhdeo et al. 2007; Doghman et al. 2008; Minke et al. 2009; Doghman et al. 2008; Minke et al. 2009). Sukhdeo et al. (2007) reported that PKF115-584 inhibited proliferation of both chemotherapy-sensitive and chemotherapy-resistant MM cells in a time- and dose-dependent manner; it also inhibited tumor growth and prolonged survival in a xenograft model of human MM. Doghman et al. (2008) examined the effectiveness of PKF115-584 in H295R ACT cells and found that it inhibited β-catenin/TCF signaling and cell proliferation in a dose-dependent manner, inhibiting entry into S phase and inducing apoptosis. They suggested that PKF115-580 may be useful in the treatment of ACT if its safety profile proves to be acceptable. Minke et al. (2009) reported that treatment with PKF115-584 and CGP049090 killed the AML cell lines Kasumi-1 and HL-60 and primary AML blast cells, with IC_{50} values of 0.14 ± 0.01 to 0.98 ± 0.12 μM. They showed that in most cases, both compounds reduced expression of all Wnt target genes and of CTNNB1(β-catenin gene) in the AML cell lines tested. They also reported that both compounds induced cell death in a dose-dependent manner with clinically acceptable EC_{50} values of 0.22 ± 0.02 to 0.65 ± 0.19 μM. Importantly, the EC_{50} values of the compounds in healthy peripheral blood mononuclear cells were 100 times higher than the EC_{50} values in AML cells, indicating that the healthy cells would be largely unaffected by the inhibitors. These results support the further development of these two inhibitors for treatment of AML. Wei et al. (2010) investigated the activity of three inhibitors (PKF115-584, CGP049090, and PKF118-310) in HCC. The three compounds downregulated the Wnt target genes c-Myc, cyclin D1, and survivin in the HCC cell lines HepG2 and Huh7 and were less cytotoxic to normal hepatocytes than to HCC cells. The compounds also suppressed tumor growth in vivo in a HepG2 xenograft model. These observations suggest that antagonists targeting β-catenin/TCF interaction are promising anticancer reagents. However, the experimental structural characterization of β-catenin or TCF in complex with small molecule inhibitors has not yet been reported, which may limit their optimization and applications in cancer treatment.

Another compound targeting β-catenin/TCF interaction is PNU-74654 (Fig. 9.1c) (Trosset et al. 2006). Because the crystal structure of the β-catenin/TCF complex is available (Graham et al. 2000; Poy et al. 2001), Trosset et al. (2006) conducted virtual screening and medium-throughput biophysical assays to identify compounds that disrupt β-catenin/TCF interaction. They first identified a "hot spot" on β-catenin that is supposedly crucial to the β-catenin/Tcf interaction; subsequently, a collection of 17,700 compounds were docked to this hot spot. The best 22 compounds were selected for further NMR and ITC assays, which showed that three compounds bind to β-catenin and compete with Tcf4. Compound PNU-74654, which bound with greatest affinity, showed a K_D of 450 nM. Although the binding between β-catenin and Tcf4 is generally considered to involve a large interface and high binding affinity ($K_D \sim 10$ nM), this study provided an alternative small-molecule approach to disruption of β-catenin/Tcf interaction. The biological effect of PNU-74654 needs to be further investigated in various cancers.

9.3.1.2 Targeting of β-Catenin and Its Cofactors

Given that Wnt activation requires the nuclear translocation of β-catenin and the formation of a complex between β-catenin and a member of the T-cell factor family of transcription factors, the discovery of small-molecule inhibitors targeting β-catenin/TCF interaction, especially in cancer cells, has been of great interest. However, biochemical and structural studies showed that the region of β-catenin that binds to TCF is overlapped by other binding partners, such as E-cadherin

(Huber and Weis 2001) and APC (Liu et al. 2006). The results indicate that small molecules targeting β-catenin/TCF(LEF) may also disrupt these other interactions, resulting in undesirable consequences (Lepourcelet et al. 2004; Takemaru et al. 2008). Importantly, structural studies showed that the β-catenin region that binds to its cofactors, such as CBP or BCL9, is distinct from the region that binds to TCF, suggesting small molecules that disrupt the interaction of β-catenin and its cofactor as an alternative therapeutic approach (Sampietro et al. 2006; Takemaru et al. 2008; Kawamoto et al. 2009).

Targeting β-catenin/CBP interaction is an example of the above approach. Emami et al. (2004) screened a small molecule library of 5,000 compounds containing peptidomimetic templates that mimic protein secondary structures, such as the α-helix and β-strand. The most potent compound, ICG-001 (Fig. 9.1c), had an IC_{50} value of 3 μM in a TOPflash reporter assay. A chemical genomics approach revealed that the binding partner of ICG-001 is the transcriptional coactivator Creb-binding protein (CBP) (Takemaru and Moon 2000; Emami et al. 2004; McMillan and Kahn 2005). Because β-catenin may also interact with the closely related CBP homolog p300 or with other components of the basal transcription machinery, the finding that ICG-001 specifically disrupts the β-catenin/CBP interaction without interfering with the β-catenin/p300 interaction is of great interest. ICG-001 block-ade of the β-catenin/CBP interaction reduces the expression of Wnt target genes (including survivin and cyclin D1) in SW480 and HCT116 colon carcinoma (CRC) cell lines and in breast and prostate cancer cells (Ma et al. 2005). ICG-001 reduced in vitro growth of CRC cells and exerted antitumor effects in both the Min mouse (which has a germline mutation in one allele of the APC tumor suppressor gene) and the nude mouse SW620 xenograft model of colon cancer. Notably, ICG-001 reduced the formation of colon and small intestine polyps in a manner very similar to that of sulindac, a cancer chemopreventive agent (Corpet and Pierre 2003; Emami et al. 2004). Emami et al. (2004) proposed that ICG-001 has significant therapeutic potential for the treatment of cancer. Subsequently, a solution-phase synthetic method was developed for the multigram-scale preparation of ICG-001, which may permit rapid analog generation to improve the compound's efficacy and safety (Piergentill et al. 2007).

In summary, targeting β-catenin protein and its interactions has been shown to be a promising approach to modulate Wnt signaling as well as to inhibit the growth of different tumor cells. These studies expanded our understanding of cell signaling and revealed new opportunities for cancer therapy.

9.3.2 Targeting of Dishevelled Proteins

In the canonical Wnt signaling pathway, binding of Wnt ligand to the Fz-LRP receptor complex triggers the formation of Dvl-Fz complex, and axin is relocalized from the β-catenin destruction complex (axin, GSK3β, and APC tumor suppressor) (Fig. 9.2) to the membrane (Bilic et al. 2007; Zeng et al. 2008). Thus, down-regulation of Dvl protein upstream of the Wnt pathway has the potential to suppress Wnt signaling. Importantly, up-regulation of Dvl has been reported in various cancers showing activation of Wnt signaling (Uematsu et al. 2003a, b; Okino et al. 2003; Nagahata et al. 2003; Mizutani et al. 2005; Wei et al. 2008). Therefore, investigation of Dvl as a potential drug target is of great interest.

Dvl proteins contain three highly conserved domains: an N-terminal DIX domain, a central PDZ domain, and a DEP domain (Wong et al. 2000, 2003; Schwarz-Romond et al. 2007; Simons et al. 2009). These domains can interact with different partners, channeling Wnt signaling into distinct pathways (Wharton 2003; Wallingford and Habas 2005). It is currently believed that about 30 Dvl-binding proteins are involved in Wnt signaling, and many of them interact or partially interact with the Dvl PDZ domain (Wharton 2003; Wallingford and Habas 2005). Among these interactions, the Fz-Dvl interaction has drawn the most attention for therapeutic intervention (Wong et al. 2003; Wang et al. 2008). Wong et al. (2003) discovered that a conserved sequence (KTxxxW) in Fz, located two residues after the transmembrane domain, binds to the Dvl PDZ domain; this interaction plays an important role in activation of Wnt signaling. Consistent with this finding, a short Fz7 peptide (GKTLQSWRRYH) that bound to the active site of the Dvl PDZ domain attenuated Wnt/β-catenin signaling induced by Wnt1 ligand at the level of Dvl (Wong et al. 2003). This finding prompted us and others to develop peptides (Lee et al. 2009b; Zhang et al. 2009) and small molecule inhibitors (Shan et al. 2005; Fujii et al. 2007; Shan and Zheng 2009; Grandy et al. 2009) that target Dvl-Fz interaction in human cancer, with the aim of counteracting the interaction's cancer-promoting effect (Fig. 9.1d, Table 9.1).

Given that the *apo* (unbound to ligand) and *holo* (bound to ligand) structures of the Dvl PDZ domain are available (Cheyette et al. 2002; Wong et al. 2003), the NCI database was virtually screened to identify compounds that may bind to the Dvl PDZ domain (Shan et al. 2005; Wang et al. 2008; Shan and Zheng 2009). The interaction of potential candidates with the Dvl PDZ domain was experimentally confirmed by NMR spectroscopy. The validated binders were further characterized in biological systems. By using this strategy, Shan et al. (2005) identified the peptidomimetic compound NSC668036 (Fig. 9.1d) as an antagonist of Wnt/β-catenin signaling.

NSC668036 can attenuate canonical Wnt signaling induced by Wnt3A, but not by β-catenin, suggesting that this compound indeed blocks Wnt signaling upstream of β-catenin (Shan et al. 2005). To improve the potential effectiveness of NSC668036 in cancer cells, Grandy et al. (2009) performed extensive NMR-assisted virtual screening and discovered an additional 50 drug-like compounds. Among them, compound 3289–8625 showed the highest binding affinity to the Dvl PDZ domain and effectively blocked Wnt3A-induced signaling in a *Xenopus* assay. In subsequent cell assays, Grandy et al. (2009) found decreased levels of β-catenin in both the cytosolic and membrane fractions, suggesting that compound 3289–8625 indeed inhibited Wnt signaling in these prostate cancer cells. Importantly, compound 3289–8625 penetrated the membrane of vascular endothelial cells, and the growth of PC-3 prostate cancer cells was reduced approximately 16%

($IC_{50} \sim 12.5$ μM) after 72 h of treatment. The effect of this compound in other cancer cells, especially those that overexpress Dvl, will be of great interest (Uematsu et al. 2003a, b; Okino et al. 2003; Nagahata et al. 2003; Mizutani et al. 2005; Wei et al. 2008).

FJ-9 is a lead compound identified by using the AlphaScreen energy transfer assay and an NMR-titration experiment (Fujii et al. 2007). In the LOX melanoma cell line and the H460 and H1703 nonsmall cell lung cancer (NSCLC) lines, FJ-9 downregulated TCF transcription, regardless of β-catenin mutation, and decreased the expression of the β-catenin target genes c-myc, cyclin D1, and survivin. In a mouse xenograft model of human NSCLC, compound FJ-9 significantly inhibited tumor growth without significant weight loss (<5%). Fujii and coworkers are now developing the chemical library to rationally generate small-molecule agents that suppress tumor cell growth by downregulating canonical Wnt signaling (You et al. 2008).

The NSAID sulindac is used to reduce fever and pain, but it also exerts activity against various cancers (Glavin and Sitar 1986; Labayle et al. 1991; Waddell 1994; Goluboff et al. 1999; Whitehead et al. 2003; Zhang et al. 2004; Webster and Leibovich 2005; Matsumoto et al. 2006; Han et al. 2008). Lee et al. (2009a) found that the NSAIDs sulindac and sulindac sulfone (exisulind) bind to the Dvl PDZ domain and thereby inhibit Wnt3A-induced signaling at the Dvl level in a *Xenopus* model. Given that both agents target Wnt signaling through the Dvl PDZ domain but that only sulindac also targets COX signaling, the efficacy and safety of the two compounds in normal and cancer cells will be of interest (Keller and Giardiello 2003; Koehne and DuBois 2004; Lee et al. 2009a).

In summary, several compounds have been identified as specific antagonists of Dvl/Fz interaction and characterized by using NMR and other biophysical methods. The biological effects of these antagonists in various cancers remain to be studied.

9.4   Targeting of Enzyme Activity to Inhibit Wnt Signaling in Cancer

Although much of the effort to develop Wnt antagonists has focused on protein–protein interactions, disruption of such interactions with a small molecule is challenging because the contact surfaces involved in protein–protein interactions are much larger (~1,500–3,000 Å) (Jones and Thornton 1996) than those involved in protein–small molecule interactions (~300–1,000 Å) (Cheng et al. 2007; Wells and McClendon 2007). Targeting of enzyme activity is an attractive strategy for development of Wnt signaling inhibitors because enzymes usually have well-defined binding pockets (Huang et al. 2009). Recent studies discovered that novel enzymes, such as TRF1-interacting ankyrin-related ADP-ribose polymerase (TNKS), porcupine, TRAF2- and NCK-interacting kinase (TNIK), and Bruton's tyrosine kinase (BTK), regulate Wnt signaling (Huang et al. 2009; Mahmoudi et al. 2009; James et al. 2009) and are therefore potentially druggable components of the Wnt-mediated pathway (Fearon 2009; Peterson 2009). Some compounds have already been developed as specific inhibitors of TNKS and porcupine by using high-throughput screening (HTS) array and chemical genomics approaches (Fig. 9.1e).

9.4.1   Targeting of Tankyrase

TNKS is a member of the poly-ADP-ribose polymerase (PARP) family that utilizes NAD$^+$ to generate ADP-ribose polymers on the target protein (Chiang et al. 2008; Hsiao and Smith 2008). TNKS1 and TNKS2 directly bind to axin and promote its ubiquitination through poly-ADP-ribosylation (PARsylation) (Huang et al. 2009). Because axin is the concentration-limiting component of the destruction complex that regulates the stability of β-catenin, inhibition of TNKS activity may provide a strategy to antagonize Wnt signaling (Huang et al. 2009; Fearon 2009; Peterson 2009).

XAV939 (Fig. 9.1e) is a small-molecule inhibitor of TNKS that was identified by using a high-throughput screen (HTS) and a Wnt-responsive Super-TOPflash (STF) luciferase reporter assay in HEK293 cells (Huang et al. 2009). Treatment with XAV939 blocked Wnt3a-induced Wnt signaling in HEK293 cells and blocked abnormally activated Wnt signaling in SW480 colorectal cancer cells. Huang et al. (2009) reported that XAV939 treatment of SW480 cells increases the level of axin-GSK3β complex and destabilizes β-catenin. In an independent HTS of ~20,000 synthetic compounds, five compounds were identified as inhibitors of the Wnt response (IWRs) (IWR 1–5; IC$_{50}$ 0.18–2.0 μM) (Chen et al. 2009a). These inhibitors blocked Wnt signaling induced by Wnt3A as well as by Wnt1 and Wnt2. The compounds also bound to and stabilized axin, partially through TNKS inhibition. To understand the structure–activity relationship of IWR1/2, the authors synthesized a series of IWR analogs and compared their ability to inhibit Wnt signaling in luciferase-based assays; they showed that the in vivo activity of the IWRs was correlated with their in vitro activity (Lu et al. 2009b).

9.4.2   Targeting of Porcupine

Porcupine (Porcn) is a member of the membrane-bound O-acyltransferase (MBOAT) family that adds the palmitoyl group to Wnt proteins (Takada et al. 2006; Bartscherer and Boutros 2008). O-acylation is important for both Wnt protein secretion and Wnt signaling ability. By screening a diverse synthetic chemical library using a β-catenin/TCF-based assay, Chen et al. (2009a) identified a set of inhibitors of Wnt production (IWPs) (Fig. 9.1e) that target Porcupine (Fig. 9.1e). Expression of Porcn but not of other members of the MBOAT family alleviated the effects of IWP-2 on both Wnt secretion and Wnt activity, suggesting that Porcn, as a Wnt protein-specific *O*-acyltransferase, interacts with IWPs (Fig. 9.2). In addition, biotinylated IWP compounds (IWP-PB) can pull down Porcn protein, and competitive binding to Porcn by IWPs and IWP-PB was observed (Chen et al. 2009a).

IWPs directly regulate Wnt protein production by selectively targeting MBOAT family members; this mechanism is completely distinct from the targeting of transducers of Wnt-mediated cellular responses (Chen et al. 2009a). Moreover, these findings suggest that the MBOAT family may be of great therapeutic interest, as Hedgehog protein and the appetite-regulating hormone ghrelin are also MBOAT substrates (Chamoun et al. 2001; Yang et al. 2008; Chen et al. 2009a). The mechanism of binding of IWPs to Porcn protein remains to be established.

In summary, the identification of enzymes involved in Wnt signaling has dramatically expanded opportunities to develop targeting agents as potential cancer treatments, and it offers an alternative to Wnt modulation. The challenge to be addressed is the specificity of these enzymes, some of which may participate in hundreds of transcriptional pathways. Structural studies of these enzymes in complex with lead compounds are urgently needed in order to optimize the compounds.

9.5 Conclusions and Perspectives

Abnormal activation of Wnt signaling has been linked to various cancers. Therefore, small molecules that regulate Wnt signaling have attracted significant attention as potential cancer treatment or chemopreventive agents. Existing drugs and natural compounds have been recognized as Wnt signaling inhibitors. Recent drug repurposing efforts have revealed many more existing drugs as antagonists of Wnt signaling. These drugs and natural compounds provide valuable clues to potential therapeutic targets and to the molecular mechanisms involved.

Several strategies to block Wnt signaling with small molecules at different levels have been proposed. Advanced technologies (structure-based screening, large-scale screening, and chemical genomics approaches) have helped to generate small-molecule inhibitors and to identify new druggable targets. In addition, these compounds have provided new tools to examine the regulation of Wnt signaling and its effects in normal and cancer cells. However, most compounds developed so far are not in clinical trials, with the exception of compound AVN316 (Clinical Data Inc.), which is in preclinical development for cancer (Edelson 2009).

Several challenges remain to be overcome in developing clinically useful Wnt pathway inhibitors. First, information about the three-dimensional structures of key components of Wnt signaling and their complex structures with their binding molecules is urgently needed. Second, the selectivity of protein–protein interaction antagonists – that is, whether they interfere significantly with interactions essential to healthy cells – remains to be characterized. And finally, the efficacy, safety, and toxicity of all developed compounds need to be optimized.

Small-molecule inhibitors of cancer-associated Wnt signaling provide a promising tool to elucidate a wide range of Wnt-related malignancies and to seek new strategies to treat them. In the near future, these compounds will certainly yield agents that are clinically useful against malignant diseases.

Acknowledgments We thank Sharon Naron for editorial help. This work is supported by the American Lebanese Syrian Associated Charities, by the Cancer Center Support Grant (CA21765) from the National Cancer Institute, and by National Institutes of Health Grant GM081492.

References

Aggarwal BB, Kumar A, Bharti AC (2003) Anticancer potential of curcumin: preclinical and clinical studies. Anticancer Res 23:363–398

Arce L, Yokoyama NN, Waterman ML (2006) Diversity of LEF/TCF action in development and disease. Oncogene 25:7492–7504

Barker N, Clevers H (2006) Mining the Wnt pathway for cancer therapeutics. Nat Rev Drug Discov 5:997–1014

Bartscherer K, Boutros M (2008) Regulation of Wnt protein secretion and its role in gradient formation. EMBO Rep 9:977–982

Batra S, Shi Y, Kuchenbecker KM, He B, Reguart N, Mikami I, You L, Xu Z, Lin YC, Clement G, Jablons DM (2006) Wnt inhibitory factor-1, a Wnt antagonist, is silenced by promoter hyper-methylation in malignant pleural mesothelioma. Biochem Biophys Res Commun 342:1228–1232

Behari J, Zeng G, Otruba W, Thompson MD, Muller P, Micsenyi A, Sekhon SS, Leoni L, Monga SP (2007) R-Etodolac decreases beta-catenin levels along with survival and proliferation of hepatoma cells. J Hepatol 46:849–857

Bengochea A, de Souza MM, Lefrancois L, Le RE, Galy O, Chemin I, Kim M, Wands JR, Trepo C, Hainaut P, Scoazec JY, Vitvitski L, Merle P (2008) Common dysregulation of Wnt/Frizzled receptor elements in human hepatocellular carcinoma. Br J Cancer 99:143–150

Bilic J, Huang YL, Davidson G, Zimmermann T, Cruciat CM, Bienz M, Niehrs C (2007) Wnt induces LRP6 signalosomes and promotes dishevelled-dependent LRP6 phosphorylation. Science 316:1619–1622

Boguski MS, Mandl KD, Sukhatme VP (2009) Drug discovery. Repurposing with a difference. Science 324:1394–1395

Boon EM, Keller JJ, Wormhoudt TA, Giardiello FM, Offerhaus GJ, van der Neut R, Pals ST (2004) Sulindac targets nuclear beta-catenin accumulation and Wnt signalling in adenomas of patients with familial adenomatous polyposis and in human colorectal cancer cell lines. Br J Cancer 90:224–229

Bos CL, Kodach LL, van den Brink GR, Diks SH, van Santen MM, Richel DJ, Peppelenbosch MP, Hardwick JC (2006) Effect of aspirin on the Wnt/beta-catenin pathway is mediated via protein phosphatase 2A. Oncogene 25:6447–6456

Cavallo R, Rubenstein D, Peifer M (1997) Armadillo and dTCF: a marriage made in the nucleus. Curr Opin Genet Dev 7:459–466

Chamoun Z, Mann RK, Nellen D, von Kessler DP, Bellotto M, Beachy PA, Basler K (2001) Skinny hedgehog, an acyltransferase required for palmitoylation and activity of the hedgehog signal. Science 293:2080–2084

Chen B, Dodge ME, Tang W, Lu J, Ma Z, Fan CW, Wei S, Hao W, Kilgore J, Williams NS, Roth MG, Amatruda JF, Chen C, Lum L (2009a) Small molecule-mediated disruption of Wnt-dependent signaling in tissue regeneration and cancer. Nat Chem Biol 5:100–107

Chen M, Wang J, Lu J, Bond MC, Ren XR, Lyerly HK, Barak LS, Chen W (2009b) The anti-helminthic niclosamide inhibits Wnt/Frizzled1 signaling. Biochemistry 48:10267–10274

Chen Z, Venkatesan AM, Dehnhardt CM, Dos SO, Delos SE, yral-Kaloustian S, Chen L, Geng Y, Arndt KT, Lucas J, Chaudhary I, Mansour TS (2009c) 2, 4-Diamino-quinazolines as inhibitors of beta-catenin/Tcf-4 pathway: Potential treatment for colorectal cancer. Bioorg Med Chem Lett 19:4980–4983

Cheng AC, Coleman RG, Smyth KT, Cao Q, Soulard P, Caffrey DR, Salzberg AC, Huang ES (2007) Structure-based maximal affinity model predicts small-molecule druggability. Nat Biotechnol 25:71–75

Cheyette BN, Waxman JS, Miller JR, Takemaru K, Sheldahl LC, Khlebtsova N, Fox EP, Earnest T, Moon RT (2002) Dapper, a Dishevelled-associated antagonist of beta-catenin and JNK signaling, is required for notochord formation. Dev Cell 2:449–461

Chiang YJ, Hsiao SJ, Yver D, Cushman SW, Tessarollo L, Smith S, Hodes RJ (2008) Tankyrase 1 and tankyrase 2 are essential but redundant for mouse embryonic development. PLoS ONE 3:e2639

Choi H, Gwak J, Cho M, Ryu MJ, Lee JH, Kim SK, Kim YH, Lee GW, Yun MY, Cuong NM, Shin JG, Song GY, Oh S (2010) Murrayafoline A attenuates the Wnt/beta-catenin pathway by promoting the degradation of intracellular beta-catenin proteins. Biochem Biophys Res Commun 391:915–20

Clement G, Guilleret I, He B, Yagui-Beltran A, Lin YC, You L, Xu Z, Shi Y, Okamoto J, Benhattar J, Jablons D (2008) Epigenetic alteration of the Wnt inhibitory factor-1 promoter occurs early in the carcinogenesis of Barrett's esophagus. Cancer Sci 99:46–53

Clevers H (2006) Wnt/beta-catenin signaling in development and disease. Cell 127:469–480

Clevers H, van de Wetering M (1997) TCF/LEF factor earn their wings. Trends Genet 13:485–489

Corpet DE, Pierre F (2003) Point: from animal models to prevention of colon cancer. Systematic review of chemoprevention in min mice and choice of the model system. Cancer Epidemiol Biomarkers Prev 12:391–400

Dashwood WM, Orner GA, Dashwood RH (2002) Inhibition of beta-catenin/Tcf activity by white tea, green tea, and epigallocatechin-3-gallate (EGCG): minor contribution of H(2)O(2) at physiologically relevant EGCG concentrations. Biochem Biophys Res Commun 296:584–588

Demerson CA, Humber LG, Abraham NA, Schilling G, Martel RR, Pace-Asciak C (1983) Resolution of etodolac and antiinflammatory and prostaglandin synthetase inhibiting properties of the enantiomers. J Med Chem 26:1778–1780

Deschner EE, Ruperto JF, Wong GY, Newmark HL (1993) The effect of dietary quercetin and rutin on AOM-induced acute colonic epithelial abnormalities in mice fed a high-fat diet. Nutr Cancer 20:199–204

Dihlmann S, von Knebel DM (2005) Wnt/beta-catenin-pathway as a molecular target for future anti-cancer therapeutics. Int J Cancer 113:515–524

Doghman M, Cazareth J, Lalli E (2008) The T cell factor/beta-catenin antagonist PKF115-584 inhibits proliferation of adrenocortical carcinoma cells. J Clin Endocrinol Metab 93:3222–3225

Dorfman DM, Greisman HA, Shahsafaei A (2003) Loss of expression of the WNT/beta-catenin-signaling pathway transcription factors lymphoid enhancer factor-1 (LEF-1) and T cell factor-1 (TCF-1) in a subset of peripheral T cell lymphomas. Am J Pathol 162:1539–1544

Duvoix A, Blasius R, Delhalle S, Schnekenburger M, Morceau F, Henry E, Dicato M, Diederich M (2005) Chemopreventive and therapeutic effects of curcumin. Cancer Lett 223:181–190

Edelson S (2009) Clearing the path to Wnt. SciBX 2(37):1

Emami KH, Nguyen C, Ma H, Kim DH, Jeong KW, Eguchi M, Moon RT, Teo JL, Kim HY, Moon SH, Ha JR, Kahn M (2004) A small molecule inhibitor of beta-catenin/CREB-binding protein transcription [corrected]. Proc Natl Acad Sci USA 101:12682–12687

Esaki M, Matsumoto T, Mizuno M, Kobori Y, Yoshimura R, Yao T, Iida M (2002) Effect of sulindac treatment for attenuated familial adenomatous polyposis with a new germline APC mutation at codon 161: report of a case. Dis Colon Rectum 45:1397–1402

Ewan KB, Dale TC (2008) The potential for targeting oncogenic WNT/beta-catenin signaling in therapy. Curr Drug Targets 9:532–547

Fearon ER (2009) PARsing the phrase "all in for Axin"- Wnt pathway targets in cancer. Cancer Cell 16:366–368

Feng R, Lentzsch S (2007) Treatment of multiple myeloma with SDX-308. Drug News Perspect 20:431–435

Feng R, Anderson G, Xiao G, Elliott G, Leoni L, Mapara MY, Roodman GD, Lentzsch S (2007) SDX-308, a nonsteroidal anti-inflammatory agent, inhibits NF-kappaB activity, resulting in strong inhibition of osteoclast formation/activity and multiple myeloma cell growth. Blood 109:2130–2138

Fournier DB, Gordon GB (2000) COX-2 and colon cancer: potential targets for chemoprevention. J Cell Biochem Suppl 34:97–102

Fujii N, You L, Xu Z, Uematsu K, Shan J, He B, Mikami I, Edmondson LR, Neale G, Zheng J, Guy RK, Jablons DM (2007) An antagonist of dishevelled protein-protein interaction suppresses beta-catenin-dependent tumor cell growth. Cancer Res 67:573–579

Gao J, Liu X, Rigas B (2005) Nitric oxide-donating aspirin induces apoptosis in human colon cancer cells through induction of oxidative stress. Proc Natl Acad Sci USA 102:17207–17212

Gao Z, Xu Z, Hung MS, Lin YC, Wang T, Gong M, Zhi X, Jablon DM, You L (2009) Promoter demethylation of WIF-1 by epigallocatechin-3-gallate in lung cancer cells. Anticancer Res 29:2025–2030

Glavin GB, Sitar DS (1986) The effects of sulindac and its metabolites on acute stress-induced gastric ulcers in rats. Toxicol Appl Pharmacol 83:386–389

Goluboff ET, Shabsigh A, Saidi JA, Weinstein IB, Mitra N, Heitjan D, Piazza GA, Pamukcu R, Buttyan R, Olsson CA (1999) Exisulind (sulindac sulfone) suppresses growth of human prostate cancer in a nude mouse xenograft model by increasing apoptosis. Urology 53:440–445

Graham TA, Weaver C, Mao F, Kimelman D, Xu W (2000) Crystal structure of a beta-catenin/Tcf complex. Cell 103:885–896

Graham TA, Ferkey DM, Mao F, Kimelman D, Xu W (2001) Tcf4 can specifically recognize beta-catenin using alternative conformations. Nat Struct Biol 8:1048–1052

Graham TA, Clements WK, Kimelman D, Xu W (2002) The crystal structure of the beta-catenin/ICAT complex reveals the inhibitory mechanism of ICAT. Mol Cell 10:563–571

Grandy D, Shan J, Zhang X, Rao S, Akunuru S, Li H, Zhang Y, Alpatov I, Zhang XA, Lang RA, Shi DL, Zheng JJ (2009) Discovery and characterization of a small molecule inhibitor of the PDZ domain of dishevelled. J Biol Chem 284:16256–16263

Gwak J, Song T, Song JY, Yun YS, Choi IW, Jeong Y, Shin JG, Oh S (2009) Isoreserpine promotes beta-catenin degradation via Siah-1 up-regulation in HCT116 colon cancer cells. Biochem Biophys Res Commun 387:444–449

Hale KJ, Manaviazar S, Lazarides L, George J, Walters MA, Cai J, Delisser VM, Bhatia GS, Peak SA, Dalby SM, Lefranc A, Chen YN, Wood AW, Crowe P, Erwin P, El-Tanani M (2009) Synthesis of A83586C analogs with potent anticancer and beta-catenin/ TCF4/osteopontin inhibitory effects and insights into how A83586C modulates E2Fs and pRb. Org Lett 11:737–740

Han EK, Arber N, Yamamoto H, Lim JT, Delohery T, Pamukcu R, Piazza GA, Xing WQ, Weinstein IB (1998) Effects of sulindac and its metabolites on growth and apoptosis in human mammary epithelial and breast carcinoma cell lines. Breast Cancer Res Treat 48:195–203

Han A, Song Z, Tong C, Hu D, Bi X, Augenlicht LH, Yang W (2008) Sulindac suppresses beta-catenin expression in human cancer cells. Eur J Pharmacol 583:26–31

Herbst A, Kolligs FT (2007) Wnt signaling as a therapeutic target for cancer. Methods Mol Biol 361:63–91

Hope C, Planutis K, Planutiene M, Moyer MP, Johal KS, Woo J, Santoso C, Hanson JA, Holcombe RF (2008) Low concentrations of resveratrol inhibit Wnt signal throughput in colon-derived cells: implications for colon cancer prevention. Mol Nutr Food Res 52(suppl 1):S52–S61

Hsiao SJ, Smith S (2008) Tankyrase function at telomeres, spindle poles, and beyond. Biochimie 90:83–92

Huang SM, Mishina YM, Liu S, Cheung A, Stegmeier F, Michaud GA, Charlat O, Wiellette E, Zhang Y, Wiessner S, Hild M, Shi X, Wilson CJ, Mickanin C, Myer V, Fazal A, Tomlinson R, Serluca F, Shao W, Cheng H, Shultz M, Rau C, Schirle M, Schlegl J, Ghidelli S, Fawell S, Lu C, Curtis D, Kirschner MW, Lengauer C, Finan PM, Tallarico JA, Bouwmeester T, Porter JA, Bauer A, Cong F (2009) Tankyrase inhibition stabilizes axin and antagonizes Wnt signalling. Nature 461:614–620

Huber AH, Weis WI (2001) The structure of the beta-catenin/E-cadherin complex and the molecular basis of diverse ligand recognition by beta-catenin. Cell 105:391–402

Huber AH, Nelson WJ, Weis WI (1997) Three-dimensional structure of the armadillo repeat region of beta-catenin. Cell 90:871–882

James RG, Biechele TL, Conrad WH, Camp ND, Fass DM, Major MB, Sommer K, Yi X, Roberts BS, Cleary MA, Arthur WT, MacCoss M, Rawlings DJ, Haggarty SJ, Moon RT (2009) Bruton's tyrosine kinase revealed as a negative regulator of Wnt-beta-catenin signaling. Sci Signal 2:ra25

Jin G, Lu D, Yao S, Wu CC, Liu JX, Carson DA, Cottam HB (2009) Amide derivatives of ethacrynic acid: synthesis and evaluation as antagonists of Wnt/beta-catenin signaling and CLL cell survival. Bioorg Med Chem Lett 19:606–609

Jones S, Thornton JM (1996) Principles of protein-protein interactions. Proc Natl Acad Sci USA 93:13–20

Kawamoto SA, Thompson AD, Coleska A, Nikolovska-Coleska Z, Yi H, Wang S (2009) Analysis of the interaction of BCL9 with beta-catenin and development of fluorescence polarization and surface plasmon resonance binding assays for this interaction. Biochemistry 48:9534–9541

Keller JJ, Giardiello FM (2003) Chemoprevention strategies using NSAIDs and COX-2 inhibitors. Cancer Biol Ther 2:S140–S149

Kelloff GJ, Boone CW, Crowell JA, Steele VE, Lubet RA, Doody LA, Malone WF, Hawk ET, Sigman CC (1996) New agents for cancer chemoprevention. J Cell Biochem Suppl 26:1–28

Kim J, Zhang X, Rieger-Christ KM, Summerhayes IC, Wazer DE, Paulson KE, Yee AS (2006) Suppression of Wnt signaling by the green tea compound (-)-epigallocatechin 3-gallate (EGCG) in invasive breast cancer cells. Requirement of the transcriptional repressor HBP1. J Biol Chem 281:10865–10875

Koehne CH, DuBois RN (2004) COX-2 inhibition and colorectal cancer. Semin Oncol 31:12–21

Koornstra JJ, Rijcken FE, Oldenhuis CN, Zwart N, van der Sluis T, Hollema H, deVries EG, Keller JJ, Offerhaus JA, Giardiello FM, Kleibeuker JH (2005) Sulindac inhibits beta-catenin expression in normal-appearing colon of hereditary nonpolyposis colorectal cancer and familial adenomatous polyposis patients. Cancer Epidemiol Biomarkers Prev 14:1608–1612

Kuo SM (1996) Antiproliferative potency of structurally distinct dietary flavonoids on human colon cancer cells. Cancer Lett 110:41–48

Labayle D, Fischer D, Vielh P, Drouhin F, Pariente A, Bories C, Duhamel O, Trousset M, Attali P (1991) Sulindac causes regression of rectal polyps in familial adenomatous polyposis. Gastroenterology 101:635–639

Lee HJ, Wang NX, Shi DL, Zheng JJ (2009a) Sulindac inhibits canonical Wnt signaling by blocking the PDZ domain of the protein Dishevelled. Angew Chem Int Ed Engl 48:6448–6452

Lee H-J, Wang NX, Shao Y, Zheng JJ (2009b) Identification of tripeptides recognized by the PDZ domain of Dishevelled. Bioorg Med Chem 17:1701–1708

Lentzsch S, Elliott G, Roodman GD (2007) SDX-308 and SDX-101, non-steroidal anti-inflammatory drugs, as therapeutic candidates for treating hematologic malignancies including myeloma. Arch Pharm (Weinheim) 340:511–516

Leow PC, Ong ZY, Ee PL (2010a) Natural compounds as antagonists of canonical Wnt/β-catenin signaling. Curr Chem Biol 4:49–63

Leow PC, Tian Q, Ong ZY, Yang Z, Ee PL (2010b) Antitumor activity of natural compounds, curcumin and PKF118-310, as Wnt/beta-catenin antagonists against human osteosarcoma cells. Invest New Drugs 28:766–782

Lepourcelet M, Chen YN, France DS, Wang H, Crews P, Petersen F, Bruseo C, Wood AW, Shivdasani RA (2004) Small-molecule antagonists of the oncogenic Tcf/beta-catenin protein complex. Cancer Cell 5:91–102

Li X, Ohtsuki T, Koyano T, Kowithayakorn T, Ishibashi M (2009) New Wnt/beta-catenin signaling inhibitors isolated from *Eleutherine palmifolia*. Chem Asian J 4:540–547

Lim JT, Joe AK, Suzui M, Shimizu M, Masuda M, Weinstein IB (2006) Sulindac sulfide and exisulind inhibit expression of the estrogen and progesterone receptors in human breast cancer cells. Clin Cancer Res 12:3478–3484

Lin YC, You L, Xu Z, He B, Mikami I, Thung E, Chou J, Kuchenbecker K, Kim J, Raz D, Yang CT, Chen JK, Jablons DM (2006) Wnt signaling activation and WIF-1 silencing in nasopharyngeal cancer cell lines. Biochem Biophys Res Commun 341:635–640

Lindhagen E, Nissle S, Leoni L, Elliott G, Chao Q, Larsson R, Aleskog A (2007a) R-etodolac (SDX-101) and the related indole-pyran analogues SDX-308 and SDX-309 potentiate the antileukemic activity of standard cytotoxic agents in primary chronic lymphocytic leukaemia cells. Cancer Chemother Pharmacol 60:545–553

Lindhagen E, Rickardson L, Elliott G, Leoni L, Nygren P, Larsson R, Aleskog A (2007b) Pharmacological profiling of novel non-COX-inhibiting indole-pyran analogues of etodolac reveals high solid tumour activity of SDX-308 in vitro. Invest New Drugs 25:297–303

Liu JJ, Wang JY, Hertervig E, Nilsson A, Duan RD (2002) Sulindac induces apoptosis, inhibits proliferation and activates caspase-3 in Hep G2 cells. Anticancer Res 22:263–266

Liu J, Xing Y, Hinds TR, Zheng J, Xu W (2006) The third 20 amino acid repeat is the tightest binding site of APC for beta-catenin. J Mol Biol 360:133–144

Logan CY, Nusse R (2004) The Wnt signaling pathway in development and disease. Annu Rev Cell Dev Biol 20:781–810

Lu D, Zhao Y, Tawatao R, Cottam HB, Sen M, Leoni LM, Kipps TJ, Corr M, Carson DA (2004) Activation of the Wnt signaling pathway in chronic lymphocytic leukemia. Proc Natl Acad Sci USA 101:3118–3123

Lu D, Cottam HB, Corr M, Carson DA (2005) Repression of beta-catenin function in malignant cells by nonsteroidal antiinflammatory drugs. Proc Natl Acad Sci USA 102:18567–18571

Lu D, Liu JX, Endo T, Zhou H, Yao S, Willert K, Schmidt-Wolf IG, Kipps TJ, Carson DA (2009a) Ethacrynic acid exhibits selective toxicity to chronic lymphocytic leukemia cells by inhibition of the Wnt/beta-catenin pathway. PLoS One 4:e8294

Lu J, Ma Z, Hsieh JC, Fan CW, Chen B, Longgood JC, Williams NS, Amatruda JF, Lum L, Chen C (2009b) Structure-activity relationship studies of small-molecule inhibitors of Wnt response. Bioorg Med Chem Lett 19:3825–3827

Lu W, Tinsley HN, Keeton A, Qu Z, Piazza GA, Li Y (2009c) Suppression of Wnt/beta-catenin signaling inhibits prostate cancer cell proliferation. Eur J Pharmacol 602:8–14

Ma H, Nguyen C, Lee KS, Kahn M (2005) Differential roles for the coactivators CBP and p300 on TCF/beta-catenin-mediated survivin gene expression. Oncogene 24:3619–3631

Mahmoudi T, Li VS, Ng SS, Taouatas N, Vries RG, Mohammed S, Heck AJ, Clevers H (2009) The kinase TNIK is an essential activator of Wnt target genes. EMBO J 28:3329–3340

Matsumoto T, Nakamura S, Esaki M, Yao T, Iida M (2006) Effect of the non-steroidal anti-inflammatory drug sulindac on colorectal adenomas of uncolectomized familial adenomatous polyposis. J Gastroenterol Hepatol 21:251–257

Mazieres J, He B, You L, Xu Z, Lee AY, Mikami I, Reguart N, Rosell R, McCormick F, Jablons DM (2004) Wnt inhibitory factor-1 is silenced by promoter hypermethylation in human lung cancer. Cancer Res 64:4717–4720

McMillan M, Kahn M (2005) Investigating Wnt signaling: a chemogenomic safari. Drug Discov Today 10:1467–1474

Minke KS, Staib P, Puetter A, Gehrke I, Gandhirajan RK, Schlosser A, Schmitt EK, Hallek M, Kreuzer KA (2009) Small molecule inhibitors of WNT signaling effectively induce apoptosis in acute myeloid leukemia cells. Eur J Haematol 82:165 175

Mizutani K, Miyamoto S, Nagahata T, Konishi N, Emi M, Onda M (2005) Upregulation and overexpression of DVL1, the human counterpart of the Drosophila dishevelled gene, in prostate cancer. Tumori 91:546–551

Moon RT, Kohn AD, De Ferrari GV, Kaykas A (2004) WNT and beta-catenin signalling: diseases and therapies. Nat Rev Genet 5:691–701

Nagahata T, Shimada T, Harada A, Nagai H, Onda M, Yokoyama S, Shiba T, Jin E, Kawanami O, Emi M (2003) Amplification, up-regulation and over-expression of DVL-1, the human counterpart of the Drosophila disheveled gene, in primary breast cancers. Cancer Sci 94:515–518

Nath N, Kashfi K, Chen J, Rigas B (2003) Nitric oxide-donating aspirin inhibits beta-catenin/T cell factor (TCF) signaling in SW480 colon cancer cells by disrupting the nuclear beta-catenin-TCF association. Proc Natl Acad Sci USA 100:12584–12589

Nath N, Vassell R, Chattopadhyay M, Kogan M, Kashfi K (2009) Nitro-aspirin inhibits MCF-7 breast cancer cell growth: effects on COX-2 expression and Wnt/beta-catenin/TCF-4 signaling. Biochem Pharmacol 78:1298–1304

Nguyen DX, Chiang AC, Zhang XH, Kim JY, Kris MG, Ladanyi M, Gerald WL, Massague J (2009) WNT/TCF signaling through LEF1 and HOXB9 mediates lung adenocarcinoma metastasis. Cell 138:51–62

Nikitakis NG, Hebert C, Lopes MA, Reynolds MA, Sauk JJ (2002) PPARgamma-mediated antineoplastic effect of NSAID sulindac on human oral squamous carcinoma cells. Int J Cancer 98:817–823

Nugent KP, Farmer KC, Spigelman AD, Williams CB, Phillips RK (1993) Randomized controlled trial of the effect of sulindac on duodenal and rectal polyposis and cell proliferation in patients with familial adenomatous polyposis. Br J Surg 80:1618–1619

Okino K, Nagai H, Hatta M, Nagahata T, Yoneyama K, Ohta Y, Jin E, Kawanami O, Araki T, Emi M (2003) Up-regulation and overproduction of DVL-1, the human counterpart of the Drosophila dishevelled gene, in cervical squamous cell carcinoma. Oncol Rep 10:1219–1223

Park CH, Chang JY, Hahm ER, Park S, Kim HK, Yang CH (2005) Quercetin, a potent inhibitor against beta-catenin/Tcf signaling in SW480 colon cancer cells. Biochem Biophys Res Commu 328:227–234

Park S, Gwak J, Cho M, Song T, Won J, Kim DE, Shin JG, Oh S (2006) Hexachlorophene inhibits Wnt/beta-catenin pathway by promoting Siah-mediated beta-catenin degradation. Mol Pharmacol 70:960–966

Pasricha PJ, Bedi A, O'Connor K, Rashid A, Akhtar AJ, Zahurak ML, Piantadosi S, Hamilton SR, Giardiello FM (1995) The effects of sulindac on colorectal proliferation and apoptosis in familial adenomatous polyposis. Gastroenterology 109:994–998

Patten EJ, DeLong MJ (1999) Effects of sulindac, sulindac metabolites, and aspirin on the activity of detoxification enzymes in HT-29 human colon adenocarcinoma cells. Cancer Lett 147: 95–100

Peterson RT (2009) Drug discovery: propping up a destructive regime. Nature 461:599–600

Petropoulos K, Arseni N, Schessl C, Stadler CR, Rawat VP, Deshpande AJ, Heilmeier B, Hiddemann W, Quintanilla-Martinez L, Bohlander SK, Feuring-Buske M, Buske C (2008) A novel role for Lef-1, a central transcription mediator of Wnt signaling, in leukemogenesis. J Exp Med 205:515–522

Piazza GA, Alberts DS, Hixson LJ, Paranka NS, Li H, Finn T, Bogert C, Guillen JM, Brendel K, Gross PH, Sperl G, Ritchie J, Burt RW, Ellsworth L, Ahnen DJ, Pamukcu R (1997) Sulindac sulfone inhibits azoxymethane-induced colon carcinogenesis in rats without reducing prostaglandin levels. Cancer Res 57:2909–2915

Piergentill A, Bello FD, Gentili F, Giannella M, Quaglia W, Vesprini C, Thomas RJ, Robertson GM (2007) Solution-phase synthesis of ICG-001, a β-turn peptidomimetic molecule inhibitor of β-catenin–Tcf-mediated transcription. Tetrahedron 63:12912–12916

Poy F, Lepourcelet M, Shivdasani RA, Eck MJ (2001) Structure of a human Tcf4-beta-catenin complex. Nat Struct Biol 8:1053–1057

Prasad CP, Rath G, Mathur S, Bhatnagar D, Ralhan R (2009) Potent growth suppressive activity of curcumin in human breast cancer cells: Modulation of Wnt/beta-catenin signaling. Chem Biol Interact 181(2):263–271

Rahman MA, Dhar DK, Masunaga R, Yamanoi A, Kohno H, Nagasue N (2000) Sulindac and exisulind exhibit a significant antiproliferative effect and induce apoptosis in human hepatocellular carcinoma cell lines. Cancer Res 60:2085–2089

Ravindranath A, O'Connell A, Johnston PG, El-Tanani MK (2008) The role of LEF/TCF factors in neoplastic transformation. Curr Mol Med 8:38–50

Reguart N, He B, Xu Z, You L, Lee AY, Mazieres J, Mikami I, Batra S, Rosell R, McCormick F, Jablons DM (2004) Cloning and characterization of the promoter of human Wnt inhibitory factor-1. Biochem Biophys Res Commun 323:229–234

Rigas B (2007) Novel agents for cancer prevention based on nitric oxide. Biochem Soc Trans 35:1364–1368

Rigas B, Kashfi K (2004) Nitric-oxide-donating NSAIDs as agents for cancer prevention. Trends Mol Med 10:324–330

Rigas B, Williams JL (2008) NO-donating NSAIDs and cancer: an overview with a note on whether NO is required for their action. Nitric Oxide 19:199–204

Roccaro AM, Leleu X, Sacco A, Moreau AS, Hatjiharissi E, Jia X, Xu L, Ciccarelli B, Patterson CJ, Ngo HT, Russo D, Vacca A, Dammacco F, Anderson KC, Ghobrial IM, Treon SP (2008) Resveratrol exerts antiproliferative activity and induces apoptosis in Waldenstrom's macroglobulinemia. Clin Cancer Res 14:1849–1858

Roose J, Clevers H (1999) TCF transcription factors: molecular switches in carcinogenesis. Biochim Biophys Acta 1424:M23–M37

Ryu MJ, Cho M, Song JY, Yun YS, Choi IW, Kim DE, Park BS, Oh S (2008) Natural derivatives of curcumin attenuate the Wnt/beta-catenin pathway through down-regulation of the transcriptional coactivator p300. Biochem Biophys Res Commun 377:1304–1308

Sakoguchi-Okada N, Takahashi-Yanaga F, Fukada K, Shiraishi F, Taba Y, Miwa Y, Morimoto S, Iida M, Sasaguri T (2007) Celecoxib inhibits the expression of survivin via the suppression of promoter activity in human colon cancer cells. Biochem Pharmacol 73:1318–1329

Sampietro J, Dahlberg CL, Cho US, Hinds TR, Kimelman D, Xu W (2006) Crystal structure of a beta-catenin/BCL9/Tcf4 complex. Mol Cell 24:293–300

Sarkar FH, Li Y, Wang Z, Kong D (2009) Cellular signaling perturbation by natural products. Cell Signal 21:1541–1547

Schwarz-Romond T, Fiedler M, Shibata N, Butler PJ, Kikuchi A, Higuchi Y, Bienz M (2007) The DIX domain of Dishevelled confers Wnt signaling by dynamic polymerization. Nat Struct Mol Biol 14:484–492

Shan J, Shi DL, Wang J, Zheng J (2005) Identification of a specific inhibitor of the dishevelled PDZ domain. Biochemistry 44:15495–15503

Shan BE, Wang MX, Li RQ (2009) Quercetin inhibit human SW480 colon cancer growth in association with inhibition of cyclin D1 and survivin expression through Wnt/beta-catenin signaling pathway. Cancer Invest 27:604–612

Shan J, Zheng JJ (2009) J Comput Aided Mol Des 23:37–47

Sharma M, Li L, Celver J, Killian C, Kovoor A, Seeram NP (2009) Effects of fruit ellagitannin extracts, ellagic acid, and their colonic metabolite, urolithin A, on Wnt signaling (dagger). J Agric Food Chem 58:3965–3969

Simons M, Gault WJ, Gotthardt D, Rohatgi R, Klein TJ, Shao Y, Lee HJ, Wu AL, Fang Y, Satlin LM, Dow JT, Chen J, Zheng J, Boutros M, Mlodzik M (2009) Electrochemical cues regulate assembly of the Frizzled/Dishevelled complex at the plasma membrane during planar epithelial polarization. Nat Cell Biol 11:286–294

Song GY, Lee JH, Cho M, Park BS, Kim DE, Oh S (2007) Decursin suppresses human androgen-independent PC3 prostate cancer cell proliferation by promoting the degradation of beta-catenin. Mol Pharmacol 72:1599–1606

Suh Y, Afaq F, Johnson JJ, Mukhtar H (2009) A plant flavonoid fisetin induces apoptosis in colon cancer cells by inhibition of COX2 and Wnt/EGFR/NF-kappaB-signaling pathways. Carcinogenesis 30:300–307

Sukhdeo K, Mani M, Zhang Y, Dutta J, Yausi H, Rooney MD, Carrasco DE, Zheng M, He H, Tai YT, Mitsiades C, Anderson KC, Carrasco DR (2007) Targeting the beta-catenin/TCF transcriptional complex in the treatment of multiple myeloma. Proc Natl Acad Sci USA 104: 7516–7521

Takada R, Satomi Y, Kurata T, Ueno N, Norioka S, Kondoh H, Takao T, Takada S (2006) Monounsaturated fatty acid modification of Wnt protein: its role in Wnt secretion. Dev Cell 11:791–801

Takahashi-Yanaga F, Sasaguri T (2007) The Wnt/beta-catenin signaling pathway as a target in drug discovery. J Pharmacol Sci 104:293–302

Takahashi-Yanaga F, Yoshihara T, Jingushi K, Miwa Y, Morimoto S, Hirata M, Sasaguri T (2008) Celecoxib-induced degradation of T-cell factors-1 and -4 in human colon cancer cells. Biochem Biophys Res Commun 377:1185–1190

Takemaru KI, Moon RT (2000) The transcriptional coactivator CBP interacts with beta-catenin to activate gene expression. J Cell Biol 149:249–254

Takemaru KI, Ohmitsu M, Li FQ (2008) An oncogenic hub: beta-catenin as a molecular target for cancer therapeutics. Handb Exp Pharmacol (186):261–284

Teiten MH, Eifes S, Dicato M, Diederich M (2010) Curcumin-the paradigm of a multi-target natural compound with application in cancer prevention and treatment. Toxins 2:128–162

Thun MJ, Henley SJ, Patrono C (2002) Nonsteroidal anti-inflammatory drugs as anticancer agents: mechanistic, pharmacologic, and clinical issues. J Natl Cancer Inst 94:252–266

Toney JH, Fasick JI, Singh S, Beyrer C, Sullivan DJ Jr (2009) Purposeful learning with drug repurposing. Science 325:1339–1340

Trosset JY, Dalvit C, Knapp S, Fasolini M, Veronesi M, Mantegani S, Gianellini LM, Catana C, Sundstrom M, Stouten PF, Moll JK (2006) Inhibition of protein-protein interactions: the discovery of druglike beta-catenin inhibitors by combining virtual and biophysical screening. Proteins 64:60–67

Uematsu K, He B, You L, Xu Z, McCormick F, Jablons DM (2003a) Activation of the Wnt pathway in non small cell lung cancer: evidence of dishevelled overexpression. Oncogene 22:7218–7221

Uematsu K, Kanazawa S, You L, He B, Xu Z, Li K, Peterlin BM, McCormick F, Jablons DM (2003b) Wnt pathway activation in mesothelioma: evidence of Dishevelled overexpression and transcriptional activity of beta-catenin. Cancer Res 63:4547–4551

Waddell WR (1994) The effect of sulindac on colon polyps: circumvention of a transformed phenotype–a hypothesis. J Surg Oncol 55:52–55

Wallingford JB, Habas R (2005) The developmental biology of Dishevelled: an enigmatic protein governing cell fate and cell polarity. Development 132:4421–4436

Wang NX, Lee HJ, Zheng JJ (2008) Therapeutic use of PDZ protein-protein interaction antagonism. Drug News Perspect 21:137–141

Webster WS, Leibovich BC (2005) Exisulind in the treatment of prostate cancer. Expert Rev Anticancer Ther 5:957–962

Wei Q, Zhao Y, Yang ZQ, Dong QZ, Dong XJ, Han Y, Zhao C, Wang EH (2008) Dishevelled family proteins are expressed in non-small cell lung cancer and function differentially on tumor progression. Lung Cancer 62:181–192

Wei W, Chua MS, Grepper S, So S (2010) Small molecule antagonists of Tcf4/beta-catenin complex inhibit the growth of HCC cells in vitro and in vivo. Int J Cancer 126:2426–2436

Wells JA, McClendon CL (2007) Reaching for high-hanging fruit in drug discovery at protein-protein interfaces. Nature 450:1001–1009

Wharton KA Jr (2003) Runnin' with the Dvl: proteins that associate with Dsh/Dvl and their significance to Wnt signal transduction. Dev Biol 253:1–17

Whitehead CM, Earle KA, Fetter J, Xu S, Hartman T, Chan DC, Zhao TL, Piazza G, Klein-Szanto AJ, Pamukcu R, Alila H, Bunn PA Jr, Thompson WJ (2003) Exisulind-induced apoptosis in a non-small cell lung cancer orthotopic lung tumor model augments docetaxel treatment and contributes to increased survival. Mol Cancer Ther 2:479–488

Winde G, Gumbinger HG, Osswald H, Kemper F, Bunte H (1993) The NSAID sulindac reverses rectal adenomas in colectomized patients with familial adenomatous polyposis: clinical results of a dose-finding study on rectal sulindac administration. Int J Colorectal Dis 8:13–17

Wong HC, Mao J, Nguyen JT, Srinivas S, Zhang W, Liu B, Li L, Wu D, Zheng J (2000) Structural basis of the recognition of the dishevelled DEP domain in the Wnt signaling pathway. Nat Struct Biol 7:1178–1184

Wong HC, Bourdelas A, Krauss A, Lee HJ, Shao Y, Wu D, Mlodzik M, Shi DL, Zheng J (2003) Direct binding of the PDZ domain of Dishevelled to a conserved internal sequence in the C-terminal region of Frizzled. Mol Cell 12:1251–1260

Yang J, Brown MS, Liang G, Grishin NV, Goldstein JL (2008) Identification of the acyltransferase that octanoylates ghrelin, an appetite-stimulating peptide hormone. Cell 132:387–396

Yang TM, Leu SW, Li JM, Hung MS, Lin CH, Lin YC, Huang TJ, Tsai YH, Yang CT (2009) WIF-1 promoter region hypermethylation as an adjuvant diagnostic marker for non-small cell lung cancer-related malignant pleural effusions. J Cancer Res Clin Oncol 135:919–924

Yasui H, Hideshima T, Hamasaki M, Roccaro AM, Shiraishi N, Kumar S, Tassone P, Ishitsuka K, Raje N, Tai YT, Podar K, Chauhan D, Leoni LM, Kanekal S, Elliott G, Munshi NC, Anderson KC (2005) SDX-101, the R-enantiomer of etodolac, induces cytotoxicity, overcomes drug resistance, and enhances the activity of dexamethasone in multiple myeloma. Blood 106:706–712

Yasui H, Hideshima T, Ikeda H, Ocio EM, Kiziltepe T, Vallet S, Okawa Y, Neri P, Sukhdeo K, Podar K, Chauhan D, Richardson PG, Raje N, Carrasco DR, Anderson KC (2007) Novel etodolac analog SDX-308 (CEP-18082) induces cytotoxicity in multiple myeloma cells associated with inhibition of beta-catenin/TCF pathway. Leukemia 21:535–540

Yeh RK, Chen J, Williams JL, Baluch M, Hundley TR, Rosenbaum RE, Kalala S, Traganos F, Benardini F, Del SP, Kashfi K, Rigas B (2004) NO-donating nonsteroidal antiinflammatory drugs (NSAIDs) inhibit colon cancer cell growth more potently than traditional NSAIDs: a general pharmacological property? Biochem Pharmacol 67:2197–2205

You L, Xu Z, Punchihewa C, Jablons DM, Fujii N (2008) Evaluation of a chemical library of small-molecule Dishevelled antagonists that suppress tumor growth by down-regulating T-cell factor-mediated transcription. Mol Cancer Ther 7:1633–1638

Zeng X, Huang H, Tamai K, Zhang XJ, Harada Y, Yokota C, Almeida K, Wang J, Doble B, Woodgett J, Wynshaw-Boris A, Hsieh JC, He X (2008) Initiation of Wnt signaling: control of Wnt coreceptor Lrp6 phosphorylation/activation via frizzled, dishevelled and axin functions. Development 135:367–375

Zhang T, Fields JZ, Ehrlich SM, Boman BM (2004) The chemopreventive agent sulindac attenuates expression of the antiapoptotic protein survivin in colorectal carcinoma cells. J Pharmacol Exp Ther 308:434–437

Zhang Y, Appleton BA, Wiesmann C, Lau T, Costa M, Hannoush RN, Sidhu SS (2009) Inhibition of Wnt signaling by Dishevelled PDZ peptides. Nat Chem Biol 5:217–219

Chapter 10
Targeting of Wnt Signaling Inside the Nucleus

Miki Shitashige and Tesshi Yamada

Abstract More than 80% of colorectal cancers have mutations in one of two genes involved in the Wnt signaling pathway: the adenomatous polyposis coli (*APC*) and β-catenin (*CTNNB1*) genes. Mutation of either gene commonly results in continuous activation of Wnt signaling, and thus Wnt signaling is considered to be the most fundamental pathway driving colorectal carcinogenesis. However, only a few "druggable" target molecules have been identified in this pathway, and the loss of function of the mutated *APC* tumor suppressor gene does not seem to be amendable with currently available medical technologies. Therefore, we have been searching for drug target molecules downstream of APC, especially in the nucleus. Our recent series of proteomic studies has revealed that various classes of nuclear proteins participate in the β-catenin and TCF-4 (T-cell factor-4) complex and modulate its transcriptional activity. In this review, we describe nuclear proteins that enhance the transcriptional activity of the β-catenin and TCF-4 complex and nuclear pore complex (NPC) proteins that mediate the nuclear translocation of β-catenin. These proteins are considered feasible targets for the development of drugs directed at the aberrant Wnt signaling pathway.

Abbreviations

APC	Adenomatous polyposis coli
CKI	Cascin kinase I
CML	Chronic myeloid leukemia
EGFR	Epidermal growth factor receptor
FUS/TLS	Fusion/translocated in liposarcoma
GSK3β	Glycogen synthase kinase 3β
HCC	Hepatocellular cancer

T. Yamada (✉)
Chemotherapy Division, National Cancer Center Research Institute,
5-1-1 Tsukiji, Chuo-ku, Tokyo 104-0045, Japan
e-mail: tyamada@ncc.go.jp

K.H. Goss and M. Kahn (eds.), *Targeting the Wnt Pathway in Cancer*,
DOI 10.1007/978-1-4419-8023-6_10, © Springer Science+Business Media, LLC 2011

LC   Liquid chromatography
LEF   Lymphoid enhancer factor
MS/MS   Tandem mass spectrometry
NPC   Nuclear pore complex
PARP-1   Poly(ADP-ribose) polymerase-1
Ran   Ras-related nuclear protein
RanBP2   Ran binding protein-2
RanGAP1   Ran GTPase-activating protein-1
SF1   Splicing factor-1
SUMO   Small ubiquitin-related modifier
TCF-4   T-cell factor-4
TNIK   Traf2- and Nck-interacting kinase
Topo II   Topoisomerase II

Colorectal cancer is becoming a major health problem all over the world. For example, in Japan alone during 2007, the number of patients registered as having died of cancers of the colon and rectum was 14,061 and 8,949, respectively (Kato et al. 2007). The number of such cancer deaths seems to be increasing rapidly, probably as a result of changes in dietary habits. The majority of colorectal cancer patients without lymph node or organ metastasis can be cured by surgical resection alone. However, the results of treatment for metastasized or recurrent disease have been disappointing. Despite recent advances in combination chemotherapy, including agents such as oxaliplatin (FOLFOX) and irinotecan (FOLFIRI) (Kelly and Goldberg 2005), the outcome for such patients still remains unsatisfactory. Therapeutic antibodies directed against vascular endothelial growth factor and epidermal growth factor receptor (EGFR) have been shown to be effective for the treatment of unresectable colorectal cancer (Tabernero et al. 2007; Saltz et al. 2008), but their efficacy is limited and only a small proportion of individuals achieves the anticipated benefits (Bokemeyer et al. 2009). It is therefore necessary to identify molecules that are fundamentally essential for colorectal cancer proliferation, and to develop new drugs capable of targeting them.

The genetic and epigenetic alterations occurring during the course of multistage colorectal carcinogenesis have been extensively explored in the last few decades (Kinzler and Vogelstein 1996; Kondo and Issa 2004; Bodmer 2006). The most noteworthy finding is that the great majority of colorectal cancers have mutations in one of two genes involved in the Wnt signaling pathway: the adenomatous polyposis coli (*APC*) (Kinzler and Vogelstein 1996) and β-catenin (*CTNNB1*) genes (Morin et al. 1997; Sparks et al. 1998). The *APC* gene product forms a cytoplasmic multiprotein complex that contains β-catenin, axin/axin2, casein kinase I (CKI), and glycogen synthase kinase 3β (GSK3β) and others (Kikuchi 2003). This complex acts as a molecular chaperone that mediates the phosphorylation of β-catenin by GSK3β. Phosphorylated β-catenin protein is subjected to ubiquitination and subsequent degradation through the proteasome pathway. Mutation of the *CTNNB1* gene is often detected at the GSK3β-phosphorylation sites of β-catenin protein, and this prevents its phosphorylation. Mutation of either the *APC* or *CTNNB1* gene commonly results in the accumulation of β-catenin protein and resembles active Wnt signaling (Peifer and Polakis 2000; Polakis 2000; Clevers 2004). The accumulated β-catenin protein is translocated into the nucleus, where it acts as a coactivator for T-cell factor (TCF)/lymphoid enhancer factor (LEF) family transcription factors (Behrens et al. 1996; Huber et al. 1996; van de Wetering et al. 1997).

10.1 Constitutive Transactivation of TCF-4 Target Genes is Essential for the Maintenance of Malignant Phenotypes

TCF/LEF transcription factors transactivate many genes involved in the regulation of cell proliferation, differentiation, and death. c-Jun (*JUN*) (Mann et al. 1999), c-myc (*MYC*) (He et al. 1998), cyclin D1 (*CCND1*) (Tetsu and McCormick 1999), multidrug resistance 1 (MDR1) (*ABCB1*) (Yamada et al. 2000, 2003), matrilysin (*MMP7*) (Brabletz et al. 1999; Crawford et al. 1999), axin2 (*AXIN2*) (Yan et al. 2001; Jho et al. 2002), and survivin (*BIRC5*) (Zhang et al. 2001) have been identified as the target genes of TCF/LEF.

The TCF/LEF transcription factor family comprises LEF-1 (*LEF1*), TCF-1 (*TCF7*), TCF-3 (*TCF7L1*), and TCF-4 (*TCF7L2*). Among them, TCF-4 has been implicated in colorectal carcinogenesis. TCF-4 is essential for the maintenance of undifferentiated intestinal crypt epithelial cells (Korinek et al. 1998). Mice lacking *Tcf7L2* show no proliferative compartment in the crypt regions. Undifferentiated cells at the bottom of the intestinal crypts accumulate nuclear β-catenin (van de Wetering et al. 2002). The constitutively accumulated β-catenin causes colorectal carcinogenesis by coactivating the target genes of TCF-4, which is commonly expressed in colorectal cancer cells (Korinek et al. 1997). Suppression of β-catenin-evoked gene transactivation of colorectal cancer cells by dominant-negative TCF-4 switches off genes involved in cell proliferation and switches on genes involved in cell differentiation (van de Wetering et al. 2002). TCF-4 lacking the N-terminal β-catenin-binding site suppresses transcriptional activity in a dominant-negative manner (Korinek et al. 1997). By using a strict tetracycline-regulation system (Gossen et al. 1995), we established colorectal cancer cells that were capable of inducing dominant-negative TCF-4. The TCF/LEF transcriptional activity, formation of piled-up foci, and formation colonies in soft agar (Naishiro et al. 2001) were significantly suppressed by induction of dominant-negative TCF-4 in colorectal cancer cells. Induction of dominant-negative TCF-4 restored the epithelial polarity of colorectal cancer cells and converted them into a single layer resembling normal columnar epithelium (Naishiro et al. 2001). These results indicate that colorectal cancer cells are highly dependent upon the continuous transcriptional activity of TCF-4 for the maintenance of proliferation, depolarization, and dedifferentiation.

10.2   Targeting of Wnt Signaling

Based on the findings described above, the Wnt signaling pathway has been considered an attractive target for therapy of colorectal cancer. Furthermore, other malignant tumors such as medulloblastoma, hepatocellular carcinoma, hepatoblastoma, gastric cancer, ovarian cancer, and uterine endometrial carcinoma also show mutations in the *CTNNB1* gene. Aberration of Wnt signaling has also been implicated in the pathogenesis of some human fibrosing diseases, such as idiopathic pulmonary fibrosis and desmoid. Any drug targeting the Wnt signaling pathway would seem to be promising for the treatment of these diseases and would be expected to have a wide range of clinical applications. However, only a few "druggable" target molecules have been identified in this pathway, and so far no treatment has been established. The loss of function of mutated *APC* tumor suppressor genes does not seem to be amendable with currently available medical technologies. β-Catenin is a molecule that mediates the physical intercellular adhesion of normal epithelia (Oyama et al. 1994). TCF-4 is essential for maintaining the undifferentiated status of intestinal epithelial cells, and this molecule also cannot be a drug target. We have therefore been searching for drug target molecules downstream of APC, especially in the nucleus.

10.3   Protein Components of the β-Catenin
and TCF-4 Transcriptional Complex

In a series of proteomic studies, we identified that fusion/translocated in liposarcoma (FUS/TLS) (Sato et al. 2005), poly(ADP-ribose) polymerase-1 (PARP-1) (Idogawa et al. 2005), Ku70 (Idogawa et al. 2007), Ku80 (Idogawa et al. 2007), DNA topoisomerase IIα (Topo IIα) (Huang et al. 2007), splicing factor-1 (SF1) (Shitashige et al. 2007), Ran (ras-related nuclear protein) (Shitashige et al. 2008b), RanBP2 (Ran binding protein-2) (Shitashige et al. 2008b), and RanGAP1 (Ran GTPase-activating protein-1) (Shitashige et al. 2008b) are putative protein components of the β-catenin and TCF-4 nuclear complex and regulate its transcriptional activity positively or negatively. Topo IIα, PARP-1, RanBP2, and RanGAP1 were activators, whereas SF1, FUS/TLS, and Ku70 were repressors (Shitashige et al. 2008a). Furthermore, we found that the protein composition of the TCF-4-containing nuclear complex is not fixed, but dynamically altered. The levels of expression of PARP-1, Topo IIα, FUS/TLS, SF1, and RanGAP1 proteins were regulated according to the differentiation status of intestinal epithelial cells, and highly dysregulated in colorectal cancer. In the following sections, we introduce proteins that interact endogenously with the β-catenin and TCF-4 complex in the nucleus of colorectal cancer cells and are considered eligible as drug targets. These include nuclear proteins that activate the transcriptional activity of the β-catenin and TCF-4 complex, and nuclear pore complex (NPC) proteins that mediate the

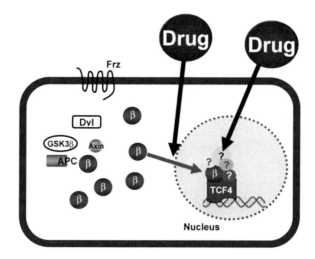

Fig. 10.1 Drug targets in the Wnt signaling pathway. In this review article, we describe nuclear proteins that activate the transcriptional activity of the β-catenin and TCF-4 complex and nuclear pore complex (NPC) proteins that mediate the nuclear translocation of β-catenin in colorectal cancer cells. *APC* adenomatous polyposis coli; *β* β-catenin; *GSK3β* glycogen synthase kinase 3β; *TCF-4* T-cell factor-4

nuclear translocation of β-catenin (Fig. 10.1). These proteins are essential for the transcriptional activity of TCF-4 and the growth of colorectal cancer cells. The expression of these proteins was increased in clinical samples of colorectal cancer, and furthermore their enzymic nature is of practical importance because it may be possible to design small chemical inhibitors that can target their catalytic activities.

10.4 PARP-1

We identified a poly-ADP-ribosylating enzyme, PARP-1, as one of the coactivators of the β-catenin and TCF-4 complex (Idogawa et al. 2005). PARP-1 is an enzyme that catalyzes the polyADP-ribosylation of acceptor proteins in response to DNA damage, and plays an important role in the maintenance of genome integrity (Masutani et al. 1999; Miwa and Masutani 2007). PARP-1 interacts with TCF-4 in the region distal to the high-mobility group box. PARP-1 is cleaved by caspase-3 during the course of apoptosis (Masutani et al. 1999; Miwa and Masutani 2007). This cleavage is likely to inhibit the interaction between PARP-1 and TCF-4 (Idogawa et al. 2005) and terminates Wnt signaling.

PARP-1 was highly expressed in intestinal adenoma cells of patients with familial adenomatous polyposis and mice with multiple intestinal polyposis (Idogawa et al. 2005). The expression of PARP-1 was closely associated with β-catenin expression and with the undifferentiated status of intestinal epithelial cells. The expression level of PARP-1 was highest in undifferentiated cells at the bottom of normal intestinal crypts and decreased gradually along the axis of cell differentiation. The expression level of PARP-1 was also increased in sporadic colorectal cancer. PARP-1 functioned as a modest enhancer for the β-catenin and TCF-4 complex, and knockdown of PARP-1 by RNA interference (RNAi) significantly suppressed both transcriptional activity and proliferation by colorectal cancer cells. Although PARP-1 has been thought to play a protective role against carcinogenesis, these expression patterns and functional properties were highly suggestive of its oncogenic activity. Recently, Huang et al. have identified a small molecule that selectively inhibits β-catenin-mediated transcription by stabilizing axin. Through proteomic analysis, this compound was found to stabilize axin by inhibiting two other poly-ADP-ribosylating enzymes, tankyrase 1 and tankyrase 2, indicating that the Wnt signaling pathway is regulated by polyADP-ribosylation at various points (Huang et al. 2009). We observed increased formation of polyADP-ribose in the nuclei of colorectal adenoma cells (Idogawa et al. 2005). These observations imply the fundamental involvement of aberrant polyADP-ribosylation in colorectal carcinogenesis.

An inhibitor of the polyADP-ribosylation activity of PARP-1, 3-aminobenzamide, did not affect TCF/LEF transcriptional activity (Idogawa et al. 2005). However, a new class of PARP inhibitors has been developed and shown to have significant activity against breast cancer in BRCA1/2 mutant carriers (Fong et al. 2009). The different mechanism of this new type of PARP inhibitor may make it applicable for targeting of Wnt signaling.

10.5 Topo IIα

Topoisomerase is an enzyme that catalyzes the relaxation of supercoiled DNA molecules, and the catenation, decatenation, knotting, and unknotting of circular DNA (Wang 2002), its expression, therefore, being closely correlated with DNA replication and cell proliferation. Topo IIα is expressed in the nuclei of epithelial cells in the suprabasal to middle region of normal large-intestinal crypts (Huang et al. 2007), where the stem and transit amplifying cells are believed to reside. Unlike PARP-1, the expression level of Topo IIα in colorectal adenoma cells is almost equal to that in normal proliferating cells. However, the expression of Topo IIα is markedly increased in adenocarcinoma cells. Double fluorescence immunohistochemistry revealed that the Topo IIα protein was colocalized with β-catenin in the nuclei of colorectal cancer cells. In normal intestinal epithelial cells, Topo IIα existed in the nucleus and β-catenin in the cell membrane, and the two proteins were not colocalized, indicating that the interaction between Topo IIα and β-catenin occurs during the process of carcinogenesis.

Topo IIα physically interacts with β-catenin and functions as an enhancer for the transcriptional activity of the β-catenin and TCF-4 complex. Topo II is a known target molecule of chemotherapeutic agents, and its inhibitors are used widely for the treatment of various cancers (Meresse et al. 2004; Sinkule 1984). We found that the TCF/LEF transcriptional activity could be inhibited by two mechanistically distinct Topo II inhibitors, merbarone and etoposide (Huang et al. 2007). Merbarone is an inhibitor for the catalytic activity of the Topo II enzyme (Khélifa and Beck 1999). By contrast, etoposide does not directly inhibit the enzymatic activity of Topo II, but stabilizes the Topo II-DNA complex (Meresse et al. 2004). The formation of stable Topo II-DNA complexes is likely to inhibit recycling of the Topo II enzyme into new substrates. However, a relatively high dose of merbarone (~200 μM) or etoposide (~100 μM) was necessary to shut down the transcriptional activity completely. These levels of concentration are considered unachievable by the current route of drug administration, and thus not applicable in a routine clinical setting. The enhancement effect of Topo IIα on TCF/LEF transcriptional activity requires its physical association with β-catenin. A new drug targeting the interaction of Topo IIα with β-catenin might therefore be applicable for the suppression of Wnt signaling. We established a mammalian two-hybrid assay that can evaluate the interaction of Topo IIα with β-catenin in a high-throughput manner. This assay might be useful for rapid screening of chemicals that antagonize the protein–protein interaction.

10.6   RanBP2, Ran, RanGAP1, and Ubc9

β-Catenin has no identifiable nuclear localization signal (Fagotto et al. 1998), and the mechanisms by which cytoplasmic β-catenin is imported into the nucleus and forms complexes with TCF/LEF nuclear proteins have not been fully elucidated.

To obtain insight into the molecular mechanisms behind the nuclear translocation of β-catenin, we searched for protein components of native complexes containing TCF-4 (Shitashige et al. 2008b). For this purpose, we used shotgun proteomics, which is an emerging concept whereby whole proteins are enzymatically digested into a large array of small peptide fragments having uniform physical and chemical characteristics. The resulting peptides are then separated by low-speed liquid chromatography (LC) and analyzed by electrospray ionization–tandem mass spectrometry (MS/MS). Separation by low-flow-rate high-performance liquid chromatography (LC) with small reverse-phase columns is known to significantly increase the sensitivity of MS/MS. Proteins of two colorectal cancer cell lines, HCT-116 and DLD1, immunoprecipitated with anti-TCF-4 antibody were analyzed directly using shotgun proteomics. The redundant LC-MS/MS data were compiled, and we found 70 proteins to be constantly immunoprecipitated with anti-TCF-4 antibody (Table 10.1).

We noticed that the 70 TCF-4-associated proteins included a large number of NPC component proteins. Ran is a nuclear GTP-binding protein required for bidirectional transport of proteins and ribonucleoproteins across the NPC (Matunis et al. 1996). RanGAP1 resides at the cytoplasmic periphery of the NPC and regulates the hydrolysis of RanGTP (Matunis et al. 1996). RanBP2 is the small ubiquitin-related modifier (SUMO) E3 ligase of RanGAP1 (Matunis et al. 1998). RanBP2, Ubc9, RanGAP1, and SUMO1 form a stable NPC complex (Reverter and Lima 2005). Ubc9 was a SUMO E2-conjugating enzyme (Desterro et al. 1997), and RanBP2 was an E3-ligating enzyme for TCF-4 (Shitashige et al. 2008b). SUMO1

Table 10.1 List of proteins immunoprecipitated with TCF-4

GI	Name (definition)
gi|13540471	Transcription factor 7-like 2 (T-cell specific, HMG-box)
gi|4503131	Catenin (cadherin-associated protein), β1, 88 kDa
gi|33946327	Nucleoporin 214 kDa; NPC protein Nup214
gi|41281437	Nucleoporin 93 kDa
gi|21264365	Nucleoporin 98 kDa isoform 1; Nup98-Nup96 precursor
gi|24497453	Nucleoporin 88 kDa; NPC protein 88; karyoporin
gi|41148144	PREDICTED: similar to NPC protein Nup205
gi|26051237	Nucleoporin 54 kDa; nucleoporin p54
gi|51467633	PREDICTED: nucleoporin 188 kDa
gi|24497603	Nucleoporin 62 kDa; nuclear pore glycoprotein p62
gi|30102928	Nucleoporin like 1
gi|6382079	RAN binding protein-2 (RanBP2); nucleoporin 358
gi|26051235	Nucleoporin 133 kDa
gi|51470875	PREDICTED: nucleoporin 160 kDa
gi|24430146	Nucleoporin 153 kDa; NPC protein hnup153
gi|24497447	Nucleoporin 50 kDa isoform a; nuclear pore-associated protein 60L
gi|9966881	NPC protein Nup107
gi|10835063	Nucleophosmin 1; nucleolar phosphoprotein B23
gi|35493987	Ubiquitin-conjugating enzyme E2I; SUMO1-protein ligase; Ubc9
gi|11415030	H4 histone family, member E
gi|4506411	RanGAP1
gi|24432016	Pre-mRNA cleavage factor I, 59 kDa subunit
gi|4758200	Desmoplakin; desmoplakin (DPI, DPII)
gi|5453555	Ras-related nuclear protein (=Ran)
gi|31745138	RAS p21 protein activator 4
gi|15487670	Nuclear RNA export factor 1 (Mex67, yeast, homolog)
gi|4506399	RAE1 (RNA export 1, *Schizosaccharomyces pombe*) homolog
gi|4557627	GLE1-like, RNA export mediator isoform 2
gi|4501955	Poly(ADP-ribosyl) transferase; poly(ADP-ribose) synthetase
gi|4758138	DEAD (Asp-Glu-Ala-Asp) box polypeptide 5
gi|10863945	ATP-dependent DNA helicase II; DNA repair protein XRCC5
gi|31543021	KIAA0893 protein
gi|16507237	Heat shock 70 kDa protein 5 (glucose-regulated protein, 78 kDa)
gi|5901926	Cleavage and polyadenylation-specific factor 5, 25 kDa subunit
gi|29728547	PREDICTED: TRAF2 and NCK interacting kinase
gi|18765750	Dual-specificity tyrosine-(Y)-phosphorylation regulated kinase 1A isoform 3
gi|24850117	Misshapen/NIK-related kinase isoform 2; GCK family kinase MINK
gi|4503471	Eukaryotic translation elongation factor 1 α1
gi|4503841	Thyroid-lupus autoantigen p70; ATP-dependent DNA helicase II, 70 kDa subunit
gi|51467100	PREDICTED: chromodomain helicase DNA binding protein 7
gi|14389309	Tubulin α6
gi|13514809	DEAD (Asp-Glu-Ala-Asp) box polypeptide 3
gi|34932414	Non-POU domain containing, octamer-binding; Nuclear RNA-binding protein, 54-kDa

(continued)

Table 10.1 (continued)

GI	Name (definition)
gi|4504451	RNA binding motif protein, X chromosome
gi|46367787	Poly(A) binding protein, cytoplasmic 1; poly(A) binding protein, cytoplasmic 2
gi|14043072	Heterogeneous nuclear ribonucleoprotein A2/B1 isoform B1
gi|14110428	Heterogeneous nuclear ribonucleoprotein C isoform a
gi|14141152	Heterogeneous nuclear ribonucleoprotein M isoform a; M4 protein
gi|14043070	Heterogeneous nuclear ribonucleoprotein A1 isoform b
gi|14110414	Heterogeneous nuclear ribonucleoprotein D isoform c
gi|4506753	TATA binding protein interacting protein 49 kDa; RuvB (*E coli* homolog)-like 1
gi|5174735	Tubulin β2
gi|11321640	Basic β1 syntrophin; syntrophin, β1 (dystrophin-associated protein A1, 59 kDa
gi|5032281	Dystrophin Dp427c isoform; dystrophin (muscular dystrophy, Duchenne and Becker types)
gi|11968182	Ribosomal protein S18; 40S ribosomal protein S18
gi|42657272	PREDICTED: similar to 40S ribosomal protein S25
gi|4506671	Ribosomal protein P2; 60S acidic ribosomal protein P2; acidic ribosomal phosphoprotein P2
gi|4885381	H1 histone family, member 5
gi|4885375	H1 histone family, member 2; histone H1d
gi|29788785	β5-Tubulin; βIb tubulin
gi|19747267	Titin isoform N2-A; connectin; CMH9, included; cardiomyopathy, dilated 1G (autosomal dominant)
gi|5730023	RuvB-like 2; erythrocyte cytosolic protein, 51-kDa; TBP-interacting protein, 48-kDa
gi|4501885	β-Actin; β-cytoskeletal actin
gi|15451763	Promyelocytic leukemia protein isoform 1
gi|41322908	Plectin 1 isoform 3; hemidesmosomal protein 1
gi|4826998	Splicing factor proline/glutamine rich (polypyrimidine tract binding protein associated)
gi|4557643	3-Hydroxy-3-methylglutaryl-coenzyme A reductase
gi|5902076	Splicing factor, arginine/serine-rich 1
gi|4506901	Splicing factor, arginine/serine-rich 3
gi|4502201	ADP-ribosylation factor 1

Proteins of two colorectal cancer cell lines, HCT-116 and DLD1, immunoprecipitated with anti-TCF-4 antibody were analyzed by nano-flow liquid chromatography (LC) and tandem mass spectrometry (MS/MS), and the 70 proteins were constantly detected in four independent experiments (two experiments using HCT-116 and two experiments using DLD1) (Adapted from Shitashige et al. (2008b) with permission (License Number: 2354110247646))

modification is known to affect the mutual interaction between proteins. Sumoylation of TCF-4 enhanced the interaction between TCF-4 and β-catenin (Shitashige et al. 2008b). Transfection of RanBP2, RanGAP1, Ubc9, or SUMO1 cDNA into colorectal cancer cells increased the amount of the TCF-4 and β-catenin proteins in the nuclear fraction. Conversely, knock-down of the NPC proteins by small interference RNA decreased the amount of nuclear β-catenin and TCF-4 proteins. Overexpression of the NPC proteins enhanced the TCF/LEF transcriptional activity and colony formation of colorectal cancer cells and increased the expression of the target genes of TCF/LEF. RanGAP1 was localized in the nuclear envelope, and its expression level was increased significantly in colorectal adenoma and adenocarcinoma in comparison with normal colon epithelium (Fig. 10.2). All these results indicate the involvement

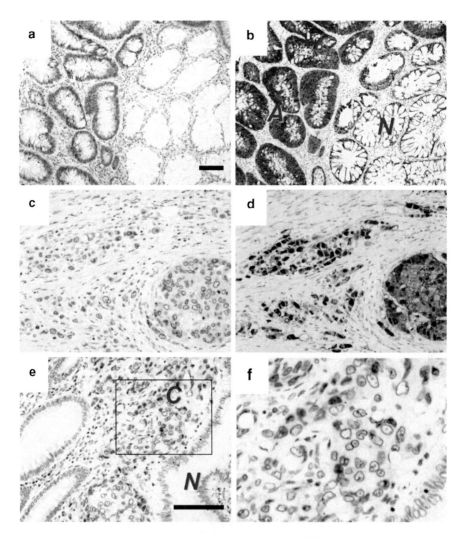

Fig. 10.2 Expression of Ran GTPase-activating protein-1 (RanGAP1) in colorectal tumors. Expression of the RanGAP1 (**a, c, e,** and **f**) and β-catenin (**b, d**) proteins in adenoma (**a, b**) and adenocarcinoma (**c–f**) tissue specimens from patients with familial adenomatous polyposis (**a, b**) and sporadic colorectal cancer (**c–f**). Figure 10.2f is an enlargement of the *boxed area* in Fig. 10.2e. Figure 10.2a and b as well as Fig. 10.2c and d are serial sections of the same blocks. *Bars,* 100 μm. *A* adenoma; *C* carcinoma; *N* normal

of aberration of NPC protein function in colorectal carcinogenesis. The sumoylation enzymes of the NPC might therefore be considered as candidate drug targets for the Wnt signaling pathway.

10.7 Traf2- and Nck-Interacting Kinase

Among the 70 proteins coimmunoprecipitated with anti-TCF-4 antibody, Traf2- and Nck-interacting kinase (TNIK) (Shitashige et al. 2008b) attracted our interest because various small-molecule kinase inhibitors have been applied successfully to cancer treatment (Druker et al. 2006; Llovet et al. 2008; Mok et al. 2009). Recently, Mahmoundi et al. (2009) also identified Tnik as a protein interacting with Tcf4 in the mouse intestinal crypt. Their data overlapped partly with ours: TNIK was an activating kinase for the TCF-4 and β-catenin transcriptional complex. HEK293 cells have the wild-type *APC* and *CTNNB1* genes. Cotransfection with hemagglutinin-tagged wild-type TNIK-WT, but not with catalytic inactive TNIK-K54R, enhanced the β-cateninΔN134- and Wnt3a-evoked TCF/LEF transcriptional activity (Fig. 10.3a, b), and β-cateninΔN134-evoked colony formation by HEK293 (Fig. 10.3c). TNIK did not significantly affect transcriptional activity or colony formation in the absence of β-cateninΔN134.

Several synthetic ATP competitors of protein kinases have been incorporated successfully into oncological practice. For example, imatinib, which blocks the Bcr-Abl fusion kinase of chronic myeloid leukemia (CML), is currently a first-line therapeutic drug for CML (Druker et al. 2006). The EGFR tyrosine kinase inhibitors, gefitinib and erlotinib, have been used in the treatment of non-small cell lung cancer (Goffin et al. 2010). A multi-kinase inhibitor sorafenib significantly improved the overall survival of patients with advanced hepatocellular cancer (HCC) (Llovet et al. 2008) and has been approved as a systemic chemotherapeutic drug for unresectable HCC. Wnt signaling is a major force driving colorectal carcinogenesis. The protein kinase TNIK was activated in colorectal cancer, and colorectal cancer cells were highly dependent upon the expression and kinase activity of TNIK for proliferation. TNIK is a feasible target for the development of drugs directed against the Wnt signaling pathway.

10.8 Conclusion

The past few decades have seen significant progress in the fields of cancer genetics and epigenetics, and we are now entering a phase in which the findings of basic science need to be translated into measures for the prevention, diagnosis, and treatment of this lethal disease. Although cancer is a disease of the genome, alterations of protein quantity, protein posttranslational modification, and protein–protein interaction impact more directly and fundamentally on the biological behavior of

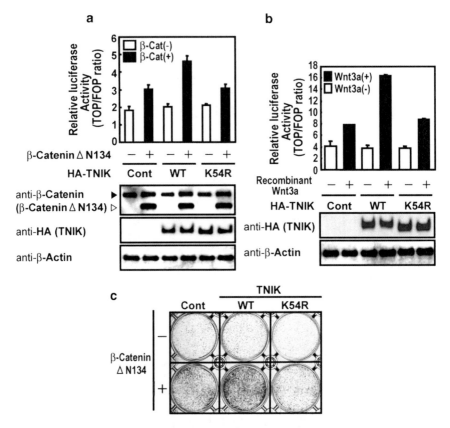

Fig. 10.3 Enhancement of TCF/LEF transcriptional activity by Traf2- and Nck-interacting kinase (TNIK). HEK293 cells were cotransfected with pFLAG-β-CateninΔN134 (+) or empty plasmid (pFLAG-CMV4) (−) and pCIneoHA-TNIK-WT, -TNIK-K54R, or empty plasmid (Cont) (**a**, **c**). HEK293 cells were transfected with pCIneoHA-TNIK-WT, -TNIK-K54R, or empty plasmid (Cont) and then treated with (+) or without (−) 20 ng/mL recombinant Wnt3a protein for 6 h (**b**). Luciferase activity and colony formation were assessed as described previously. The expression levels of β-catenin, HA-tagged TNIK-WT or -K54R, and β-actin (loading control) proteins were analyzed by immunoblotting

cancer. Starting from the genetics of colorectal carcinogenesis, we have identified proteins that are essential for the activation of Wnt signaling at various levels. These proteins are considered feasible targets for drugs aimed at this signaling pathway. Translation of these findings into the development of actual drugs will require closer collaboration with industry.

Acknowledgments This study was supported by the "Program for Promotion of Fundamental Studies in Health Sciences" conducted by the National Institute of Biomedical Innovation of Japan, the "Third-Term Comprehensive Control Research for Cancer" and "Research on Biological Markers for New Drug Development" conducted by the Ministry of Health, Labor and Welfare of Japan.

References

Behrens J, von Kries JP, Kuhl M et al (1996) Functional interaction of beta-catenin with the transcription factor LEF-1. Nature 382:638–642

Bodmer WF (2006) Cancer genetics: colorectal cancer as a model. J Hum Genet 51:391–396

Bokemeyer C, Bondarenko I, Makhson A et al (2009) Fluorouracil, leucovorin, and oxaliplatin with and without cetuximab in the first-line treatment of metastatic colorectal cancer. J Clin Oncol 27:663–671

Brabletz T, Jung A, Dag S et al (1999) Beta-catenin regulates the expression of the matrix metalloproteinase-7 in human colorectal cancer. Am J Pathol 155:1033–1038

Clevers H (2004) Wnt breakers in colon cancer. Cancer Cell 5:5–6

Crawford HC, Fingleton BM, Rudolph-Owen LA et al (1999) The metalloproteinase matrilysin is a target of beta-catenin transactivation in intestinal tumors. Oncogene 18:2883–2891

Desterro JM, Thomson J, Hay RT (1997) Ubch9 conjugates SUMO but not ubiquitin. FEBS Lett 417:297–300

Druker BJ, Guilhot F, O'Brien SG et al (2006) Five-year follow-up of patients receiving imatinib for chronic myeloid leukemia. N Engl J Med 355:2408–2417

Fagotto F, Glück U, Gumbiner BM (1998) Nuclear localization signal-independent and importin/karyopherin-independent nuclear import of beta-catenin. Curr Biol 8:181–190

Fong PC, Boss DS, Yap TA et al (2009) Inhibition of poly(ADP-ribose) polymerase in tumors from *BRCA* mutation carriers. N Engl J Med 361:123–134

Goffin J, Lacchetti C, Ellis PM et al (2010) First-line systemic chemotherapy in the treatment of advanced non-small cell lung cancer: a systematic review. J Thorac Oncol 5:260–274

Gossen M, Freundlieb S, Bender G et al (1995) Transcriptional activation by tetracyclines in mammalian cells. Science 268:1766–1769

He TC, Sparks AB, Rago C et al (1998) Identification of c-MYC as a target of the APC pathway. Science 281:1509–1512

Huang L, Shitashige M, Satow R et al (2007) Functional interaction of DNA topoisomerase II alpha with the beta-catenin and T-cell factor-4 complex. Gastroenterology 133:1569–1578

Huang SM, Mishina YM, Liu S et al (2009) Tankyrase inhibition stabilizes axin and antagonizes Wnt signalling. Nature 461:614–620

Huber O, Korn R, McLaughlin J et al (1996) Nuclear localization of beta-catenin by interaction with transcription factor LEF-1. Mech Dev 59:3–10

Idogawa M, Yamada T, Honda K et al (2005) Poly(ADP-ribose) polymerase-1 is a component of the oncogenic T-cell factor-4/beta-catenin complex. Gastroenterology 128:1919–1936

Idogawa M, Masutani M, Shitashige M et al (2007) Ku70 and poly(ADP-ribose) polymerase-1 competitively regulate beta-catenin and T-cell factor-4-mediated gene transactivation: possible linkage of DNA damage recognition and Wnt signaling. Cancer Res 67:911–918

Jho EH, Zhang T, Domon C et al (2002) Wnt/beta-catenin/Tcf signaling induces the transcription of Axin2, a negative regulator of the signaling pathway. Mol Cell Biol 22:1172–1183

Kato H, Sobue T, Katanoda K et al; Editorial Board of the Cancer Statistics in Japan (2007) Cancer statistics in Japan 2007. Foundation for Promotion of Cancer Research, Tokyo

Kelly H, Goldberg RM (2005) Systemic therapy for metastatic colorectal cancer: current options, current evidence. J Clin Oncol 23:4553–4560

Khélifa T, Beck WT (1999) Merbarone, a catalytic inhibitor of DNA topoisomerase II, induces apoptosis in CEM cells through activation of ICE/CED-3-like protease. Mol Pharmacol 55:548–556

Kikuchi A (2003) Tumor formation by genetic mutations in the components of the Wnt signaling pathway. Cancer Sci 94:225–229

Kinzler KW, Vogelstein B (1996) Lessons from hereditary colorectal cancer. Cell 87:159–170

Kondo Y, Issa JP (2004) Epigenetic changes in colorectal cancer. Cancer Metastasis Rev 23:29–39

Korinek V, Barker N, Morin PJ et al (1997) Constitutive transcriptional activation by a beta-catenin-Tcf complex in *APC*⁻/⁻ colon carcinoma. Science 275:1784–1787

Korinek V, Barker N, Moerer P et al (1998) Depletion of epithelial stem-cell compartments in the small intestine of mice lacking *TCF-4*. Nat Genet 19:379–383

Llovet JM, Ricci S, Mazzaferro V et al (2008) Sorafenib in advanced hepatocellular carcinoma. N Engl J Med 359:378–390

Mahmoudi T, Li VS, Ng SS et al (2009) The kinase TNIK is an essential activator of Wnt target genes. EMBO J 28:3329–3340

Mann B, Gelos M, Siedow A et al (1999) Target genes of beta-catenin-T cell-factor/lymphoid-enhancer-factor signaling in human colorectal carcinomas. Proc Natl Acad Sci U S A 96: 1603–1608

Masutani M, Nozaki T, Nishiyama E et al (1999) Function of poly(ADP-ribose) polymerase in response to DNA damage: gene-disruption study in mice. Mol Cell Biochem 193:149–152

Matunis MJ, Coutavas E, Blobel G (1996) A novel ubiquitin-like modification modulates the partitioning of the Ran-GTPase-activating protein RanGAP1 between the cytosol and the nuclear pore complex. J Cell Biol 135:1457–1470

Matunis MJ, Wu J, Blobel G (1998) SUMO-1 modification and its role in targeting the Ran GTPase-activating protein, RanGAP1, to the nuclear pore complex. J Cell Biol 140:499–509

Meresse P, Dechaux E, Monneret C et al (2004) Etoposide: discovery and medicinal chemistry. Curr Med Chem 11:2443–2466

Miwa M, Masutani M (2007) PolyADP-ribosylation and cancer. Cancer Sci 98:1528–1535

Mok TS, Wu YL, Thongprasert S et al (2009) Gefitinib or carboplatin-paclitaxel in pulmonary adenocarcinoma. N Engl J Med 361:947–957

Morin PJ, Sparks AB, Korinek V et al (1997) Activation of beta-catenin-Tcf signaling in colon cancer by mutations in beta-catenin or APC. Science 275:1787–1790

Naishiro Y, Yamada T, Takaoka AS et al (2001) Restoration of epithelial cell polarity in a colorectal cancer cell line by suppression of beta-catenin/T-cell factor 4-mediated gene transactivation. Cancer Res 61:2751–2758

Oyama T, Kanai Y, Ochiai A et al (1994) A truncated beta-catenin disrupts the interaction between E-cadherin and alpha-catenin: a cause of loss of intercellular adhesiveness in human cancer cell lines. Cancer Res 54:6282–6287

Peifer M, Polakis P (2000) Wnt signaling in oncogenesis and embryogenesis – a look outside the nucleus. Science 287:1606–1609

Polakis P (2000) Wnt signaling and cancer. Genes Dev 14:1837–1851

Reverter D, Lima CD (2005) Insights into E3 ligase activity revealed by a SUMO-RanGAP1-Ubc9-Nup358 complex. Nature 435:687–692

Saltz LB, Clarke S, Diaz-Rubio E et al (2008) Bevacizumab in combination with oxaliplatin-based chemotherapy as first-line therapy in metastatic colorectal cancer: a randomized phase III study. J Clin Oncol 26:2013–2019

Sato S, Idogawa M, Honda K et al (2005) Beta-catenin interacts with the FUS proto-oncogene product and regulates pre-mRNA splicing. Gastroenterology 129:1225–1236

Shitashige M, Naishiro Y, Idogawa M et al (2007) Involvement of splicing factor-1 in beta-catenin/T-cell factor-4-mediated gene transactivation and pre-mRNA splicing. Gastroenterology 132:1039–1054

Shitashige M, Hirohashi S, Yamada T (2008a) Wnt signaling inside the nucleus. Cancer Sci 99:631–637

Shitashige M, Satow R, Honda K et al (2008b) Regulation of Wnt signaling by the nuclear pore complex. Gastroenterology 134:1961–1971

Sinkule JA (1984) Etoposide: a semisynthetic epipodophyllotoxin. Chemistry, pharmacology, pharmacokinetics, adverse effects and use as an antineoplastic agent. Pharmacotherapy 4:61–73

Sparks AB, Morin PJ, Vogelstein B et al (1998) Mutational analysis of the APC/beta-catenin/Tcf pathway in colorectal cancer. Cancer Res 58:1130–1134

Tabernero J, Van Cutsem E, Diaz-Rubio E et al (2007) Phase II trial of cetuximab in combination with fluorouracil, leucovorin, and oxaliplatin in the first-line treatment of metastatic colorectal cancer. J Clin Oncol 25:5225–5232

Tetsu O, McCormick F (1999) Beta-catenin regulates expression of cyclin D1 in colon carcinoma cells. Nature 398:422–426

van de Wetering M, Cavallo R, Dooijes D et al (1997) Armadillo coactivates transcription driven by the product of the Drosophila segment polarity gene dTCF. Cell 88:789–799

van de Wetering M, Sancho E, Verweij C et al (2002) The beta-catenin/TCF-4 complex imposes a crypt progenitor phenotype on colorectal cancer cells. Cell 111:241–250

Wang JC (2002) Cellular roles of DNA topoisomerases: a molecular perspective. Nat Rev Mol Cell Biol 3:430–440

Yamada T, Takaoka AS, Naishiro Y et al (2000) Transactivation of the multidrug resistance 1 gene by T-cell factor 4/beta-catenin complex in early colorectal carcinogenesis. Cancer Res 60:4761–4766

Yamada T, Mori Y, Hayashi R et al (2003) Suppression of intestinal polyposis in $Mdr1$-deficient $Apc^{Min/+}$ mice. Cancer Res 63:895–901

Yan D, Wiesmann M, Rohan M et al (2001) Elevated expression of axin2 and hnkd mRNA provides evidence that Wnt/beta-catenin signaling is activated in human colon tumors. Proc Natl Acad Sci U S A 98:14973–14978

Zhang T, Otevrel T, Gao Z et al (2001) Evidence that APC regulates survivin expression: a possible mechanism contributing to the stem cell origin of colon cancer. Cancer Res 61:8664–8667

Index

A
Abaan, H.O., 100
Acute lymphoblastic leukemia (ALL)
   B-and T-cell lineage, 129–130
   BTK, defective expression, 133
   subtypes, 132
Acute myeloid leukemia (AML)
   B-and T-cell lineage, 130
   CSCs, 39
   hypermethylation, 135
   leukemia-initiation, 134
   leukemogenic fusion transcription factor, 135
   oncogenic fusion genes, 134
   stem cell maintenance
      β-catenin, 136
      phenotype, 135
   WNT/β-catenin signaling, 132
Adenocarcinoma
   mammary carcinoma, 66
   prostaglandin E2 pathways, 65
   squamous cell carcinomas, 89
   Wnt activity, 63
Adenoma
   Apc^{Min}, 157
   proliferation rate, 151
   TNF-α, 69
   Wnt signaling, 61
Adenomatous polyposis coli (APC)
   and β-catenin, 212–213
   defined, 6
   inactivation, 7
   sporadic colorectal cancers, 3
   tumor-suppressive activity, 6
Adenosine monophosphate-activated protein
      kinase (AMPK), 151
Adrenal tumors, 103
Aggarwal, B.B., 187
Ahnen, D.J., 187

Ailles, L.E., 130, 137
Akhtar, A.J., 187
Akt
   colorectal and prostate cancer, 66
   levels, 66
   phosphorylation and regulation, 67
   translocation, 152
Akunuru, S., 188, 197
Alberts, D.S., 187
Alferez, D., 147
ALL. See Acute lymphoblastic leukemia
Alpatov, I., 188, 197
Amatruda, J.F., 188, 199
AML. See Acute myeloid leukemia
Anderson, K.C., 187, 194
Aoki, K., 146, 151
Aoki, M., 143
APC. See Adenomatous polyposis coli
Arber, N., 187
Arimura, S., 153
Armadillo
   additional coactivator, 10
   β-catenin, 54
   crystal structure, 11
   Drosophila, 6
   intracellular distribution, 3
   loss-of-function mutations, 2
Armstrong, S.A., 136
Attali, P., 187
Augenlicht, L.H., 187
Axin
   APC, 8
   axis-forming activity, 7
   β-catenin destruction complex, 8
   interaction maps, 5
   levels, 8
   plasma membrane, 9
   potential therapeutic drug target, 11